Advance Praise for Low-Fat Living
by Robert K. Cooper, Ph.D., with Leslie L. Cooper

"*Low-Fat Living* is an excellent summary of state-of-the-art thinking about what a powerful difference lifestyle choices can make in helping you live better, not just longer. Highly recommended."

—Dean Ornish, M.D.

Founder and president of the Preventive Medicine Research Institute in Sausalito, California, assistant clinical professor of medicine at the University of California, San Francisco, School of Medicine and author of *Dr. Dean Ornish's Program for Reversing Heart Disease* and *Eat More, Weigh Less*

"An impressive collection of firepower for America's war on fat."

—Tom Ferguson, M.D.

Medical editor of *The Millennium Whole Earth Catalog* and author of *Health OnLine: The Complete Guide to Finding Health Information through Your Computer*

"Inspirational—and filled with great tips! *Low-Fat Living* is a book we *all* need to help ourselves live healthier and live longer."

—Holly McCord, R.D.

Nutrition editor, *Prevention* magazine

"*Low-Fat Living* is an excellent guidebook. . . filled with highly practical, realistic suggestions to help Americans improve the quality of their lives."

—Bill Hettler, M.D.

Cofounder of the National Wellness Institute and director of health services at the University of Wisconsin

"The very best book I've ever read on the subject—written by two health experts who are living examples of its day-to-day effectiveness for busy people. An immensely practical guide!"
—Harold H. Bloomfield, M.D.
Psychiatrist and author of *Making Peace with Yourself*

"A wise and wonderful program for an active 'low-fat lifestyle.' My family has new favorite recipes and now knows that *Low-Fat Living* is no sacrifice!"
—Sirah Vettese, Ph.D.
Co-author of *Lifemates: The Love Fitness Program for a Lasting Relationship* and author of *Reinventing Love*

Low-
Fat
Living

Low-Fat Living

Turn *off* the fat-makers
Turn *on* the fat-burners
for Longevity
Energy
Weight Loss
Freedom from Disease

Robert K. Cooper, Ph.D., with Leslie L. Cooper

Rodale Press, Inc.
Emmaus, Pennsylvania

Cover Designer: Debra Sfetsios
Book Designer: Christopher R. Neyen
Illustrators: Pat Alexander, Michael Gellatly and Mark Murphy

Library of Congress Cataloging-in-Publication Data
Cooper, Robert K.
    Low-fat living : turn off the fat-makers, turn on the fat-burners
for longevity, energy, weight loss, freedom from disease/Robert K.
Cooper, with Leslie L. Cooper.   p.   cm.
    Includes index.
    ISBN 0–87596–295–5 hardcover
    ISBN 1–57954–021–X paperback
    1. Weight loss.   2. Low-fat diet.   3. Health.   I. Cooper, Leslie L.
II. Title.
RM222.2.C617   1996
613.2′8—dc20   95–38190

Distributed in the book trade by St. Martin's Press

          18 20 19   hardcover
    6 8 10 9 7   paperback

---- OUR PURPOSE ----

*"We inspire and enable people to improve
their lives and the world around them."*

Notice

This book is intended as a reference volume only, not as a medical manual. The information given here is designed to help you make informed decisions about your health. It is not intended as a substitute for any treatment that may have been prescribed by your doctor. If you suspect that you have a medical problem, we urge you to seek competent medical help.

For Chris, Chelsea and Shanna, with our love and encouragement
for a lifetime of vibrant health and for the continued achievement
of your dreams

Contents

Acknowledgments xvii

Part I: Phase Out Fat— With Skillpower, Not Willpower

Chapter I
Making It Easier to Get the Fat Out 3

Chapter 2
What Low-Fat Living Will Do for You 11

Chapter 3
The Best Place to Begin: Turning Off Your
Body's Ten Fat-Maker Switches 27

Fat-Maker Switch #1: High-Fat Meals or
Snacks 29

Fat-Maker Switch #2: Stuffing Yourself—
Even with Low-Fat or Nonfat Foods 41

Fat-Maker Switch #3: Low-Fiber or No-Fiber
Meals or Snacks 45

Fat-Maker Switch #4: Vanishing Muscle Tone 48

Fat-Maker Switch #5: Alcohol—Two or More
Drinks per Day 50

Fat-Maker Switch #6: Skipping Meals or
Snacks 55

Fat-Maker Switch #7: Hidden Dehydration 58

Fat-Maker Switch #8: Inactivity 60

Fat-Maker Switch #9: Poor-Quality Sleep 62

Fat-Maker Switch #10: Mismanaged Stress 63

Part 2: Your Ten Fat-Burner Switches

Chapter 4
Fat-Burner Switch #1: Quick-Start Your
Morning Metabolism 69

Chapter 5
Fat-Burner Switch #2: Eat Low-Fat,
High-Fiber Snacks 79

Chapter 6
Fat-Burner Switch #3: Drink Water and
Other Fat-Fighting Beverages 91

Chapter 7
Fat-Burner Switch #4: Enjoy Do-It-
Anywhere Active Minutes and
Low-Intensity Aerobics 99

Chapter 8
Fat-Burner Switch #5: Have a
Fat-Fighting Lunch 121

Chapter 9
Fat-Burner Switch #6: Use On-the-Spot
Distress Blockers 131

Contents

Chapter 10
Fat-Burner Switch #7: Count on Fast
Firm-Ups: Quick and Easy
Muscle-Toning 155

Chapter 11
Fat-Burner Switch #8: Catch a Late-Day
Second Wind 183

Chapter 12
Fat-Burner Switch #9: Reverse Your
Dinner Habits: Make It Early—And Get
a Fresh Start on Your Evening 191

Chapter 13
Fat-Burner Switch #10: Get Deeper,
High-Metabolism Sleep and Awaken
Invigorated 203

Part 3: Reprogram Your Kitchen and Fight Fat When You Dine Out

Chapter 14
Meals in Minutes: Low-Fat Fast Food
at Home 211

Chapter 15
Phase Out Fat in Every Meal 225

Chapter 16
Fight Fat When You Eat Out 247

Chapter 17
Restock Your Pantry 255

Contents

Part 4: Fresh-Start Recipes for Low-Fat Living

Chapter 18
Fresh-Start Recipes for Low-Fat
Lunches 265

Chapter 19
Fresh-Start Recipes for Low-Fat
Dinners 309

Chapter 20
Fresh-Start Recipes for Low-Fat Snacks
and Desserts 355

Chapter 21
Fresh-Start Recipes for Homemade Yeast
Breads 383

References 427

Subject Index 449

Recipe Index 462

For an interactive experience, visit our web site
at http://www.lowfatliving.com

Contents

Acknowledgments

We wish to express our special gratitude to those individuals who provided us with ongoing professional support in researching and writing this book. Pat Corpora, president, and Bill Gottlieb, senior vice-president and editor-in-chief of Rodale Books, created and championed the general concept of this Low-Fat Living initiative from the start. Ed Claflin, managing editor, worked many highly focused hours crafting the book into shape for the broadest range of readers, and Jane Sherman guided the manuscript through the final editing stages.

Jennifer Haigh, associate writer for Rodale Health and Fitness Books, provided detailed assistance in establishing the latest scientific and medical rationale for low-fat living—and helped us present and clarify the many health benefits of a low-fat living program. Anita Small and Valerie Edwards-Paulik provided medical and scientific reference searches, as did Lisa Schoppmann, our research assistant at the University of Michigan Medical Library. Linda R. Yoakam, R.D., conducted the nutritional analyses on all recipes, and Linda Miller and Jean Rogers provided editorial supervision of the recipe section of the book. From time to time throughout the writing process, others at Rodale Books—Dudley Jahnke, Lois Hazel, Linda Johns, Mary Lengle and Bernadette Sauerwine—offered us their encouragement and expertise.

We are deeply grateful to many professionals who have influenced our thinking and inspired our efforts over the years: Liz Applegate, Ph.D.; George L. Blackburn, M.D., Ph.D.; Steven N. Blair, P.E.D.; Harold H. Bloomfield, M.D.; Kelly D. Brownell, Ph.D.; C. Wayne Callaway, M.D.; Thomas F. Cash, Ph.D.; Kenneth H. Cooper, M.D.; Ellington Darden, Ph.D.; Robert S. Eliot, M.D.; William Evans, Ph.D.; Tom Ferguson, M.D.; Peter Hauri, Ph.D.; Sheldon Saul Hendler, M.D., Ph.D.; William Hettler, M.D.; Michael F. Jacobson, Ph.D.; Lawrence E. Lamb, M.D.; Wayne C. Miller, Ph.D.; Martin Moore-Ede, M.D., Ph.D.; Joyce D. Nash, Ph.D.; Esther M. Orioli; Dean Ornish, M.D.; James Perl, Ph.D.; Judith Rodin, Ph.D.; Irwin H. Rosenberg, M.D.; Ernest Lawrence Rossi, Ph.D.; Bryant A. Stamford, Ph.D.; Robert E. T. Stark, M.D.; Robert L. Swezey, M.D.; Robert E. Thayer, Ph.D.; Art Ulene, M.D.; Peter D. Vash, M.D.; Wayne L. Westcott, Ph.D.; and Redford Williams, M.D.

Finally, we want to thank the many other dedicated researchers, educators and clinicians throughout the world who regularly bring forth vital health revelations that give hope to our collective future and wings to our personal dreams.

Acknowledgments

Phase Out Fat—With Skillpower, Not Willpower

Fat isn't something that just shows up on your exterior. Instead it becomes part of your life in much the same way it becomes part of your cells. It alters the function of your body and may impair its immune power. When you begin low-fat living, you change your cells—which means that you also change your body and your mind. And as you do that, you're changing your life.

You know, of course, that you're not the only person worried about excess fat. If you're like millions of other Americans, you're ready to be rid of it once and for all. But it's worth taking a moment to get some perspective on your own dilemma. For instance:

■ Are you an over-30 woman who has gained weight with each pregnancy and can't take it off?

■ Are you an over-30 man who is worried because you can already see the "spare tire" or potbelly look beginning to grow on you?

■ Are you working longer hours—and finding that you have scarcely any time to exercise?

Part

1

■ Are you concerned about preventing heart disease and cancer?

■ Are you struggling to look and feel younger as you get older?

■ If you're overeating high-fat foods, do you suspect that stress is driving you to do it?

■ Do you like to dine out—but feel sabotaged by all of the "hidden fats" in restaurant meals?

■ Do you find it harder than ever to stay in shape?

■ Do you have an expanding midriff—the classic "middle-age spread"—that won't disappear no matter how hard you try to tighten your abdomen and lose pounds?

The good news is that whoever you are, whatever your fat-fighting dilemma, the Low-Fat Living Program is practical enough to fit your lifestyle. And this program is universal: It's targeted at the most common, precise causes of fat gain and uses the simplest, most effective fat-burning strategies discovered by physicians and scientists from around the world.

Chapter One

Making It Easier
to Get the Fat Out

First of all, let's begin by recognizing that we're each fighting an uphill battle against our own biology. You have to deal with your day-to-day hunger and stress levels, for example. These two formidable forces make high-fat foods so irresistible and exercise so, well, resistible that you might be a bit dismayed. And if you've tried valiantly to "starve" your fat cells by skipping meals or dieting for weeks on end, you've discovered the real truth: It doesn't work.

Why? Because the brain and body have an ancient, inherent drive to form and store fat. This drive seems to shift into high gear with maddening ease whenever you try some of those old, well-intended techniques for losing weight. If you try to slash calories, carve out time for hour-long exercise sessions and skip crucial meals like breakfast, lunch or between-meal snacks, you're not really losing fat forever. You're just fighting a battle of the bulge that you'll probably have to fight again.

Although nationwide surveys indicate that today millions of us want to succeed—permanently—at losing fat, it just plain isn't happening—and we're frustrated.

The Low-Fat Living Program will, quite simply, help you unravel two mysteries that boggle most fat-fighters: how to turn *off* the switches for fat-making and how to turn *on* the switches for fat-burning. Throughout this book you'll discover practical new ways to become healthier and stay that way. You'll find out how to outsmart your innate cravings for high-fat foods. You'll be able to reduce—or turn off—your body's ancient biological tendencies to form fat and store fat.

At the same time, the program will enable you to take greater, hour-to-hour control over your metabolism—the energy-burning processes that go on in your cells 24 hours a day.

You'll learn a variety of specific and practical techniques to healthfully raise your own metabolism. You'll master the various ways your body can burn calories to produce energy to carry out essential functions. And when you switch on those metabolic processes, you'll be switching on a fat-burner. It's that simple.

Why "Switches"?

If you think fat's your fault, it's time to reconsider. You don't have to blame yourself. The fact is, we're overfat because fat-makers are part of our lifestyle and fat-burners are not.

Few of us actually have the right tools to help us win. And that's why the Low-Fat Living Program gives you tools rather than tricks.

It's *skill*power, not *will*power, that really makes the difference. You don't have to master a big, complicated plan for fighting fat. You can choose your tactics from a whole menu of possibilities.

And to use your skillpower, I recommend very specific action steps. Each of the action steps is based upon sound theories about the body's processes—theories that are being researched extensively.

You can do these action steps on the spot, throughout the day, anytime, anywhere. Each one represents what scientists call a leverage-point skill. It's a small, well-focused choice that requires awareness and timing rather than brute-force struggle. And none of these steps has anything to do with deprivation.

According to researchers, we don't achieve permanent self-change by setting lofty goals. It's nice to have those goals, but that's not what matters most. Instead we need to make well-timed choices. No matter how insignificant each one of these choices may seem, they add up to the most powerful way to achieve immediate and lasting results.

Small Steps to Big Changes

With the Low-Fat Living Program, you'll be using the powers inherent in your brain and body to trim down and get healthier. The result: more lifelong vigor and a far greater sense of well-being. As soon as you practice low-fat living, you'll find that it easily becomes a natural part of your days. Before long, you won't even need to think about it.

Unlike other programs you may have tried in the past, the actions that I recommend in the Low-Fat Living Program focus on the crux of the problem—the way your brain and body adjust your energy and metabolism in response to the choices you make.

All day long, from the moment you awaken in the morning until you climb into bed at night, switches are going on and off—making fat or burning it. Not just at mealtimes, and not only during formal fitness sessions, but all day, every day.

And that includes right now.

Yes, whether you know it or not, you are now sending specific cues or "signals" to billions of your body cells. You are telling those cells to do one of two things—to form and store more body fat or to burn more fat for energy and healing.

Which are you choosing? As you read these words, are you sitting or lying down? When was the last time you ate? What, specifically, will you be doing during the next ten minutes?

Your decisions aren't passive—you're making active choices.

To help you learn how to activate the Fat-Burner Switches, I encourage you to practice the "Switchbreaks" you'll find throughout this book. Each of these Switchbreaks describes an immediate and easy way to start burning more fat.

Want an example? Just read the Switchbreak on page 6.

But reading about it is just the first step. Then you have to take a real break and do it.

Switchbreak
SKILLPOWER
---▶ NOT
WILLPOWER

Is there some ice in your refrigerator? A glass nearby? You have everything you need to switch on a fat-burner right now.

Take a moment to get some ice from the tray, put it in a glass and fill the glass with cold water. As you're reading the rest of this chapter, pause every now and then to take a sip.

As simple as this action seems, your body is responding in two very important ways. First of all, it's spending some extra energy to warm up the ice-cold water. And second, any time you drink liquids, you're helping to "fool" your stomach into feeling full. That, of course, is an instant damper to appetite.

You'll find out more about the power of staying hydrated when you read about Fat-Burner Switch #3 (page 91). But right now, take a break and get that glass of ice water before you go on.

It won't take long. And if you can practice each Switchbreak while you're reading this book, you'll start to swing into the habits that can change your life.

Why Skillpower Counts More Than Willpower

According to the results of more than 50 research studies involving over 30,000 subjects, effective self-change depends on doing the right things at the right times.

One review of more than 80 research articles indicated that a leading element in successful self-change is perceived control, a sense that you can take charge of the steps required. According to one leading research team, "People who rely solely upon willpower set themselves up for failure." That's why the Low-Fat Living Program is based on the theme of skillpower, not willpower.

Whenever you learn new skills, of course, you're more likely to make a habit of using them if you understand why they're so effective. The skills of low-fat living are no different. What happens to your body when you switch off the fat-makers and switch on the fat-burners? Why are your cells storing fat sometimes and releasing it other times? Why do you have to be careful about eating carbohydrates as well as fat? And why do you have to keep an eye on calories as well?

Not surprisingly, if you've previously put your faith in willpower, you may not know the answers to these questions. When we rely on willpower, we're more likely to test ourselves, constantly saying things like "If I can only skip this meal or stop this craving, I'll prove to myself I can do it, and that will help me cut fat from my diet and shed fat from my body for ever and ever."

But your body really doesn't care about your win/lose battles with willpower. In fact, if you're locked in a daily power struggle with your will, your body may be waiting for you to give up and pay attention to your fat switches instead.

Nor does it make sense to focus on one aspect of fat-burning at the expense of another. Why fight fat by going off on a tangent with an exercise-only or nutrition-only program? And yet many people do just that. According to one study, most people who watch their diets are physically inactive. And conversely, many people who focus on exercise simply disregard the need to eat healthy low-fat meals and snacks.

If you eat certain foods, exercise in specific ways, rest and awaken in particular patterns, you automatically program your efficient and responsive body to burn more fat rather than making or storing it. Understand that program, and you no longer have to think about success or failure in terms of losing weight or gaining it, overeating or undereating, feasting or starving. In fact, you never have to use such words again.

Timing may not be everything in life, but when it comes to success, it's difficult to think of another single factor that makes or breaks more people's lives. Everything ultimately happens at a point in time . . . and when your timing is right, success is at last within reach.

—Denis Waitley, Ph.D., author of
Timing Is Everything

Cook Up Something Good

The Low-Fat Living Program will help you make sure you don't get on a gain-again/lose-again program. The principles in this book are based on theories that have been developed from a wide range of the latest research. And that research encompasses not only medicine and nutrition but also exercise science, psychology, chronobiology (the influence of daily biological rhythms in the body and brain), sleep patterns, neuroscience, environmental factors, stress dynamics and much more.

Along with the other skills required for low-fat living, it's critical to learn low-fat cooking skills. Whether or not you're the person who starts the steamer and wields the spatula in the household, you need to know how to stock your pantry with delicious low-fat fare, how to cook low-fat meals everyone in your family will love and how to browse a menu for fat-free flavors when you're dining out.

Low-fat cooking techniques are not complicated, but it's essential to learn them. Shop smart, substitute wholesome low-fat ingredients for high-fat ones, measure serving sizes and tip-toe around the fast-food traps. Beyond that, you need low-fat meals that include a variety of fruits, vegetables, grains and other nutrient-rich ingredients. These foods help bring out the very best flavors, so every meal is an experience to enjoy.

In parts 3 and 4 of this book, you'll find information on the skills you need to begin mastering a complete low-fat cooking program. There's a practical guide to help you shop and eat low-fat whether you're dining in or out, along with scores of recipes for implementing the Low-Fat Living 3-plus-4 Eating Plan—low-fat meals, desserts and snacks that take off from traditional favorites and offer a panoply of new flavors.

Best of all, you'll discover that there's nothing elaborate about switching to the low-fat kitchen. As you'll see, all it takes are a few extra kitchen tools and a few easily learned, basic low-fat cooking techniques.

In fact, low-fat shopping, food preparation and cooking are among the most pleasurable pastimes you can discover. Far from avoiding food—the dead-end route of so many restricted diets of past popularity—low-fat eating gives you the very best meals to look forward to. Once you've tried some of these recipes and you're hooked on the bonus of more flavors with less fat, you'll be eating so well and enjoying it so much that you'll never look back.

First-Person Testing

The program you'll discover on the pages ahead is the one I've followed with my own family for more than a dozen years, and I have shared it with my professional colleagues and many friends. Each aspect of this program is based on scientific or medical research or the advice of specialists, and I've provided hundreds of references to substantiate the guidelines you'll be learning.

I credit low-fat living with making a major difference in my own life—improving my health, fitness and levels of energy and work effectiveness. Over the past decade, this program has transformed my family's weight-control efforts into something surprisingly easy and automatic, a plan that literally takes care of itself, without so much as a second thought.

My wife, Leslie, has experienced lasting benefits from this program. While we were developing the Low-Fat Living Program, she was steadily shedding excess body fat—so much so that she gradually changed from a dress size of 12 in 1984 to a size 5 (her natural size) just two years later. Even after her pregnancies in 1990 and 1993, she restored her natural weight and figure—and, even more important, her energy level and stamina. Ever since we've made low-fat living an ongoing part of our lifestyle, she has maintained her weight and energy—and she still wears a size 5.

All the recipes you'll find in part 4 were created by Leslie, right here in our kitchen. We love them all, and so do our children—including our picky 16-year-old and the even-choosier 5-year-old. (*Note:* We also have a 2-year-old, but she's not ready for low-fat eating. Nutritionists agree that children under 2 should not be on a very low fat diet.) The advantage of right-at-home, family testing is that these meals and snacks have all been tried by stern critics—and revised whenever necessary.

So they're not just low-fat—they're also delicious. And nearly all of them can be prepared in a hurry.

Making It Easier to Get the Fat Out

Chapter Two

What Low-Fat Living Will Do for You

Trimming the fat from your diet and including more nutrient-packed foods such as fruits and vegetables offers both short-term and long-term benefits. Once you succeed at low-fat living, your quality of life improves immediately. Your mood lifts. Your grocery bills shrink. You're more alert and energetic.

Some of the benefits of low-fat living are the result of weight loss. Less fat in your diet means less fat on your body: If you're overweight, sensible low-fat eating combined with regular activity is a safe, natural way to lasting weight loss—without starving, feeling deprived or obsessing about eating. Once you put the Low-Fat Living Program into practice, you can stop worrying about your weight and start enjoying the benefits of a lean, healthy body.

Here are some of the benefits, confirmed by the most recent studies.

■ Better self-esteem

■ Less joint pain

■ Lower blood pressure and cholesterol

■ A lower risk of developing gout, varicose veins and work-related injuries like carpal tunnel syndrome

■ A decrease in your risk of heart attack, stroke, diabetes and cancer—four of the top ten leading causes of death in the United States

But weight loss isn't the only reason to cut the fat from your diet. Even if your weight is normal, adopting a low-fat diet still reduces your risk of serious illness. It can also lead to fewer backaches and a stronger immune system to ward off colds and recover from injury. And since good eating habits are as contagious as bad ones, your spouse and children will benefit from your example. Teaching your family healthy habits is a sound investment in their future health—one that will continue to pay off for the rest of their lives.

Weight Loss: A National Obsession

Knowing the benefits of a lean life is one thing. Putting them into practice is a whole different ball game—one that Americans, by and large, are losing. Ten years ago, about one in four Americans was seriously overweight, says Wayne Miller, Ph.D., director of the Weight Loss Clinic at the University of Indiana in Bloomington. Today it's one in three—and climbing.

Obesity is a complex condition with genetic, psychological and behavioral components, so there's no easy explanation for why so many people can't seem to shake the excess weight. Many of us assume that heavy people simply eat too much, but studies show that overweight people, as a group, don't eat any more than thin people do. They do eat differently, however: Thin people get most of their calories from carbohydrates and lean proteins. Overweight people get more of their calories from fat.

This key difference goes a long way toward explaining why some struggle with their weight while others seem to stay trim with little effort. Fat in the diet is more likely to end up as fat on the body, says Dr. Miller. "We've known for a long time that there's something about dietary fat that just promotes body fat accumulation."

That "something" is the body's natural tendency to store fat calories on your belly or hips instead of burning them for energy. Researchers know that the body has a much easier time storing fat than carbohydrates or protein. "Storing fat is very energy-efficient," says Dr. Miller. "It has been estimated that you burn up only about 3 to 5 percent of the calories in fat to store it, whereas for carbohydrates it's 25 to 27 percent."

Better Burn for Your Bucks

Replacing fats with carbohydrates or lean protein also has a terrific effect on your metabolism. Every time you eat, you initiate the thermic effect of food (TEF)—a temporary increase in your metabolism to help you digest and absorb nutrients.

The TEF is greatest following a meal or snack containing lots of complex carbohydrates and a moderate amount of protein and much lower after a high-fat meal. This is why many scientists consider complex carbohydrates and protein "heat-generating" foods. And eating these "hotter" foods means you burn more calories, says Elliot Danforth, M.D., director of clinical research at the University of Vermont College of Medicine in Burlington.

As far as your metabolism is concerned, eating a high-carbohydrate snack is like tossing a load of dry, crackling leaves on a campfire: The flame leaps up and consumes the fuel quickly and efficiently. If you have a snack that's high in fat, it's like using kindling that's damp: The fire has to struggle to burn it, and you end up with more smoke than heat.

Day after day, low-fat meal after low-fat meal, that extra calorie burn can translate into slow but significant weight loss. In fact, some researchers believe that by switching from a diet that gets 40 percent of its calories from fat (the current American average) to one that's 20 to 25 percent fat, an average, active person can lose body fat without cutting back on total calories.

Lean for Life

This brings us to the greatest benefit of the Low-Fat Living Program: Unlike restrictive diets, it's an eating strategy you can follow for the rest of your life.

An L Ride for Cholesterol

When someone says "My cholesterol is too high," it's usually with a frown of concern—and rightfully so.

Usually, they're talking about total cholesterol, the full amount of cholesterol in the blood, which is measured in milligrams per deciliter. And it's true that high total cholesterol raises the specter of added risk for stroke and heart disease.

But your risk actually depends to a great extent on the type of blood transports—called lipoproteins—that tote cholesterol around the body. There are three major types of lipoproteins.

HDL (high-density lipoprotein). Often referred to as good cholesterol, this is the protective type. It actually draws cholesterol away from the coronary arteries and transports it elsewhere. In general, therefore, the higher your HDL level, the better you're protected against heart disease.

LDL (low-density lipoprotein). This type is generally regarded as the predominant culprit in heart disease. Teaming up with other bloodborne chemicals, LDL adheres to the walls of the coronary arteries, especially those near the heart, contributing to formation of a complex artery-clogging substance called plaque. The higher the LDL level in the blood, the greater the risk of heart disease.

VLDL (very-low density lipoprotein). This type of cholesterol is manufactured by the liver to transport various fatty substances through the body. These substances include triglycerides, the free fatty acids that are linked in groups of three and stored in the body as fat. VLDL also transports LDL. The higher the VLDL level, the more LDL the liver can produce. So, directly or indirectly, VLDL contributes to fat transport and storage and to the production of "bad" cholesterol.

An ideal total serum cholesterol reading is 200 milligrams per deciliter, according to the American Heart Association and the National Institutes of Health in Bethesda, Maryland. Some studies, however, indicate that lower may be better, with the ideal total cholesterol level for the average adult in the range of 180 to 190 milligrams per deciliter.

Many health organizations now advise that the most important number is the ratio of total cholesterol to HDL—and the "safe" ratios are different for men and women. The recommended ratio is below 4.6 for men and below 4.0 for women.

By staying in these recommended ranges, you help protect yourself against coronary heart disease. Also, reducing elevated levels of serum cholesterol reportedly may reduce the risk of colorectal cancer.

A study at the University of Minnesota in Minneapolis compared the weight loss of two groups of overweight women. One group stuck to a low-calorie diet—1,200 calories a day, with no more than 40 grams of fat. The women in the other group could eat as much as they wanted—as long as they kept their daily fat intakes to under 20 grams a day. After six months on the plan, both groups lost the same amount of weight, but the lower-fat eaters reported more energy and were more satisfied with their food than the calorie-cutters.

What's more, when the researchers contacted the women a year later, the low-fat eaters had kept off more than twice as much weight as the calorie-cutters.

"The women on the low-fat diet were more satisfied with their quality of life than the women on the calorie-restricted diet," says Meena Shah, Ph.D., a research fellow at the Center for Human Nutrition at the University of Texas at Dallas and one of the authors of the study. "A low-fat diet isn't an excuse to overeat, but it does allow you to eat more, especially if you concentrate on the complex carbohydrates, like fruits, vegetables and whole grains."

Keeping a lid on total calories can also be very important, as you'll see when we look at some Fat-Maker Switches. But there's no way you can lose fat and keep it off just by counting calories—as people did on old-style diet plans. The route to success in losing body fat can be followed only by controlling dietary fat. Furthermore, low-fat eaters are less likely to feel hungry and deprived than people who simply cut back on calories, and they are less likely to throw in the towel out of frustration.

Dodging the Ups and Downs

With a low-fat diet, you also avoid the pitfall of weight cycling—dieting and losing weight, only to put it back on within a few months. Besides the emotional toll of constantly worrying about your weight, weight cycling has another hidden cost: Research shows that people who continually lose weight only to regain it actually accumulate more abdominal fat than those who reach a weight and stay there.

Any way you look at it, excess abdominal fat is bad news. A potbelly isn't just unattractive, it's downright dangerous. Experts know that the infamous "spare tire" is much more dangerous than fat on the hips and thighs: It's linked to a higher risk of diabetes, heart disease and cancer.

And if research is any indication, abdominal fat may have other health effects scientists aren't aware of yet. A "spare tire" seems to be associated with a higher risk of gallstones, while fat on the hips and thighs isn't as significant a factor. Some research even suggests that excess abdominal fat might be connected with infertility in women.

If you've ever tried starving yourself on a very low calorie diet, you'll find low-fat eating much less difficult. And here's more good news: Living the low-fat life actually gets easier with time. Research indicates that once you reduce the fat in your diet for several months, you and other family members may actually lose your taste for fat. Over half the women in one study reported that they started to dislike the taste of fat, and nearly two-thirds said that within a few months of being on a low-fat menu, they felt physically uncomfortable after eating high-fat foods.

Fight Disease and Build Bones

Up until now, we've focused on how low-fat living can improve your life and your health by helping you lose weight. But what if you're not overweight? Is there any reason for you to give up your high-fat diet if your weight is already right on target?

The answer is an emphatic yes. Even if you're one of the lucky few who can stay trim while eating fat-filled foods, chances are that your body doesn't look quite as good on the inside as it does on the outside. Even if your weight is normal, a steady diet of high-fat foods is bound to catch up with you, weakening your immune system and increasing your risk of health problems, from impotence and gallstones to heart disease and cancer.

Research shows that a low-fat diet increases the number of disease-fighting white blood cells, your body's first line of defense against infection. These immune system benefits may be the reason that people who eat less fat are less prone to certain types of cancer.

Studies also suggest that low-fat eating can prevent gallstones—pebblelike particles that form in the gallbladder, a pear-shaped organ located below the liver. Most common in men and women over 35, gallstones can cause jaundice and severe abdominal pain if they escape from the gallbladder—a serious condition that often requires surgery.

A low-fat diet may even be a weapon in the fight against osteoporosis, the "brittle-bone disease" that incapacitates thousands of elderly people each year. Results are preliminary, but one study shows that women who eat lean are less likely to suffer bone fractures than those who eat fat.

There is even some evidence that a low-fat diet may reduce the severity of complications associated with multiple sclerosis.

Matters of the Heart

Perhaps the best-known benefit of a low-fat diet is its effect on your heart and blood vessels. Heart disease is the leading cause of death among American men and women. How many times have you heard that someone had a "sudden heart attack"?

The irony, of course, is that most heart attacks are the result of gradual changes in the circulatory system that develop over many years. These changes include atherosclerosis, a gradual hardening and thickening of the blood vessels due to an accumulation of plaque, a fatty, waxy substance that builds up over years of sedentary living and poor eating. Plaque restricts the flow of blood through your arteries. At the same time, people with heart disease are more prone to forming blood clots, and in an artery that's already narrowed by plaque, one of these clots can be enough to stop blood flow entirely. The result is a myocardial infarction—what we call a heart attack.

Doctors have long known that a diet high in saturated fat is a primary cause of atherosclerosis and that cutting the fat from your diet can slow the process or even reverse it.

Lower Pressure plus More Potency

A low-fat diet can also reduce your risk of high blood pressure, which is another major risk factor for heart disease. If you're overweight, one of the most reliable ways for you to

The Fat You Need Is the Fat You Get

True, we've got a lot of uncomplimentary things to say about fat in this book. But not all fat should be vilified. On the contrary, there's some you absolutely need for good body function.

Polyunsaturated fats, which are the kinds found in grains, seeds, nuts, soy foods (such as tofu) and some vegetables, are essential to body function, because without them the body can't utilize fats properly. This group of fats provides essential fatty acids called alpha-linoleic acid and linoleic acid.

Linoleic acid is readily converted in the body to arachidonic acid, which is important to the makeup of cell membranes. So you need polyunsaturated fats both to help you store fat—which you have to do to survive—and to help build cell membranes.

But although this fat is necessary, it's unlikely you'll ever need to worry about getting enough of it. These days, with such a wide variety of whole foods available, you get all the linoleic acid you need—whether you're on a low-fat, high-fat or ignore-the-fat diet. It's simply not something you have to worry about, since we rarely need to obtain it from extra vegetable oil in our diets.

bring down your blood pressure is to shed some of those excess pounds of body fat.

But even if your weight is normal, trimming the fat from your diet may still help control your blood pressure. Some research shows that a low-fat diet can reduce blood pressure, with or without weight loss. Epidemiologists (those who study disease in populations of people) have observed that high blood pressure is much less common in many less-developed countries, where people generally eat less fat and more complex carbohydrates than Americans do.

People who eat a high-fat diet also have a greater tendency to form blood clots that can block the coronary arteries—another major risk factor for heart disease. This is one area where cutting back on fat brings quick results.

In a small study of young women with high cholesterol, switching to a low-fat diet for only five months reduced their chances of forming blood clots, thus cutting their risk of dying from a heart attack by about 30 percent.

Good circulation has other, less obvious benefits. Regardless of age, men who follow a low-fat diet are less likely to experience impotence than those whose arteries are gunked up with plaque. Clogged arteries have even been implicated in backaches: Autopsies show that people whose abdominal arteries are thick with plaque tend to have deterioration in the disks of the lower back, which is associated with lower back pain.

The Cancer Connection

Fat, whether it's marbling your steak or comfortably nestled around your waist, may also increase your risk of developing certain types of cancer.

Prostate cancer, the second most common cancer among American men, has been linked to fat intake. Researchers have known for a long time that prostate cancer is much less common in countries where the traditional diet is low in saturated fat—the kind found in animal products like meat, cheese, butter and whole milk. They also know that when men from Poland or Japan, where saturated fat intake is low and prostate cancer is rare, move to North America, their risk increases dramatically. The culprit, experts believe, is our all-American, extra-cheese-please, high-fat diet.

What's more, our let-the-good-times-roll approach to eating may even contribute to cancers with obvious environmental causes, like skin cancer and lung cancer. Two of the most common cancers in the United States, both of these are linked to dangerous behaviors—excessive sun exposure and cigarette smoking. Yet these may not be the only factors that determine who develops them.

A study of 76 people with skin cancer found that those who ate a low-fat diet were much less likely to develop new precancerous lesions than those who ate a high-fat diet.

Guarding Your Innards

While quitting smoking is far and away the best strategy for preventing lung cancer, scientists know that thousands of nonsmokers die of lung cancer every year. It's too soon to say for sure why some are struck while others are spared, but at least one study suggests that fat might be a factor.

When researchers compared the eating patterns of 429 nonsmoking women who had lung cancer with the diets of 1,021 healthy, cancer-free women, they found that the more saturated fat the women consumed, the greater their risk of developing lung cancer.

Dietary fat also plays a role in cancers of the digestive tract. The most common of these is colorectal cancer, which strikes over 100,000 American men and women every year—almost as many as lung cancer.

Like lung cancer, colorectal cancer may be prevented with the help of a few lifestyle changes. The formula is actually pretty simple: Cut back on fat, especially saturated fat, and eat foods high in fiber, like fruits, vegetables and whole grains. All of those foods are kitchen staples for anyone who's following the Low-Fat Living Program. As luck would have it, this is exactly the kind of diet—low in fat and high in complex carbohydrates—that may also help protect you from oral, esophageal and pancreatic cancers.

Beating Breast Cancer

While cutting dietary fat is important for anyone concerned about cancer prevention, it's particularly urgent for women. Research shows that breast, ovarian and endometrial cancers may all be linked to dietary fat intake.

Ask a roomful of women about their greatest health concerns, and chances are that breast cancer will be near the top of everyone's list. The most common cancer among women, breast cancer strikes more than 175,000 a year.

Until recently, there didn't seem to be much women could do to improve their odds and reduce their risk of getting breast cancer. Now a growing body of research suggests that reducing dietary fat intake may give women a real advantage over this dreaded killer.

True, scientists still haven't reached a consensus on how large a role dietary fat plays. But animal studies show a definite link between the amount of fat in the diet and the risk of breast cancer, and some studies suggest a similar connection in humans. And we do know that like prostate cancer, breast cancer is rare in countries where the fat consumption is lowest and high where the diet contains a lot of fat.

Not only does dietary fat seem to increase the risk of breast cancer, it may also affect the prognosis of women who develop it. A study of 678 Canadian women with breast cancer found that the more saturated fat a woman's diet contained, the more likely she was to die of the disease.

Some research even shows that a high-fat diet may be an obstacle to early detection of breast cancer: At least one study suggests that mammograms are less accurate in women who eat a fatty diet. While scientists continue to study this development, add this to the list of reasons why switching to a low-fat diet is a sensible step for women concerned about breast cancer.

Lowering Women's Risk— The Estrogen Factor

There's yet another incentive for women to follow a low-fat diet: A diet high in fat increases the risk of endometrial and possibly ovarian cancers, says Nancy L. Potischman, Ph.D., staff fellow at the environmental epidemiology branch of the National Cancer Institute in Bethesda, Maryland. In a study of 399 women with endometrial cancer and 296 healthy controls, Dr. Potischman found that the women with cancer consumed significantly more fat, particularly animal fat.

"There's quite a bit of evidence that a high-fat, Western-style diet is associated with higher estrogen levels, and we know that high estrogen levels are associated with endometrial cancer," says Dr. Potischman.

And it's not just the fat you eat that increases your cancer risk. It also makes sense to be concerned about the excess fat you wear.

First, being overweight affects your immune system, your body's built-in defense against all types of illness, including cancer. A number of studies indicate that overweight people have weaker immune systems than people of normal weight. The overweight person generally takes longer to recover from surgery than a person of average weight. And most ominously, someone who's overweight may be less successful at killing off the abnormal cells that, if allowed to run rampant, develop into cancer.

And for women, abdominal fat poses a particular threat. It affects production of a protein called sex hormone–binding globulin, which binds tightly with estrogen and carries it in the bloodstream, explains Dr. Potischman. "A woman with abdominal obesity produces less of this protein, so more of her estrogen is carried on other proteins that aren't as tightly bound.

The result is that more estrogen is available in the blood, which seems to increase the risk of cancer."

Defeating Diabetes

A low-fat diet can also be an important tool in preventing or managing diabetes, a metabolic disorder that affects over 13 million Americans. In people with diabetes, the pancreas doesn't produce enough insulin, a hormone that's needed to control blood sugar levels in your body and to convert food to energy.

While Type I (insulin-dependent) diabetes is fairly common, most people with diabetes develop it after age 40. This is known as Type II, or non-insulin-dependent, diabetes. Without proper treatment, Type II diabetes can lead to serious complications, including heart disease, kidney failure and blindness.

If Type II diabetes runs in your family, you have a greater risk of developing it. But biology isn't destiny: Experts point out that even if both your parents had Type II diabetes, your risk is only about 1 in 20. In most cases, whether or not you develop diabetes is pretty much in your hands.

A deciding factor? Body fat—specifically, too much of it. Being 20 or 30 percent overweight increases your risk threefold, whether or not diabetes runs in your family. This is one of the best reasons there is for maintaining a normal, healthy weight.

A growing body of research shows that besides contributing to excess weight, a high-fat diet might contribute to your risk of diabetes in other ways. Studies suggest that some people who eat too much fat are more likely to have impaired glucose tolerance, in which the body has trouble metabolizing carbohydrates. And impaired glucose tolerance increases your risk of developing diabetes.

How much fat is too much? A study at the University of Colorado Health Sciences Center in Denver estimates that for every 40 grams of fatty food you eat each day—the equivalent of a large fast-food hamburger and fries—your risk for Type II diabetes increases threefold. (But some people who have diabetes don't do well on a high-carbohydrate, low-fat diet, so if you have diabetes, you should definitely be monitored by your doctor to see what works for you.)

By cutting back on fat and maintaining a healthy weight, people who already have diabetes can take an active role in controlling the condition and preventing serious complications. With the right diet, many people with Type II diabetes can reduce or eliminate their need for insulin. And because people with diabetes are at increased risk for heart disease, adopting a low-fat lifestyle is crucial for protecting their hearts and blood vessels.

Note: If you already have diabetes, proper nutrition plays a crucial role in managing your condition. The Low-Fat Living Program may have many benefits for you, but you should always consult with your doctor before making any changes in your diet.

Someday They'll Thank You

If you've got children in the house, you may hear some howls of protest when you tinker with familiar recipes or come back from the grocery store without their favorite snacks. Don't view their resistance as an obstacle, though; consider it an added incentive to live the low-fat life.

The reasons to get your kids on the healthy track have never been more compelling. Between the early 1960s and the late 1970s, childhood obesity increased 54 percent, and the problem continues to worsen. Today experts say that one in four American children is overweight.

In a society obsessed with thinness, overweight kids have a rough time of it. Research shows that obese kids have lower self-esteem and more emotional stress than their normal-weight classmates. Chubby children also run a greater risk of weight problems later in life: One study of overweight 10- to 13-year-olds found that about 80 percent remained heavy as adults. They also tend to have more severe adult obesity than those who plump up later in life.

Unfair as it is, excess weight puts kids at a disadvantage socially and professionally. A number of studies have found that obese children earn less money when they grow up and are less likely to marry than their normal-weight peers.

Even if your children look slim enough, they aren't immune to the dangers of a high-fat diet and sedentary lifestyle. During the Korean War, military doctors were stunned to find a high prevalence of atherosclerosis in young, apparently healthy soldiers who were killed in action. For today's kids, who are less physically active than any generation in history, the situation is even more serious. Autopsies performed on teenagers show that virtually all of those between 15 and 19 have fatty streaks in their coronary arteries.

Your Kids Need the Benefits, Too

How is it possible that children barely old enough to drive already show signs of heart disease? Blame it on poor nutrition, a high-fat diet and a sedentary lifestyle, says Jack P. Strong, M.D., head of the Department of Pathology at Louisiana State University in New Orleans.

Kids today watch over 20 hours of television a week, which leaves 20 hours less for more active pursuits like playing sports, riding bicycles and helping around the house. While they watch, many put away snacks that are high in fat and calories and low in nutrition and view hundred of hours of commercials that push fast foods and other fatty fare.

All of this has a disastrous effect on kids' eating habits. A study of 209 fourth- and fifth-graders in the Baltimore area found that those who watched the most television were most likely to drink soda, go to fast-food restaurants, eat fatty snacks and have sugary cereals for breakfast.

But television isn't the only place kids learn poor eating habits: They're getting the same messages at school. A study of the lunch program in a Washington school district found that kids could get a lunch that met guidelines for fat and cholesterol only about one in every seven school days. The rest of the time, all the available choices were high in artery-clogging fat.

But before you give up and surrender your child to a short, sedentary life of drive-through windows and relaxed-fit jeans, you should know that the most important influence on children's eating patterns is the way their parents eat.

Studies show that consciously or unconsciously, overweight parents tend to teach their high-fat eating habits to their children. And that works both ways: If you provide nutritious, low-fat, high-fiber foods and set a positive example, you can influence your kids' eating habits for the better, says Ann Shattuck, R.D., a research nutritionist at the Fred Hutchison Cancer Center in Seattle. "If you're the main cook, meal planner and grocery shopper in your household, you have a very important role in what the rest of the family eats."

Now, it's true that children should not be on a low-fat diet during the first couple of years. In fact, nutritionists say that kids need that fat in their meals until the age of two—and you should follow your pediatrician's guidance. But after that, contrary to what many of us learned in health class, kids don't need heaping helpings of whole milk and well-marbled steak to grow up strong and healthy: Research shows that kids on a low-fat diet grow just as fast as kids who eat fatty food.

Children, like adults, are creatures of habit; repeated exposure, more than anything else, determines what they like and what they don't.

The Emotional Payoff

If you look at the big picture, it's clear the lean life is the best way to ensure your future health and well-being. But low-fat living offers plenty of immediate benefits as well.

Besides the confidence that comes from knowing you're doing everything you can to safeguard your health, you may also notice an improvement in your emotional state once you settle into your new low-fat habits. That's what happened to 165 Oregon men and women who followed a cholesterol-lowering low-fat diet as part of the Family Heart Study. Those who stuck to the eating plan for five years tested lower in depression and hostility than a control group that continued to eat a traditional high-fat diet.

"We believe it has to do with the notion of self-efficacy," says Gerdi Weidner, Ph.D., associate professor of psychology at the State University of New York at Stony Brook and one of the authors of the study. "People who succeed at making lifestyle changes have a sense of accomplishment that carries over into other areas of their lives."

And that's not all. The emotional and physical payoffs of low-fat living aren't just for you—they can actually spill over onto the rest of your family. A study at the Fred Hutchison Cancer Center shows that when one partner makes positive lifestyle changes, the other often follows that healthy example.

When researchers helped a group of 156 women make the switch to a low-fat diet, they discovered that the benefits of healthy living were contagious. For 15 months the women met regularly to learn about low-fat nutrition, shopping and cooking techniques. A year later, the researchers contacted the women's husbands and compared their eating habits with those of 148 men whose wives hadn't changed their diets. They found that even though the low-fat husbands hadn't attended meetings or gotten any other instruction in low-fat living, their fat intakes were about 10 percent lower than the control group's.

"We found a strong connection between how much fat the women were eating and how much fat their husbands ate," says Shattuck, one of the authors of the study. "Even though the husbands didn't seem to be making any special effort to choose low-fat foods when they weren't eating with their wives, the fact of having lower-fat foods available at home was enough to make a significant difference in their fat intakes."

Trimming Fat Means Trimming Bills

Many people are surprised to find that trimming the fat from the family's diet trims their grocery bills as well. Researchers at the Mary Imogene Bassett Hospital Research Center in Cooperstown, New York, kept track of the grocery bills of people on a traditional, all-American (that is, high-fat) diet and those on a low-fat diet. When the results were in, the average low-fat eater spent $2.24 less over the three-day period than a person in the high-fat group.

And if you can get your spouse and kids to jump on the bandwagon, the savings are even greater: A study at the George Washington University Lipid Research Clinic in Washington, D.C., found that a family of four on a very low fat diet (10 percent of calories from fat) spent $40 less per week than another family who ate a typical American diet (37 percent fat). That's over $2,000 a year to put toward a new car, a family vacation or new (and probably smaller) clothes for everyone in the family!

Chapter Three

The Best Place to Begin: Turning Off Your Body's Ten Fat-Maker Switches

Look out! If, like many Americans, you consider each of your body's fat cells "the enemy," then it seems they're everywhere—because you probably have about 30 billion of them. And right now these cells are capable of storing as many as 150 pounds of fat.

For years now, most of us have been coming at the enemy—fat—with well-intended but ultimately ineffective tactics. Or we attack it in a piecemeal fashion that, biologically speaking, has doomed us to failure.

Research shows that doing more of the same, only harder, isn't the way to succeed. You're not going to shed fat with more exercise, more deprivation, more dieting, more willpower and more guilt about eating "bad" or "forbidden" foods.

But if more effort isn't the answer, that means it's time to shift gears and break out of old routines.

But how?

If we're still gaining girth despite heroic efforts, one of the primary reasons is that our Fat-Maker Switches are turned on. So we need to find a way to turn them off.

Realistically, you probably are aware that the tendency to rapidly gain large amounts of excess body fat may be, to some extent, inherited. But that knowledge shouldn't be a deterrent to low-fat living.

No matter what our genes, all of us have to contend with the same potential fat-makers—especially the ten that I've identified as the key Fat-Maker Switches.

It's important to note that not all ten are of equal power. You may already be turning some of them off—by avoiding deep-fried foods, for example. But even so, there are many other ways the fat-makers are sabotaging your attempts to get the fat out of your body.

You'll discover there's almost a one-to-one correlation between the fat-makers that you need to turn off and the fat-burners you need to turn on. The skillpower you use to turn off the fat-makers is the same skillpower that will help you turn on the fat-burners.

All these skills may require some practice on your part. So here's what I suggest. As you're reading about the ten Fat-Maker Switches in this chapter, identify the one that seems the most important for you. Chances are that's the one that will seem the hardest to turn off—yet that's the very one you need to begin turning off today.

When you begin, however, remind yourself that it is the hardest. And that's good news, because once you switch off that fat-maker, you'll find it's easier to turn off the others. And each one will get easier, until you'll find yourself switching off the last few fat-makers with the greatest of ease.

Fat-Maker Switch #1

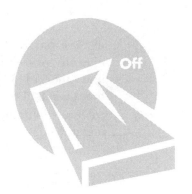

High-Fat Meals or Snacks

It's the end of the workday, and you're starved. You can hear your stomach grumbling. But you worked late, and it's past dinnertime. You won't have the chance to cook tonight, so you ordered pizza. It's on the way.

I'll bet you can already taste it. With a two-for-the-price-of-one deal, you decided to go for the works—extra cheese, olives and pepperoni. Coming right up.

And even though you thought about the fat in those extra ingredients, maybe you decided "What's the big problem? This is dinner, after all. The largest meal of the day."

Okay, let's look at another scenario.

You are rushing to work and don't have time for breakfast, so you grab a muffin. It's a big muffin, sure. But why not? Muffins are healthy, right? And this is your first, energizing meal of the day.

But wait a minute. What if you plan to eat only part of a muffin for breakfast and part of a pizza for dinner? Can't you get away with it—if you eat only a very small portion of the fat-packed pizza and nibble only a corner off that monster muffin?

Well, yes. We might intend to eat modest amounts of these high-fat foods. Yet for many of us, it's all but impossible to re-sist eating more. And when dietary fat, the fat in food, crosses from your stomach and intestines into your bloodstream, your brain and body are programmed to trigger the "store-it" sig-nal. They stuff most of the fat into body fat cells, where it's tucked away as fuel for future lean times.

In our long-ago hunting-and-gathering past, that fat was used during "emergencies"—life-or-death marches through hostile terrain and seasons of grueling heat and cold when there was little to eat. But many of our ancient needs went out with the saber-toothed tiger and woolly mammoth.

The fat stored in our cells is much less needed by most of

us these days. In terms of pulling out fat and using it, a vicarious adventure in front of the television just doesn't measure up to the bad old days of periodic starvation. Even the chores that people did a century ago on the farm—such as chopping wood or pumping water—have gone out with the horse and buggy.

Most of us today simply get up from the lounge chair, stretch, yawn, turn out the lights and go to bed. Even on the busiest mornings, it doesn't tap our fat reserves to face morning traffic or get the kids off to school.

Trade-Offs and Cell-Offs

Your body must either burn or store all the fat that you eat. But even if you're doing a lot of sitting around, your brain—following an ancient code to help preserve you—keeps signaling your cells to store fat instead of burn it.

Now it's true that we all need some dietary fat every day—and our bodies are equipped to utilize small amounts of fat at every meal or snack. But when we consume a lot of high-fat food in the evening, for example, there's not much the body can do with it.

Many of us eat huge "deal meals" at fast-food restaurants or eat high-fat foods at suppertime without paying much attention to how much fat we're eating. And we're doing it just at the hours when the body's ability to make energy and burn fat takes a major downturn.

Dietary fat is already pure fat that's ready to glide effortlessly into your fat-storing cells. For this reason, it "costs" very little energy—only about 3 calories—to convert 100 calories of fat into new body fat.

But what are the alternatives?

Well, unlike smooth-flowing dietary fat, the complex carbohydrates found in many whole-grain foods and fresh fruits and vegetables take much more energy to digest and incorporate in your body. It "costs" more than eight times as many calories to turn a food that's rich in complex carbohydrates into body fat as it does to turn dietary fat into body fat, estimates Jean-Pierre Flatt, Ph.D., professor of biochemistry at the University of Massachusetts Medical Center in Worcester. In other words, if you're eating a food that's rich in complex carbohydrates—such as a fresh vegetable salad, a bowl of old-fashioned oatmeal or a piece of whole-grain bread—your body has to work eight times as hard to turn the food into body fat.

Bacon, Fries and Other Bummers

It's not that much of an oversimplification to say that a couple of doughnuts, a double bacon-cheeseburger, a large tub of buttered popcorn or a bag of traditional potato chips may move from your stomach to your bloodstream like a heavy-laden tanker filled with fat. And when the tanker-full spills into your bloodstream, it's an easy, automatic oil spill that seeps into the fat cells in your abdomen or thighs.

In short, gaining new body fat from large doses of dietary fat can be amazingly easy. And every time you eat high-fat foods, you decrease the rate at which your body burns fat for energy, making it harder and harder for you to lose body fat and keep it off.

Also, your body dramatically increases its production of the hormone insulin when you gulp down high-fat foods. One of the effects of insulin is to increase your appetite and the rate at which your body stores fat. At the same time, insulin makes it more difficult for your body to burn fat. Net result: When you eat high-fat foods, you'll probably just want to eat more high-fat foods in the hours that follow.

Switchbreak
SKILLPOWER NOT ◄-- WILLPOWER

Pause to consider what you're going to have for your evening meal tonight. In a normal meal, some of the sources of fat might be oil, butter, margarine, cheese, sour cream, whole milk, any kind of beef or pork, potato chips or salad dressing. If you're used to having dessert, maybe you're contemplating pie, ice cream or cookies. Or maybe you'll have cream in your coffee.

Now, as you are thinking of this meal, decide on one specific change. Maybe you'll go light on the cheese or skip sour cream on your potato. You can reduce the amount of oil or margarine, eat a smaller portion of meat or have some rye crackers instead of potato chips. Instead of a regular salad dressing, choose low-fat or nonfat. For dessert, try low-fat ice cream. And use skim milk or a nonfat creamer for your coffee.

Pick one specific change. That's all. Begin there. That's less fat coming into your body—and less fat-making and fat-storing to follow.

Where Fat Sneaks In

Aren't most of us already cutting back on fat in the diet? Well, yes and no.

Although we Americans are eating less beef and butter, we're more than making up for those slight deficits with other high-fat foods. Between 1993 and 1994, for example, sales of super-premium ice cream grew more than 17 percent. But if you're one of the secret supreme-ice-cream buyers, you should know that you're getting 60 percent of your calories from fat with every single bite.

For most of us, the craving for high-fat foods isn't out of control. On the other hand, there are some body signals that might be urging us on to the next bite. For years neurobiologists have been studying a specific area of the brain called the hypothalamus that plays a key role in appetite, metabolic rate and fat storage. They've discovered that the hypothalamus produces a chemical called galanin that triggers a specific craving for fat.

Galanin levels start out low in the morning. Then they begin to rise, reaching a higher level at midday and remaining high through suppertime and on into the evening.

To make matters worse, galanin not only increases our hunger for the taste of fat, it also affects other hormones that influence fat storage. When your galanin level is up, you can be almost sure that the excess fat you eat is being stored as body fat. Researchers at Rockefeller University in New York City have discovered in studies on rats that eating fat seems to promote even more fat-eating.

"The mechanisms that enhance the appetite for fat appear more potent than those that curb it," says Sarah Leibowitz, Ph.D., the neurobiologist at Rockefeller University who headed the research team. As Dr. Leibowitz's animal studies have shown, once rats begin to eat fat, they seem to crave even more of it. It seems likely that the same influences on appetite also hold for humans.

So are we stuck with being dominated by fat cravings that begin at lunchtime and go on for the rest of the day?

Maybe not. Even though a brain-generated chemical like galanin can be powerful, it isn't the only influence, according to biological anthropologist Stephen Bailey, Ph.D., of Tufts University in Medford, Massachusetts. "Though it's clear that compounds like galanin play an important role in controlling our appetites, it's also true that we're capable of generating a great variety of responses to the brain's cues or signals to eat fat," observes Dr. Bailey.

Shifting Your Weight

There is growing evidence that the longer you eat a high-fat diet, the more your body actually begins to shift toward *storing* fat instead of *burning* it for energy. In other words, your metabolism may actually change in the direction of storing more and using less.

This undesirable transformation involves an enzyme that is called lipoprotein lipase (LPL). The job of LPL is to break down fat molecules into components called fatty acids, which are small enough to pass through the walls of your body's fat cells.

As you eat more fat, the body sends out stronger signals, activating this fat-storing enzyme. More dietary fat gets stuffed into your body's fat cells.

The most potent fat promoting foods seem to be those that are high in both fat and sugar, which describes some of America's most popular foods. Just think of cake, ice cream, doughnuts and chocolate candy—all ponderous mixtures of fat and sugar.

The sugar in those foods stimulates the production of insulin at the same time that large amounts of fat are entering the bloodstream. And it can substantially boost the activity of the fat-storing LPL enzyme.

In fact, any kind of refined sweetener calls up insulin in your bloodstream. Almost instantly, the insulin readies the fat cells for storage. It also encourages calories from any food source (not just fat calories) to be stored as fat rather than burned for energy. The cells appear to "open up," and the LPL essentially drives the circulating fat molecules right in the open door. The result can be dramatically increased fat storage. And in many people, that fat tends to be stored primarily in the waist and stomach areas.

In addition to actual fat gain, research has shown, the fat in high-fat foods causes mental and physical fatigue. After

Avoiding Hydro Power

Twiddling with the internal molecular patterns of certain fats, the manufacturers of processed foods sometimes come up with new substances that can pose health risks.

Such is the case with hydrogenated fats, oils that have hydrogen artificially pumped in to "stiffen" them and make them more spreadable. Since the molecular structure changes from a "cis" pattern into a "trans" pattern when hydrogen is injected, these oils are often called trans-fatty acids.

Margarine, which is produced from hydrogenated polyunsaturated oil, has been widely adopted as a cholesterol-free substitute for butter. But the hydrogenation process used in creating margarine could be leading to other health problems, researchers believe.

And margarine isn't the only source of hydrogenated oil. Other possible sources include:

- Breads and breadings
- Cakes and cookies
- Candies
- Crackers and snack chips
- Fried foods
- Frostings
- Mayonnaise and salad dressings
- Puddings
- Shortenings

There is research to suggest that excessive consumption of trans-fats may cause health problems. Partial hydrogenation may raise total cholesterol levels and may interfere with several of the body's protective mechanisms.

high-fat meals or snacks, "the viscosity (thickness) of the blood measurably increases," according to Neil Barnard, M.D., faculty member at George Washington University School of Medicine in Washington, D.C., president of the Physicians Committee for Responsible Medicine and author of *Food for Life*.

As your blood becomes thicker or more viscous, inevitably it turns sluggish. "This may be a contributor to the mental and physical after-eating slowdown that many people feel," says Dr. Barnard.

Deciding on Daily Fat Grams

To turn off the Fat-Maker Switch, you need to figure out how much fat you can take in every day. The goal is to store little if any of that dietary fat as body fat. But if you want to reach that goal, you need to set a maximum in terms of the percentage of total calories that can come from fat.

Government health agencies, the National Cancer Institute in Bethesda, Maryland, and the American Heart Association have arrived at the same figure. All say that your daily diet should not have more than 30 percent of total calories from fat.

Yet this recommendation is conservative and probably allows for too much fat in the diet. In the view of many independent nutritionists and health care experts, getting down to 30 percent is probably not enough.

Studies suggest that 30 percent fat may slow but does not stop the development of heart disease, for instance. In a Harvard University study of female nurses, researchers reported that those who had 27 to 30 percent fat in their diets had virtually the same rate of breast cancer as those who ate diets that were 40 percent fat.

Other studies indicate that one of the most important health benefits—weight loss—occurs when the dietary limit of fat is under 30 percent. In a two-phase study conducted by researchers at Cornell University in Ithaca, New York, and the University of Gotenberg, Sweden, a group of women were placed first on an unlimited-fat diet and then on a reduced-fat diet to measure the impact of low-fat eating.

During the early phase of the study, the women ate typical American fare with about 35 to 40 percent of calories coming from fat. This phase continued for 11 weeks, during which most of them gained body fat. Then came the shift to a low-fat diet. For the next 11 weeks the same women continued to eat as much food as they wanted—but the foods they could choose were only 20 to 25 percent fat.

The result? At the end of the second 11-week phase, each of the women had lost, on average, 5½ pounds of body fat. Clearly, since the amount of food was unrestricted in both phases, the difference was in the percentage of fat calories. When fewer calories were from fat, the weight came off.

Fat-Watching Made Easy

Want the lowdown on fats in your kitchen cupboard? Here's a quick reference guide to common dietary fats.

Fat	Saturated (%)	Monounsaturated (%)	Polyunsaturated (%)
Butter	68	24	4
Canola oil	7	60	30
Coconut oil	86	6	2
Corn oil	13	24	59
Olive oil	14	72	9
Peanut oil	19	46	30
Safflower oil	9	12	74
Sesame oil	15	40	40
Soybean oil	15	23	58
Sunflower oil	11	21	68

Setting Your Target

Most of us do have to cut back on dietary calories from fat if we want to turn off the Fat-Maker Switch.

For low-fat living, you'll want to target a daily diet with about 20 percent—and not more than 25 percent—of total calories from fat. Your eventual target, or a realistic future ideal, may be even less.

In truth, the human body needs only 4 to 6 percent of daily calories as fat. And there is evidence that extremely low fat diets with only 10 to 15 percent of calories from fat are very helpful for people who have certain medical conditions such as severe heart disease. But studies have not yet proven the long-term benefits of extremely low fat diets. Indeed, some research suggests a kind of rebound effect, indicating that very low fat diets may stimulate the body to produce more fat from blood sugar and increase appetite.

Until we have further evidence to the contrary, the optimal range seems to be somewhere between 10 and 25 percent. And for most of those on a standard American diet, just getting under 30 percent of calories from fat may seem like a stretch.

If you use the menus and snacks in this book, you can reasonably reach a dietary goal averaging about 20 percent of

Fast Facts on Fighting Fat

We usually lump fats together in a single category—and that makes sense if you're generally watching your fat intake. But in fact, there are different kinds with different health effects.

More than 90 percent of dietary fat is composed of complex molecules consisting of three fatty acids: saturated, monounsaturated and polyunsaturated. Animal fats usually contain a high percentage of saturated fatty acids, while most vegetable fats contain mainly unsaturated fatty acids.

These three kinds of fat play different roles in our diet and definitely affect our health in a variety of ways. Here's how.

Saturated fats. These come primarily from animal sources like beef, veal and pork and also from dairy products like eggs, butter and cheeses. Coconut oil and palm oil are also high in saturated fats. When you get more than about 5 percent of your total daily calories from these kinds of fats, you run the risk of elevating LDL levels (that's the "bad" cholesterol) and promoting disease. Also, a high intake of saturated fats is thought to increase the need for essential fatty acids, which can lead to the creation of excess body fat as well as other health problems.

Monounsaturated fatty acids. These are found in large proportions in canola oil, olive oil, peanut oil and sesame oil. Oils that are high in monounsaturates have been found by researchers to help lower LDL cholesterol levels while not affecting HDL (the "good" cholesterol).

Polyunsaturated fats. These fats are found in grains, seeds, nuts, soy foods such as tofu, and some vegetables. They're needed for adequate fat storage and for cellular health—but you get plenty in a normal diet. In some scientific studies of animals, researchers have linked polyunsaturated oils to the formation of cancerous tumors and the original damage in coronary artery disease.

These three types of fatty acids are in various combinations in different types of oils. The table below shows a comparison of the saturated, monounsaturated and polyunsaturated fats in each type of oil—with a comparison to the fats found in butter.

daily calories from fat. And as you'll see when you read about those foods, staying within that range doesn't involve any deprivation at all. In fact, you may be eating better—and probably more economically—than you ever have.

But there's something else to consider when you're calculating fat intake—and that's the kind of fat you're getting. Ideally, your daily dietary fat intake should be no more than one-third polyunsaturates, one-third or less saturates and the balance monounsaturates. At first cutting back on saturated fats may be especially important for many people. The recipes and menus in this book are carefully designed to help you maintain that balance.

Find Your Starting Points

If you have no idea how many calories you're consuming every day or what your fat target should be, you can start with a clean slate to work up a program. Here are the steps to arrive at a starting point—your goal for total daily fat intake.

1. Estimate your ideal healthy weight. Chances are you already have some idea what this is, but many Americans set unrealistic goals.

You may want to discuss your ideal healthy weight with your physician or dietitian. It's essential to realize that as you increase muscle tone and trim fat, you'll probably look much thinner than your weight on the scale may indicate.

For many years, health professionals relied on the 1959 "ideal" weight figures calculated by the Metropolitan Life Insurance Company. The standards of "ideal" were created by figuring out which group of male and female policyholders, based on their heights and weights, had the lowest mortality rates. The statistics showed that people who were in "undesirable" weight categories were more likely to die early than people in the "desirable" weight groups. But height was the only other factor taken into account when making these assessments.

Over the years, the Metropolitan Life weight tables were criticized for failing to account for body type, age, ethnicity and body fat percentage. The tables were revised in 1983 by simply adding 10 percent to the "desirable" weights listed for each height.

Now the National Institutes of Health in Bethesda, Maryland, cautions against using either the 1959 or 1983 Metropolitan Life tables as the sole indicator of your ideal weight. After reviewing 25 major studies on weight and longevity, a Harvard research team reported that most of the studies used to estab-

Approximate Daily Calorie Limit

The table below will help you calculate your daily calorie limit, taking into account your level of exercise and your target weight.

Select the category that best describes you, based on your activity level and sex. Then write your estimated ideal healthy weight in the second column. Finally, multiply by the number in the third column to arrive at an estimate of your daily calorie limit.

Post this number on your cupboard or refrigerator. Remember—this is your daily goal.

If You Are ...	And Want to Weigh ...	Multiply by ...	For Your Daily Calorie Limit
A sedentary woman	___lb.	12	_____
A sedentary man	___lb.	14	_____
A moderately active woman	___lb	15	_____
A moderately active man	___lb.	17	_____
A very active woman	___lb.	18	_____
A very active man	___lb.	20	_____

lish these weight tables in the first place underestimated the risk of being overweight. According to this review, the weight tables also contain biases that allow "desirable" weights to creep up. That's why you should check with your physician rather than consulting a table of "standards" to find out whether you're in a desirable weight range for your sex, age, height and other factors.

2. Once you know how much you want to weigh, you need to calculate your daily calorie limit. The table in "Approximate Daily Calorie Limit" will help you estimate it.

Note that the table has different daily calorie limits that depend on your sex and your lifestyle. A very active man, for instance, can consume many more calories than someone who's sedentary. That makes sense, of course, since the active individual is going to burn off more calories during the day than the sedentary individual.

If you're not sure whether you fall into the category of "moderately active" or "very active," use the moderately ac-

Your Daily Dietary Fat Budget

Calorie Limit	Fat (g.)	
	(20% Goal)	(25% Goal)
1,200	27	33
1,300	29	36
1,400	31	39
1,500	33	42
1,600	36	44
1,700	38	47
1,800	40	50
1,900	42	53
2,000	44	56
2,100	47	58
2,200	49	61
2,300	51	64
2,400	53	67
2,500	56	69
2,600	58	72
2,700	60	75

tive category as a start. If you increase your exercise level and find that you do need more calories in your diet, you can always increase the calorie content of your meals and snacks.

3. Estimate Your Daily Dietary Fat Budget. You can calculate target fat grams by multiplying 20 percent (0.20) or 25 percent (0.25) by total calories. Then divide by 9 (the number of calories in a fat gram) to calculate the maximum number of fat grams you should be getting every day. To save you some time at the calculator, here's a table with instant answers.

Of course, Your Daily Dietary Fat Budget should be divided as evenly as possible throughout the day. For instance, if you figure out that your daily maximum should be 55 grams of fat, here's how you might divide your intake among meals and snacks. But remember, these are just examples of maximum numbers, and they're also approximate.

- Breakfast: 8 grams of fat
- Midmorning snack: 4 grams of fat
- Lunch: 18 grams of fat
- Midafternoon snack: 4 grams of fat
- Supper: 18 grams of fat
- Light evening snack: 3 grams of fat

Once you've learned to recognize where fat is hidden in the foods you eat, monitoring your intake is relatively easy. You don't need to keep a calculator in hand just to figure out whether you're under your daily fat-gram target.

Later in this book, we'll provide some shortcuts to guarantee that you stay within your budgeted amount. And of course, all the meal plans and recipes in part 4 fit this basic fat-gram budget model.

Fat-Maker Switch #2

Stuffing Yourself— Even with Low-Fat or Nonfat Foods

You're preparing to relax in front of the TV with a bag or box of your favorite chips or cookies.

No, wait, you don't want to stuff yourself with high-fat goodies! So you reach instead for a bag of low-fat or fat-free snacks—potato chips, flavored rice cakes or fat-free devil's food cookies.

A healthy choice—right? No way you can get fat from nonfat foods, even if you eat a whole bagful. Right?

Well, if you grab the fat-free goodies and settle down again, you've just made a slight strategic error. While it's true that high-fat foods are the most fattening and that the more you eat at a single sitting, the more fat you pack into the body's fat cells, this is not the whole story. When eaten to excess, even nonfat foods can turn on your body's Fat-Maker Switches.

"What?" you say.

No, I'm not kidding. Chocolate-dipped cream-filled caramel-laced mini-cakes that are labeled "100% Fat-Free!!!!" do not, in fact, have a bit of fat. But they can be fattening!

And before you get set to polish off that bag of fat-free rice cakes or nonfat potato chips, you should realize that these foods can actually be fat-makers in the body. That's because they trigger hormone and enzyme reactions that can turn non-fat calories into fat and then pack it into your fat cells.

The bottom line is this: Overeating is a boon to fat cells, even if the package says low-fat or no-fat. Whenever a meal tops a limit of some 500 to 700 calories, the excess calories, even from nonfat foods, stimulate fat-forming and fat-storing.

One 20-week study found that people who restricted both fat and calories lost significantly more weight and a higher percentage of body fat than people who restricted fat intake alone.

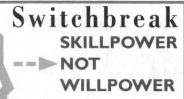

Switchbreak
SKILLPOWER
---► NOT
WILLPOWER

Does all this talk of food have you ready to make a trip to the kitchen for a bag of low-fat popcorn?

Wait a second. Once you start eating popcorn, can you stop?

Whenever you feel an urge to stuff yourself with food, turn to a drink of ice water.

Water has zero calories, which means there's no chance that it will switch on the insulin. And if you're not switching on insulin, you're turning *off* that Fat-Maker Switch.

Now think ahead to the evening meal and keep in mind what happens if you go overboard on calories. It takes about 20 minutes from the start of any meal for your body to feel satisfied and full. Turn this to your advantage by slowing down while you're eating. Plan on taking more moderate bites. Think about how you can add extra minutes throughout the meal. This is the simplest way to keep Fat-Maker Switch #2 turned off.

"We're eating fat-free foods but in industrial-size portions," observes nutritionist Joan Horbiah, R.D., author of *50 Ways to Lose Ten Pounds*.

The Secret Storage System

When you're eating a large meal, your body begins releasing insulin—and the more you eat, the more insulin that gets into your system. Insulin causes your body to try to reduce the level of excess blood sugar (glucose) any way it can. One way is to use any excess glucose that's in your blood instead of using stored fat. With insulin interfering in the process, your fat cells are very sluggish about breaking down fat and releasing it into the bloodstream, where it could be burned as fuel.

At the same time, insulin essentially helps turn your fat cells into magnets for more fat storage. That's because insulin sweeps blood sugar out of the bloodstream and helps convert it into fat that's stored in your cells.

So if you're sitting in front of the TV eating two low-fat rice cakes as a snack, that's probably okay. You're taking in about 70 calories and less than half a gram of fat.

But if you're on the verge of finishing off the package, you're turning on a fat-maker. That rush of extra calories is going to switch on excess insulin, resulting in less fat burning and more fat storage. That's why it's so important to turn *off* Fat-Maker Switch #2.

In recent years, one of the questions most often asked by

Carbs That Boost Fat-Making

Carbohydrates provide essential blood sugar—glucose—which is the fuel used for energy production in the brain and every cell of the body. Glucose also helps maintain body temperature, digestion, movement, breathing, tissue repair and immune system functions—so it's one of the most important compounds coursing through your body.

There are three basic types of carbohydrates, labeled according to the complexity of their molecular structure: monosaccharides (simplest), disaccharides and polysaccharides (most complex). Polysaccharides consist of many sugar units, bonded together by nature to form complex carbohydrates (starches).

Starches either may be left unrefined or may be refined, as happens when we process them to make certain foods. Unrefined complex carbohydrates come associated with lots of fiber, vitamins, minerals and other nutrients. Most of us need to eat more foods like whole-wheat bread and brown rice in order to get enough of these unrefined complex carbohydrates in our diets.

By contrast, foods like white bread and white rice are both less filling and less nutritious because they have refined carbohydrates. In the process of refining, such as the milling of wheat to make white flour, the fiber and many vitamins and minerals are lost.

In general, unrefined complex carbohydrates are digested slowly and efficiently, providing a steady source of energy without the biochemical roller-coaster effect of concentrated sugars. So eating foods with complex carbs helps stabilize your sugar levels.

Refined white sugar—sucrose—tops the list of "empty calories," along with its counterparts corn syrup, brown sugar, dextrose, maltose and cane syrup. High intake of refined sugar has been linked to a variety of health problems, including elevated levels of cholesterol and other blood fats, a deficiency of chromium, a trace mineral associated with heart disease and diabetes, and development of breast cancer.

The simple sugar molecules in sucrose require very little digestion, entering the bloodstream and quickly raising blood sugar levels far above normal. In response, the body's insulin secretion mechanism is activated to remove the excess glucose from the blood, causing a downswing in blood sugar levels.

Even "natural sugar alternatives" such as maple syrup, honey and fruit juice are no panacea. The fact is, no sweetener used excessively is healthful.

failed dieters at weight-loss clinics has been "How did I gain weight on a low-fat diet?"

The truth is, when you choose foods with little or no fiber, nonfat doesn't necessarily mean nonfattening. Many people who went on low-fat diets were still reaching for simple, refined carbohydrates such as sugar, white rice and white flour. At Johns Hopkins University in Baltimore, weight-loss researcher Barbara Rolls, Ph.D., has found that when reduced-fat and fat-free foods replace their high-fat counterparts, people tend to compensate by eating more.

Many clinicians and obesity researchers, including Stephen Gullo, Ph.D., who has treated over 10,000 overweight patients as director of the Institute for Health and Weight Sciences in New York City, say that switching from low-fat to high-carbohydrate foods is not enough. It's important to replace dietary fat with complex-carbohydrate, fiber-rich foods such as vegetables, fruits, whole grains and legumes such as beans, peas and lentils.

For years, researchers have known that consuming large amounts of refined sweeteners such as sugar, honey and syrup is linked to gaining body fat. "People simply do not stop gaining weight by eating large quantities of pasta or white rice," says Louis Aronne, M.D., director of the Comprehensive Weight Control Center at the New York Hospital–Cornell Medical Center in New York City.

Dr. Aronne and many other clinicians are not advocating a return to high-protein foods, however. Instead they would like to see people make a transition away from large quantities of simple carbohydrates—such as sugar, honey, white flour and alcohol—to a low-fat diet that is high in fiber and complex carbohydrates and includes fruits, vegetables, whole grains and legumes.

When you're substituting low-fat or nonfat foods, be sure you're still eating the same amount. A tablespoon of salad dressing is about 100 calories, for instance, but a tablespoon of its nonfat version can be as low as 16. So you really are reducing calories with the nonfat version—but not if you start multiplying the amount you use.

Another way to avoid overloading is to stay away from all-you-can-eat buffets in restaurants. Even if you just eat low-fat foods, you're likely to eat too much.

Fat-Maker Switch #3

Low-Fiber or No-Fiber Meals or Snacks

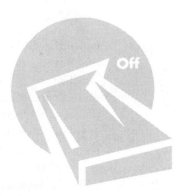

One of the other principal benefits of complex carbohydrates is fiber. The different kinds of fiber all come from the cell walls of plants. They play a major role in keeping digestion moving smoothly, making it less likely that cancer-causing toxins and other disease-promoting substances will come into prolonged contact with the digestive tract or be absorbed. High-fiber diets have been shown to help prevent heart disease, obesity and colon cancer. High fiber intake has also been shown to aid in losing excess body fat and may even help lower blood pressure by about 10 percent.

Dietary fiber encompasses all plant material that's resistant to digestion. Some people call it roughage, but fiber actually helps to produce a smooth, prompt transit through the digestive tract.

To turn *off* Fat-Maker Switch #3, you need two kinds of fiber.

Insoluble fibers include cellulose, found in foods such as wheat bran; hemicellulose, found in whole grains and vegetables; and lignin, which is the "glue" in the walls of plant cells. These fibers absorb water, which means they swell up and add bulk, making it easier for the intestines to pass along waste products.

Soluble fibers include pectin, which is in apples, citrus fruits, legumes and certain vegetables; mucilage, found in oats and legumes; and gums, which are gel-like substances in plants. These fibers have very different activities from the crude, water-insoluble fibers.

All fibers are bound to digestible carbohydrates, so they help slow down the absorption of glucose into the bloodstream. Pectin and gums slow sugar absorption from the intestines. Because these fiber properties appear to keep blood sugar levels more even, they can reduce fat-making processes in the body.

To turn *off* Fat-Maker Switch #3, most Americans need to increase their intakes of both soluble and insoluble fiber by getting a widely varied diet of fresh whole foods. Fresh fruits and vegetables, whole-grain breads and side dishes and beans and legumes are good choices.

How much total fiber should you consume per day? The average American consumes only about 10 grams. The National Cancer Institute, however, recommends 20 to 35 grams daily, and other authorities suggest that an average-size adult should consume between 30 and 60 grams of total fiber per day.

Where Insulin Gangs Up on You

When you have low-fiber or no-fiber meals and snacks along with too much sugar and starch in your diet, the hormone insulin can begin to play a huge role in fat-making.

That's because as scientists have discovered, a diet high in refined carbohydrates can trigger insulin resistance. This resistance occurs when the body responds to starches and sugars by overproducing glucose, which in turn triggers the overproduction of insulin.

This hormone generally controls glucose, but in a nimble variety of ways. First of all, it determines how much of the glucose will be used immediately as energy and how much will be converted to and stored as fat.

It also stimulates your appetite, which of course is a way of telling you that your body needs more energy. And it regulates triglycerides, which are "stored fats" in the body.

As I've mentioned, insulin also helps prevent your fat cells from breaking down stored fat and releasing it into the bloodstream, where it could be burned as fuel. And it helps turn your fat cells into "magnets" for any dietary fat that's been absorbed into your bloodstream.

Insulin resistance is linked to a wide range of factors from glucose intolerance to high blood pressure, according to Gerald Reaven, M.D., professor at Stanford University School of Medicine, who has studied insulin for more than 30 years. Though it is also linked to one kind of diabetes (Type II), you don't necessarily have diabetes just because you're insulin-resistant. In fact, Dr. Reaven says that insulin resistance affects about 25 percent of Americans who do not have diabetes.

For these people, "it is nearly impossible to lose weight by replacing a proportion of dietary fat with simple carbohydrates," explains Artemis P. Simopoulos, Ph.D., former chairwoman of the Nutritional Coordinating Committee of the National Institutes of Health and current co-chairwoman of an institute panel on insulin resistance and chronic disease.

But for many of these people, replacing dietary fat with complex carbohydrates can make a difference. That's just one more reason why eating fresh fruits, vegetables, whole grains and legumes is so important.

Switchbreak
SKILLPOWER
NOT ←--
WILLPOWER

Are you hungry right now?

If it's between meals or you're feeling that you need something sweet, reach for an apple, orange or pear. Researchers have found that these and other fruits are rich in natural fiber.

Also, a dose of the sweetness in fruit—from the fructose—may well help you feel satisfied without craving fat or refined sugars.

Turn Your S'mores to No-Mores

Here's one more point to remember: Low-fiber, high-fat meals and snacks don't switch off the "eat more" message as effectively as foods that are high in complex carbohydrates and fiber, says James Kenney, R.D., Ph.D., nutrition research specialist at the Pritikin Longevity Center in Santa Monica, California. That's because dietary fat cannot be converted into glycogen, a form of sugar that's stored primarily in the liver and muscles.

Glycogen, particularly that stored in the liver, seems to be the trigger that switches off the appetite signal and tells you that you're not hungry anymore.

In an experiment with overweight men and women, a research team at the University of Leeds in Great Britain found that individuals ate twice as much when sampling high-fat foods like pastries, cheeses, fatty meats and creamy casseroles as when eating high-fiber, high-carbohydrate foods such as whole-grain breads, cereals, fresh fruits and vegetables. Apparently, eating large amounts of high-fat foods does not stimulate the body-to-brain "signal" of satiation (feeling full) as effectively as high-fiber, low-fat foods.

So you're actually improving the accuracy of your appetite signal when you eat salads, whole-grain breads, bean soups and casseroles and virtually all the delicious meal and snack recipes you'll find in this book. All these foods not only help you feel full and satisfied while eating less fat but at the same time help increase fat-burning instead of fat-storing.

Fat-Maker Switch #4

Vanishing Muscle Tone

Most of us consider ourselves to be physically active, and we're proud of it.

But here's a surprise: Even though you're running around on the job or going flat-out with household chores and errands, you're not doing much to add firmness to your thighs and fanny.

And you're doing almost nothing to maintain the tone of hundreds of other muscles in your body. Every week—in fact, every single day—that you fail to use any of your muscles, they steadily get slacker and weaker.

Fading muscle tone is a powerful fat-maker. Toned muscle fibers help your body hold the line against fat by producing fat-burning enzymes and using fat to fuel the action of each muscle fiber.

When your muscles start to atrophy—which is literally what happens when you begin to lose muscle tone—the signal that tells those muscles to produce fat-burning enzymes gets steadily fainter. As that happens, the easier it becomes for dietary fat to be stored as body fat. And once stored, it's likely to stay there, rather than being released into the bloodstream for burning in your increasingly less active muscles.

Burning for Maintenance

For each extra pound of muscle you add to your body, you automatically burn an extra 75 calories a day to maintain it.

In contrast, if you add a pound of fat to your body, you're calling on just 2 calories a day to maintain that extra body mass.

It all depends on metabolic activity, which is the rate at which the body makes energy or burns fat. When you compare the metabolic activity of muscle and fat, it's apparent that muscle is 37½ times more metabolically active than fat. Of all the calories burned in the body, 50 to 90 percent are burned by your muscles. And that fat-burning activity occurs even when you sleep.

The decline of muscle tone, therefore, is an important Fat-Maker Switch. And to turn that switch *off*, you have to make sure your muscles get toned up and stay active.

When Muscle Goes Downhill

Unfortunately, most adults begin losing muscle starting in their midtwenties. Of course, if you are physically active and regularly do some aerobic activity such as walking, jogging or cycling, your muscles will stay in much better tone than those of the average sedentary adult. But even so, you're bound to start losing some muscle—up to a pound

Switchbreak
SKILLPOWER
NOT ◀ - -
WILLPOWER

There's no time like right now to start tuning up your muscle tone!

Think for a moment: Which major muscle areas do you use every day? By "major muscle area," I mean a group of muscles in a general part of your body—your thighs and legs, for instance, or your arms and shoulders.

Now pick one of the muscle areas that you use the least and devise a simple exercise for it.

Let's say, for example, that you don't use your shoulders very much during the day. That's the area you might choose to develop. And here's a simple way to begin.

Hold this book out to the side of your body. With your arm fully outstretched, slowly lift the book to shoulder height. Then gradually lower it again. After you've done this several times, repeat with the other arm.

As simple as this seems, you've just added some "sustained tone" to your shoulder muscles. And that's all it takes to begin a tone-maintenance program. Doing a few extra toning movements each day can help you maintain firmness and keep your muscles from atrophying. With such minor tone-up exercises, you start to turn off Fat-Maker Switch #4.

each year—after you wave good-bye to your midtwenties.

This steady decline in muscle tissue, or lean mass, has a measurable effect on your resting metabolism— that is, the rate at which you burn energy when you're lounging, reading, watching TV or sleeping. As a result of this decline, and because your body needs fewer and fewer calories to function, the excess calories are more easily stored as body fat. When they're not called upon to pump fuel into your muscle fibers, they start to build up your fat cells like honey filling a honeycomb.

Yet there doesn't seem to be any reason why we have to lose muscle tone so rapidly and drastically. New evidence shows that few if any of us need to be losing much before the age of 90, according to studies published in the *Journal of the American Medical Association*. And even if some atrophy has already occurred, evidence shows that the decline can start to reverse in a matter of just a few weeks of toning exercises.

Fat-Maker Switch #5

Off

Alcohol— Two or More Drinks per Day

Beer? Wine? Cocktails? Well, maybe. But you might want to consider some of the consequences first.

Whenever you drink alcohol, your body burns less fat and burns it more slowly than usual. Alcohol does something else as well: It actually increases your appetite. A study at the Mayo Clinic in Rochester, Minnesota, for instance, suggests that when having alcohol at a meal, a person will consume, on average, 350 extra calories. That's a big swig of extra calories. If you're a person who usually has 1,800 to 2,000 calories a day, that would mean you're increasing your consumption by more than one-sixth—just because you have some beer or wine with your meal.

A drink is usually defined, in most studies, as 1½ ounces of hard liquor, 4 to 5 ounces of dry table wine, 3 ounces of sherry or port wine or 12 ounces of beer. All those quantities of different beverages deliver the equivalent amount of alcohol. Some people believe that a glass of beer or a glass of wine has much less alcohol than a whiskey sour or a gin-and-tonic. It seems like a natural assumption, since the concentration of alcohol is much higher in hard liquor than in beer or wine.

But when you compare mixed drinks with beer or wine, you realize why they're so close in alcohol content. One jigger of hard liquor is equal to about 1½ ounces. So if a mixed drink has a jigger of hard liquor in it, and the rest is tonic, soda or some other nonalcoholic beverage, you're getting just about the same amount of alcohol that you get from beer or wine.

Fat from Firewater?

Any two drinks can have a huge impact on the way your body deals with dietary fat. In one study published in the *New England Journal of Medicine*, for example, researchers found that three ounces of an alcoholic drink reduced the body's ability to burn fat by about one-third. Alcohol can dramatically raise your blood sugar response—and insulin levels—thus revving up your body's fat-forming processes. In addition, two or more drinks may dramatically trigger high levels of insulin, which can stimulate the conversion of carbohydrate to fat and increase the gain of body fat.

For people who have more than two drinks a day, alcohol consumption has a drastic effect on the intake of calories. It's been estimated, for instance, that someone who drinks six beers a day takes in an extra 900 calories. Because drinking alcohol also leads to increased food consumption, not all of those extra calories come directly from alcohol—but many do. An alcoholic drink has 7 calories per gram—very close to fat's 9 calories per gram. That's almost twice as many calories as you get from a gram of protein or a gram of carbohydrate.

Fuel for Controversy

For many years, researchers assumed the calories from alcohol were similar to the ones from carbohydrates, since all alcohol is derived from sugar, fruit and grains and is water-soluble. But this is not the case, according to Dr. Jean-Pierre Flatt of the University of Massachusetts Medical Center. Dr. Flatt has found that when alcohol is added to the diet, it acts in the body as if you were eating more fat.

Why?

It appears that the alcohol, while it's being burned for energy in place of fat calories, also prevents the burning of fat. So essentially, it's promoting more storage of extra fat in the body's fat cells, according to a study conducted at the Institute of Physiology at Switzerland's University of Lausanne.

In the study, researchers measured the energy expenditures of eight men during two 48-hour sessions. To make the measurements, the researchers used an indirect-calorimetry chamber. They were able to calculate changes in the body's glycogen (stored sugar), fat and protein contents while measuring the amounts of oxygen consumed, carbon dioxide produced and urinary nitrogen excreted.

There were two sessions. During the first 24 hours of each session, the men ate a normal diet with 30 percent fat. Then their energy expenditures were measured, using the indirect-calorimetry chamber. The measurements from this 24-hour period—the control period—became the basis for comparison.

On the second day of the first session, the men had 25 percent more calories in their diet, all of which came from alcohol. On the second day of the second session, alcohol was substituted for an equal number of calories. Thus, in the first session, energy intake (calories consumed) was 25 percent above that of the control period, while in the second session the men consumed the same number of calories as in the control period.

In both cases, fat burning, referred to as fat oxidation, was reduced by about 50 grams, or 36 percent. The researchers drew the conclusion that alcohol certainly favored increased fat storage. And adding the extra alcohol to the control diet resulted in even further fat storage. The significance of this new data, says Dr. Flatt, is that alcohol probably needs to be added to fat when calculating overall fat intake in the diet.

If you consume a normal diet, you can assume that every extra ounce of pure alcohol is the equivalent of about ½ ounce of dietary fat, observes Dr. Flatt. So you're drinking what amounts to ½ ounce of fat if you down two beers, two cocktails or two glasses of wine. Drinking like that for a month is about the equivalent of consuming an extra 550 grams of fat or 2½ cups of oil.

The Swiss research suggests that people who wish to control or lose weight without giving up alcohol should decrease their fat intakes to compensate for the additional calories provided by the alcohol.

Where Do You Add It On?

If you're wondering where the extra alcohol-contributed fat is likely to go in your body, medical studies in both the United States and Switzerland suggest that alcohol contributes to abdominal fat gain. To measure this factor, researchers looked at the waist-to-hip ratios of people in the study. If your waist measurement is large relative to your hip measurement, it's an indication that you have more abdominal fat—translated, that means potbelly.

In a study conducted at the Stanford University School of Medicine and the University of California, San Diego, researchers found that men and women who had more than two drinks a day also had the largest waist-to-hip ratios. The drinkers had roughly twice as many large ratios among them as did the nondrinkers.

What about Wine's Pluses?

But, you may be wondering, what about those studies suggesting that several glasses of wine per day may help reduce the risk of heart disease? If that's true, you might be asking, do the health benefits of drinking wine outweigh the drawbacks of putting on a little more fat?

Switchbreak
SKILLPOWER NOT ◄-- WILLPOWER

If you're in the habit of enjoying a beer, some wine or a cocktail before dinner and another drink with your meal, you can switch on a fat-fighting tactic this very evening.

Instead of pouring a whole beer, just pour half—and save the balance to sip slowly with dinner. If you plan to have table wine with dinner, measure out two ounces beforehand. Taste it slowly while you're preparing dinner. Then have two more ounces with your meal, if you like—but don't fill the glass any more than you did the first time.

As for cutting back on a mixed drink, it's simple. When you make a mixed drink, just use a half-jigger of alcohol instead of a full one.

How Smoking Backfires

For some people, smoking and drinking literally go hand *and* hand—a drink in one hand, a cigarette in the other. And despite statistics showing that cigarette smoking claims the lives of some 400,000 Americans annually, some smokers rationalize the habit by saying it helps keep their weight under control.

Not so, experts say.

"Smoking is a terrible and potentially lethal weight-control strategy," observes Robert C. Klesges, Ph.D., professor of psychology at the University of Memphis and an international research authority on weight and smoking. "Not everyone who smokes does so in an attempt to control weight, but a large minority of smokers do."

Ultimately, the smoke-to-control-weight strategy backfires. Research suggests, for example, that for some smokers, puffing on cigarettes actually promotes body fat gain.

Swedish physicians have reported in the British journal *Lancet* that in addition to its numerous other harmful effects, smoking can produce a sudden rise in blood sugar—a reaction that, as we've seen, increases the formation of body fat. And researchers at both Stanford University and the University of California, San Diego, have reported that nearly twice as many smokers as nonsmokers have potbellies.

But so many smokers say they gain weight every time they try to quit. What's going on?

Many people who kick the habit do crave more fat and sugar, and it's true they may gain some weight at first. But this, in fact, turns out to be a relatively minor concern compared with the dramatic health benefits that come from not smoking.

In fact, if you're a smoker now, and you're planning to stop, you'll get an added benefit from low-fat living. The principles that help you turn off fat-makers and turn on fat-burners—used in combination with the low-fat recipes in the last section of this book—guarantee that you'll minimize extra body fat even while you're giving up the habit.

The fact is, any benefits of alcohol need to be compared with potential drawbacks. A study reported in the British journal *Lancet*, for instance, found that any supposed benefits that the French gain from drinking wine are offset by ailments related to the population's overindulgence in alcohol. Researchers at the University of California, San Diego, Medical Center found that while a glass or two of wine a day may offer some protection against heart disease, the people who are healthiest and live longest tend to be those who eat the most fresh fruits and vegetables rather than those who drink the most wine.

The bottom line is this: If you choose to drink alcohol, you must do it in moderation. According to an American Cancer Society study of 275,000 middle-age men, those who had four drinks a day were 30 to 35 percent more likely than those who did not drink to die prematurely of cancer.

Another study, this one including 89,000 women, showed that those who took between three and nine drinks per week were 30 percent more likely than nondrinkers to develop breast cancer.

And in a combined analysis of 12 case-controlled studies published in the *Journal of the National Cancer Institute*, medical reviewers found that even one drink a day can increase breast cancer risk by 50 percent compared with the risk for nondrinkers. More recently, a Harvard research team reported in the same journal that more than two drinks a day may increase a woman's risk of colon or rectal cancer by 78 percent.

Fat-Maker Switch #6

Skipping Meals or Snacks

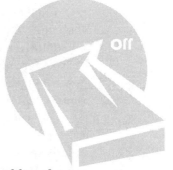

One of the most popular strategies for shedding fat is to skip breakfast and between-meal snacks in an attempt to "save calories."

Seems like the most obvious tactic in the world, right? If eating less fat is the goal, why not eat none? If fewer calories is better, then no calories is best of all . . . right?

Well, it doesn't work that way. In fact, the tactic of skipping meals actually guns the engine on your body's internal demand. When you replace a modest meal or a feeding frenzy with a big zero, your body craves to fill the loss. It just wants to make and store more body fat.

Metabolic Mutiny against Skippers

Studies have shown that skipping meals can lower your basal (baseline) metabolic rate. This rate is your normal, ho-hum, just-sittin'-there, average economical pace of ordinary fuel consumption.

To burn the maximum number of calories during the day, you want this rate to stay as high as possible. When you skip a meal and the basal metabolic rate falls, you're beginning to cancel out any meal-skipping benefits.

Let's say on a normal day you have lunch and then go about your normal afternoon chores—and on average, you burn 200 calories. But suddenly, you're seized by a new weight-loss resolution. So you decide to skip lunch.

Well, of course you take in fewer calories for lunch—zero, in fact. But studies show that you burn less—say, 180 or 190 calories—during the course of the afternoon. As you're burning fewer total calories, you're also burning fewer calories that come from fat. And since there's nowhere else for the unburned fat to go, that means you store it away.

So maybe you get a temporary advantage from skipping lunch, but you lose some ground in the afternoon. And then, if you compensate for the missing lunch by eating a bigger dinner, you're really tossing the fat to your cells, because research shows that the body is more efficient at storing fat in the evening than during the day.

"The truth is, if you eat most of your low-fat calories earlier in the day—at breakfast and lunch, for example—you'll actually stoke your internal metabolic fire to burn hotter," says Pat Harper, R.D., a spokesperson for the American Dietetic Association.

And if you skip breakfast, you're just asking for pounds of trouble. "The vast majority of overweight people are far more likely than thinner people to skip breakfast and get at least half, if not three-quarters, of their daily calories after 6:00 in the evening," observes Dr. James Kenney of the Pritikin Longevity Center.

Small and Frequent Sets the Pace

A study in the *New England Journal of Medicine* reported that frequent, small low-fat meals and snacks may be good for you in a variety of ways. To find out the impact of well-planned snacks, researchers randomly selected 14 men of average weight. They were divided—again, randomly—into two groups. Men in the first group ate three large meals a day, while those in the second group ate the same total number of calories with the identical overall percentages of protein, fat and carbohydrates in each meal. But the second group had their meals divided into 17 snacks per day.

In this study, the frequent eaters achieved significant benefits in just two weeks.

- Blood cholesterol levels plummeted 15 percent. (Lower cholesterol reduces your risk for heart disease and stroke.)
- Cortisol levels fell more than 17 percent. (Cortisol is a stress-driven, fat-forming, fat-storing hormone produced by the body when you're under increased pressure.)
- Insulin dropped nearly 28 percent. (Insulin, as noted, pulls fat molecules from the bloodstream and deposits them in your body's fat cells.)

In other words, it's not snacking that turns on your fat-makers—it's skipping snacks. But remember, we're recommending the kind of low-fat snacks you'll find in "A Quality Cornucopia: The Best Energy-Boosting, Fat-Fighting Snacks" on page 88 and in the recipe section of this book.

Switchbreak
SKILLPOWER
NOT ◄---
WILLPOWER

Take a moment right now to think about the meals you skipped or shortchanged during the past week. Did you forget about breakfast one morning because you were flying out the door? Did you gobble down a bunch of crackers for lunch because you couldn't leave your desk? Did you give up on dinner one evening and just order a late-night pizza?

Small details—right? They shouldn't matter.

Well, as you now realize, each of those missed meals was a missed opportunity to turn off Fat-Maker Switch #6.

Now think about the meals coming up in the next week. Can you say what you're going to do for breakfast, lunch and dinner each day? Do you have low-fat snacks in your cupboard and refrigerator? In your car? In your desk drawer or refrigerator at work? Remember, every time you have your low-fat meals and low-fat snacks on schedule, you're turning *off* this Fat-Maker Switch!

Fat-Maker Switch #7

Hidden Dehydration

More than 75 percent of your body is composed of water. This powerful liquid performs a crucial role in the fat-burning, fat-forming and fat-storage processes.

Water is a medium for every chemical reaction, including the burning of fat. When you don't drink enough water, your body will secrete the hormone aldosterone, which causes tissues to hold on to almost every molecule of liquid, according to Peter Lindner, M.D., in *Fat, Water Retention and You*. And several researchers suggest that a decrease in water may cause fat deposits to increase.

You'd think a cry of thirst would automatically go out from your cells. When your body needs water, doesn't it send a direct, clear signal?

The answer is yes and no. Yes, your thirst alarm will ring loud and clear if you're marathoning across Death Valley on a summer's day. But if you're running errands, making calls, clacking away at the word processor or just hanging out, the thirst alarm is likely to be very faint, distant and easily mistaken for some other kind of signal.

Signs of Dry Gulch

"The fatigue, simple headaches, lack of concentration and dizziness you feel at the end of a workday can result simply from not drinking enough water," says Liz Applegate, Ph.D., nutritional science lecturer at the University of California, Davis. "It starts every day as soon as you awaken. When you open your eyes in the morning, your body is already facing a water deficit."

Sometimes we run a deficit all day without even knowing it. Dehydration occurs when you don't take in enough water to replace all that's lost through perspiration, respiration and urination. Dehydration reduces blood volume, creating thicker, more concentrated blood, which may stress the heart and is less capable of providing muscles with oxygen and nutrients. Also, thicker blood doesn't eliminate accumulated wastes as well.

"Even a tiny shortage of water disrupts your biochemistry," says Michael Colgan, Ph.D., nutritional researcher and visiting scholar at Rockefeller University. "Dehydrate a muscle by only 3 percent, and you lose 10 percent of contractile strength and 8 percent of speed. Water balance is the single most important variable in lifelong good health and top performance."

Out to Quench

There's another side effect of hidden thirst: You may think you're hungry when actually you're not—you're just thirsty. As a result, you might eat too many snacks or fill your plate a second time at a meal when what you really need is a tall glass of water. You end up putting more food calories (both fat and nonfat) into your body when your body is just calling out for zero-calorie liquids.

But if most of us are so dehydrated, you may ask, why don't we just shrivel up and wither away?

Well, the dehydration isn't that drastic. You get adequate water from food and the few beverages you nor-

Switchbreak
SKILLPOWER
NOT ◄- -
WILLPOWER

If you've ever watched a long-distance cycling event, you have probably noticed the water bottles used by super-cyclists as they streak down the open road at 60 miles per hour.

Or maybe you've seen the tall jugs, complete with long plastic straws and emblazoned with logos, that are seized by the eager hands of aerobics instructors. Or the oversize sports-drink bottles that stand like referees alongside the tennis court, waiting to be grabbed between sets.

The hydration business has hit the big time for athletes. And now it's time for you to do some easy water bottle shopping, whether you're a part-time athlete or not.

Visit any sporting goods store, pharmacy or discount store and pick out the largest easy-to-hold, easy-to-open water container you can find. You probably won't have to spend more than $5— and it's an investment that pays out in a very big way when it comes to switching off this fat-maker.

Why? Because if you want to end hidden dehydration, you need to have water nearby almost all the time.

mally have during the day. It's just not the optimal amount that you really need to thrive.

Getting used to life with less water is like getting accustomed to constant stress or tension: It can undermine your energy and weaken your health. The solution takes some getting used to, but it's well worth the effort.

Of course, it's easy enough to turn *off* Fat-Maker Switch #7: All you have to do, as you'll see, is turn *on* Fat-Burner Switch #3. There are literally hundreds of ways to do that. But for now, you can switch off the hidden dehydration with the Switchbreak on page 59.

Fat-Maker Switch #8

Inactivity

On average, how much of the day and evening do you spend sitting?

Is it unusual for you to be sitting down for an hour? Or two? Maybe three?

The human body is biologically designed for movement, and when you're not busy moving, your body gets busy storing. Whenever you are inactive for more than 60 minutes or so, it's likely that your body is sending an ancient signal to your brain to decrease fat-*burning* and increase fat-*making*. And when you eat a big meal and then sit for an hour or longer, there's more chance you will end up storing calories from the meal as body fat.

According to studies by researchers at the National Center for Chronic Disease Prevention and Health Promotion at the Centers for Disease Control and Prevention in Atlanta, the less active people are, the more overweight they are. As you age, there's an even closer correlation between the amount of time you spend sitting and the amount of body weight you're likely to gain. So daily physical activity becomes an even more important factor as we grow older.

The Leisure Seizure

We are surrounded by manifold temptations to be sluggish. After a big dinner, many people just move from table to TV, then watch until they go to sleep. Americans watch, on average, about 4 to 4½ hours of television each day—and that's just television, not including VCR time. Evidence suggests that this prolonged evening television-watching lowers your metabolism. And there's no doubt that sitting still after a hearty meal will turn on your Fat-Maker Switch.

For some people, in fact, the TV makes more fat than multiple servings of double bacon-cheeseburgers. In a study of 6,000 working men with an average age of 40, researchers found that those who spent more than three to four hours a day watching TV doubled their risk of becoming obese—that is, acquiring 20 to 30 percent extra body fat.

The unhealthy relationship between TV and weight seems to get magnified at the three-hour-a-day mark, observe Larry A. Tucker, Ph.D., professor and director of health promotion at Brigham Young University in Provo, Utah, and Glenn M. Friedman, M.D. The researchers found that men who watch television an average of only an hour a day are half as likely to be unhealthily overweight as the three-hour-a-day watchers.

These findings seem to hold for women as well, according to a study by Dr. Tucker and Marilyn Bagwell, R.N., Ph.D. In a population of nearly 5,000 working women whose average age was 35, the researchers found that those who watched three to

Switchbreak
SKILLPOWER
NOT ◄- -
WILLPOWER

Right now, with book in hand, stand up and move your shoulders in a gentle shrugging motion.

Now pass the book from hand to hand, alternately opening and closing each hand as you pass it back and forth.

While you do this, find something natural to look at—a living plant, a flower or a nature scene outside. Now head back to your chair and sit down. Adjust your posture for greatest reading comfort.

Lift your feet. With your legs straight out in front of you, wiggle your feet in every direction.

Mission accomplished?

If so, you have just "signaled" your brain to reduce the fat-maker tendencies brought on by inactivity. For a half-hour or an hour, you have helped to turn off Fat-Maker Switch #8. It's that simple.

four hours (or more) of TV a day were twice as likely to be obese.

In addition to the weight gain that comes from just sitting still, TV seems to produce an additional fattening effect, possibly because just watching it has a depressing effect on metabolism. In a study of nearly 800 adults, published in the *Journal of the American Dietetic Association*, researchers surmised that not all the weight gain that they observed could be explained by the amount of time spent sitting, even if they took extra snacking into account. In the group they studied, the incidence of obesity among those who watched four hours or more of TV per day was quadruple that of people who watched an hour or less daily. The multihour viewers were putting on extra body fat at an accelerated rate.

Fat-Maker Switch #9

Poor-Quality Sleep

Efficient fat loss and energy building depend on your body receiving deep rest and getting a chance to recover during sleep.

Poor-quality sleep can hurt your health. When you're restless at night, the sleep/wake pattern interferes with nighttime metabolic processes. The next day, you'll find it's more difficult to stay physically active and alert—and to make good hour-by-hour choices.

When, night after night, you're getting less sleep than you need, you are significantly more likely to overeat as you attempt to prop yourself up. "People eat more when they are tired," observes Donald Bliwise, Ph.D., director of the Sleep Disorders Center at Emory University School of Medicine in Atlanta. And if you're just grabbing whatever food is available to reboot your system, it's likely you'll favor unhealthy foods that are high in fat.

A study of both laboratory animals and humans, reported

in the *Tufts University Diet and Nutrition Letter*, demonstrated that appetite increases when we're deprived of good-quality sleep. These findings may turn out to be very important in weight-control efforts. Americans now get less sleep—and poorer-quality sleep—than ever before. Research has shown that sleep-deprived people tend to increase their caloric consumption by more than 10 to 15 percent per day, according to Allan Rechtschaffen, Ph.D., professor of psychiatry and director of the Sleep Research Laboratory at the University of Chicago.

Fat-Maker Switch #10

Mismanaged Stress

How many times a day do you get frustrated or angry? How often do you feel anxious or upset? Do you often feel guilty about things you haven't done or about people you've forgotten?

All these are stress symptoms. Usually, they vanish quickly. But if they hang on, the stress not only tenses your body, it also adds to general feelings of being under nonstop pressure. In the struggle and strain of

Switchbreak
SKILLPOWER NOT ← - - WILLPOWER

Exactly how did you fall asleep last night and the night before? Were you in front of the TV? Did you nod off in midpage while you were lying on the sofa trying to read?

Many people wait for these nod-off signals before they head for bed. But whenever you fall asleep with lights on or in an awkward position, you sabotage the overall quality of your rest.

To break from this pattern—and turn off Fat-Maker Switch #9—do something different tonight. Plan to get ready for bed 15 minutes before you usually do. Don't wait for a loud commercial or the clunk of a falling book to stir you into bed-directed action. Kill the TV. Turn off the lights. Head for the bedroom.

If you get all tucked in and are not quite drowsy enough, pick up a bedside copy of a magazine that highlights wildlife or nature photography rather than calamity-of-the-week features. When you're ready to drift off, you hardly have to stir—just turn off the light. It's a much better entry into dreamland than the frenzied echo of the last late-night commercial.

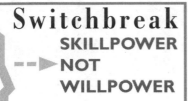

Switchbreak
SKILLPOWER
---▶ NOT
WILLPOWER

Take a long, deep breath, then release it slowly. Feel more relaxed?

The way you breathe can have a major impact on how you feel.

When you feel distressed, you tend to breathe more shallowly. The level of carbon dioxide, the primary waste product in your blood, goes up. Your oxygen level rapidly descends. If this pattern continues, anxiety increases as your body tries to breathe harder to eliminate carbon dioxide. Meanwhile, your diaphragm tenses up and you lose your ability to breathe deeply.

And that's exactly the kind of stress reaction that can turn on Fat-Maker Switch #10.

While pressure-related situations can't be avoided, good breathing technique is just one of the tools you can use to break the distress/tension cycle. Medical experts report that even a single smooth, deep breath can ease tension and increase your sense of calmness and control.

dealing with those feelings, your body pays a considerable price.

Of course, people's attitudes toward stress differ. Some view stress as a challenge to grow and develop. But if there are times when you find it difficult to cope or adapt to change, stress can turn into distress.

Under these conditions, very strong reactions are triggered. Your heartbeat becomes more rapid, blood pressure rises and muscle tension increases. It's not unusual for anxiety and fatigue to increase, and you may even feel mentally distracted.

Why Get Unstressed?

A lot of the reactions set off by stress-related hormones can translate directly into increased body fat, researchers have found. When we're reacting to stress rather than meeting it and growing from it, many of us overeat, consuming foods high in fat and refined sugar, and also skip exercise. Studies also report distress-related triggering of the "starvation response"—that is, an unconscious tendency to store food as if our bodies were preparing for famine. Not only that, distress sets fat-making processes into overdrive, so we end up storing a great deal of added body fat.

Fat-making is further increased by the hormones that are released in stressful situations, including cortisol and epinephrine. These hormones, studies have shown, may actually jolt your body into storing more body fat.

It seems that overall, the more minutes of each day you are

frustrated, impatient or angry, the more likely that distress is contributing to fat-making in your body. When your distress levels are high, blood sugar is routed away from chemical pathways that would burn it. Instead of serving your energy-burning muscles, much of the blood sugar is converted into fat and stored in fat cells.

Extended periods of distress also make it more difficult for you to listen to the brain/body signals that guide you toward healthy low-fat eating—and help guide you away from tempting high-fat foods.

Reminder List: Turn Off the Fat-Makers

Fat-Maker Switch #1: High-Fat Meals or Snacks

Fat-Maker Switch #2: Stuffing Yourself—Even with Low-Fat or Nonfat Foods

Fat-Maker Switch #3: Low-Fiber or No-Fiber Meals or Snacks

Fat-Maker Switch #4: Vanishing Muscle Tone

Fat-Maker Switch #5: Alcohol—Two or More Drinks per Day

Fat-Maker Switch #6: Skipping Meals or Snacks

Fat-Maker Switch #7: Hidden Dehydration

Fat-Maker Switch #8: Inactivity

Fat-Maker Switch #9: Poor-Quality Sleep

Fat-Maker Switch #10: Mismanaged Stress

Your Ten Fat-Burner Switches

urning on Fat-Burner Switches is quick and simple to do once you learn how. As you read about these switches in the next ten chapters, be sure to take advantage of the Switchbreaks by giving them a try. It's good practice. And the Switchbreaks will help you find out how easy it is to flick on all ten switches.

When you switch on all the fat-burners, you're taking care of your whole mind and body—digestion, muscles, circulation, heart, brain and every other system in your body. These make up a complete and integrated whole. And if you care for one exclusively, ignoring or slighting other parts of your mind or anatomy, you imperil the entire balance.

Conversely, when you switch on one fat-burner and begin to experience increased circulation or alertness or fat-burning power, you enhance the results you get from the other nine. And as I've emphasized, the time and energy it takes to flip these switches on can be adjusted to fit any lifestyle. Whether you're a mom with a thousand chores, errands and obligations or a career-driven professional who's swamped with tasks, meetings and

Part

2

messages—and spending stressful time away from home—you still have opportunities to turn on these switches.

Of course, you will want to modify these switches if you need to be cautious because of your age or medical condition. If you have a preexisting condition and the doctor has already given you guidelines for nutrition and exercise, you'll want to review those guidelines before making any drastic change in your routine. And if any of these switches causes you pain, discomfort or significant mood changes, consult your physician as soon as possible. The problem is likely to be temporary, but it never hurts to check—and it can hurt a lot if you don't. The low-fat living skills work best when they're combined with the insights and advice of your personal physician and other health professionals. As long as you follow those commonsense guidelines, you'll find that these switches can be highly effective. You're in for a treat—not a treatment.

Chapter Four

Fat-Burner Switch #1

Quick-Start Your Morning Metabolism

By simply turning on this one switch, you can increase your energy level and fat-burning patterns for the rest of the day.

Sound impossible? Actually, it's extraordinarily easy.

Stop for a moment to reflect: What are your mornings like? Are you rushing around, feeling frantic? Or is it more your style to get up feeling draggy and lethargic?

This morning when the alarm went off, did you switch on one dim light as you climbed out of bed? Did you skip breakfast—or gulp down a cup of coffee as you flew out the door?

There are as many ways to get out of bed in the morning as there are people in the world who get out of bed. You have your own style; we all do. And since it has probably been a pattern with you for many years, it's not something you often reconsider.

Maybe you should, because research has shown that you can turn on a Fat-Burner Switch the moment you get up in the morning.

Begin with Any Switch!

The ten Fat-Burner Switches are not arranged in order of importance or power. For instance, Switch #7—muscle-toning—may burn more total fat than any of the others, but they each have a role to play.

So read about all ten, then begin with any one and gradually add the other nine.

Lights—Action!

In a moment, we'll look at some ways you can instantly switch on your fat-burning metabolism and energy. But first consider the reasons that this Fat-Burner Switch works so well when you turn it on.

From the moment you get out of bed, your brain begins cuing your body to match current and anticipated physical demands. If your morning ritual takes place in low light and in slow motion, your brain gets a low signal. With that signal trudging through your nervous system on leaden paws, your body has little incentive to push your metabolism much higher than what seems near-hibernation rate.

Now suppose you extend this "sleepwalk" activity level into the morning—that is, your mind is moaning "I wish, I wish, I wish I were back in bed." And suppose you decide to skip breakfast while you're trudging around trying to get things together.

In the process, you unwittingly fail to turn on your Fat-Burner Switch #1. And you may even stimulate fat-preserving and fat-storing processes instead.

Cock-a-Doodle Do's—And Don'ts

With the Low-Fat Living Program, you can reverse this trend. There are three key elements of giving an effective wake-up call to your metabolism.

1. Turn up the lights.
2. Get at least five minutes of easy physical activity.
3. Enjoy a great-tasting, low-fat breakfast.

These three simple actions combine to turn on your body's "thermic switch" and move your natural biological rhythms into higher revs.

If these three steps already make up your morning routine, congratulations. You don't have to give a second thought to this switch—though maybe I can suggest a few variations that may help speed your metabolism even more.

If, on the other hand, you're from the I-wish-I-were-hibernating school of morning rituals, you'll need to consider what you can do differently—beginning tomorrow morning—to put these methods in motion.

Let's consider the morning strategies one by one.

It's calorie-burning, not calorie-cutting, that gives you the metabolic power you've been missing.

—Dietitians Victoria Zak, R.D., and Cris Carlin, R.D., and Peter D. Vash, M.D., eating disorders specialist at UCLA Medical Center

Turn Up the Lights

On sunny mornings, do you step outside for a breath of fresh air and soak in the brightness? Many of us do embrace this roosterlike routine on vacations but somehow neglect it the rest of the year.

Of all the signals the human brain responds to, one of the most powerful is light. The body has hundreds of biochemical and hormonal rhythms, all keyed to light and dark. Here are some ways to brighten your morning.

Get your good lux. Research has demonstrated that there's a direct link between the retina of the eye—where the light-receptor nerves are located—and a small portion of the brain that focuses our attention. In one study, a Harvard medical team took some volunteers through a series of light-exposure tests, experimenting with intensities ranging from 7,000 to 12,000 lux. This was comparable to the amount of light you'd get if you stepped outside the door into full daylight just after dawn.

By measuring the change in brain-wave patterns immediately following this exposure, scientists established the link between the retina and an area of the brain known as the suprachiasmatic nuclei. What this means, according to professors Richard Kronauer, Ph.D., and Charles Czeisler, M.D., the two scientists who headed the three-year Harvard study, is that there is a direct connection between light exposure and the part of the brain that is thought to play a key role in attention focus and energy production.

Blaze away in the morning. When your alarm sounds tomorrow morning, flick on the light you usually turn on, then look around for other light switches. The hall light? The extra lights in the bathroom? The lamp on the bureau?

Switchbreak
SKILLPOWER
‑‑► NOT
WILLPOWER

For that morning wake-up call that turns on Fat-Burner Switch #1, sun power is even better than bulb power.

Even if it's just dawn's early light, you get higher luxes from the sun than from all the lights in the house.

So tomorrow morning, throw open the curtains or pull up the blinds as soon as you get up. If the sun's already peeking in your window, take a minute to stand there and enjoy the view.

A little later, find any excuse to step outside for a couple of minutes. Take a brief stroll around the yard (perimeter inspection!) to flood your eyes with daylight. If you have a dog to walk (canine attention!), head for a sunlit patch of street or lawn—and give Bowser plenty of time to do what needs to be done. That blast of morning sun is as energizing for you as Bowser's relief is for him.

That's right—they should all go on in the morning. For many people, the added light triggers an instantaneous alertness-booster in the brain that shifts physiology away from sleep and toward a new day filled with more energy and higher metabolism.

Get at Least Five Minutes of Easy Physical Activity

I don't know about you, but a rigorous, marine-style morning sit-up routine has never seemed like much fun to me.

Fortunately, it's not necessary, either. All you need is five minutes of activity, and it doesn't have to be the kind of effort that builds abs or pecs—or tests the limits of human endurance.

Easy activity should be just that—easy. Studies show that most of us are quite sedentary in the morning hours, and this keeps our metabolism sluggish. But if you can just squeeze in $\frac{1}{12}$ of an hour of morning physical activity—either before or after breakfast—you'll definitely increase your morning metabolism.

Get in the exer-habit. If you're just starting to do morning activities, don't worry about whether you'll be able to continue the routine. In all probability, you will. A study by the Southwestern Health Institute in Phoenix found that three out of four people who did some morning exercise continued the exercise habit one year later.

In fact, the morning exercise routine is easier to make habit-forming than a later-in-the-day routine. When researchers at the health institute contrasted a morning exercise pattern with the behavior of people who usually wait until midday or evening to get their exercise, they found that only half of the midday-exercise crowd continued their routines for more than a year. And only one in four of the evening exercisers kept it up that long.

If you rev up your metabolism and energy early in the day, you're establishing a pattern without even thinking about it. If you leave exercise until later in the day, you'll probably find it's easier to make up excuses like "I'm too tired" or simply "Whoops—I ran out of time."

Move on out. Should you exercise before breakfast or after?

It's up to you. There's some evidence, however, that moderate exercise in the morning before breakfast may give you a head start in burning off excess body fat. After a full night's sleep, you don't have as much stored carbohydrate (glycogen) in your muscles. So when you get up to exercise, the fuel that's pulled from your cells is more likely to be fat than glycogen.

Whether or not this applies to all kinds of exercise, it's certainly true for runners who work out regularly before breakfast. For regular runners, two-thirds of the calories burned in prebreakfast workouts come from fat, according to a study directed by Anthony Wilcox, Ph.D., at Kansas State University in Manhattan. By contrast, in the runners' afternoon workouts, less than half the calories they burn come from fat.

Respect your pace. If you're a slow riser, someone who simply doesn't like early-morning exercise, be honest with yourself. Make it a daily habit to get out of bed slowly, get dressed at a leisurely pace and gradually increase your activity level.

Before or after eating breakfast, go through a gentle warm-up period and then do a few minutes of light physical activity. Take five minutes to stroll around the yard or neighborhood.

Equip yourself. For a good morning start, an exercise bicycle, cross-country ski machine or rowing machine comes in very handy. You can watch the morning news as you pedal at a relaxed, moderate pace on the stationary cycle, pull out some smooth, balanced oar strokes on your rowing machine or go on an imaginary cross-country ski loop.

For variety you might do some moderate strengthening or abdominal-toning exercises like those shown beginning on

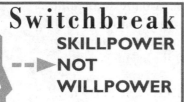

Switchbreak
SKILLPOWER
- - ▶ NOT
WILLPOWER

To make morning exercise easier, plan ahead.

Tonight before you go to bed, pull your "physical activity" clothes out of the drawer and put them on top of the bureau or on a bedroom chair. Simply seeing them there in the morning helps remind you to get moving.

These should be clothes you can slip on in an instant. Loose sweats are best. If they're ready to go, you don't even have to think about the "getting dressed" part of your morning routine.

page 155. You may soon enjoy this "active time" so much that on some days it will stretch into 10 or 15 or even 20 minutes. That's even better, of course—but don't push yourself. It should never be a strain to turn on Fat-Burner Switch #1.

Enjoy a Great-Tasting, Low-Fat Breakfast

Breakfast is the meal that matters most. Even when you're in a hurry, there are ways to grab a great-tasting morning meal on the run.

As I've described, what you do eat or don't eat first thing in the morning can throw on the Fat-Maker Switches and throw *off* the Fat-Burner Switches for your entire day.

Here's why: When you eat even a small serving of a low-fat breakfast, you switch on your energy and fat-burning power. At the same time, you turn off Fat-Maker Switch #6, the one that kicks into high gear every time you miss a meal.

"Always remember that skipping a meal leads to bingeing," explains Kathy Stone, R.D., author of *Snack Attack*. "Eating breakfast is also essential to help control eating after dinner. Surprising, but true. What you eat in the morning affects how full you feel at the end of the day. If you think that breakfast makes you hungrier, that you are actually better off on the days when you go as long as possible without eating, think again. What happens when you finally start eating? Most times you lose control."

"We can't overstress the importance of breakfast," says Peter D. Vash, M.D., endocrinologist and internist on the faculty of the University of California, Los Angeles, Medical Center, who specializes in obesity and eating disorders, and dietitians Cris Carlin, R.D., and Victoria Zak, R.D.

These researchers call the fat-burning process a thermic

switch, and they've found that it's the key to the right start. "When you wake up and get started on a new day, you must have breakfast to turn on your thermic switch, moving your body's rhythm from low ebb to high tide," the researchers say.

Don't skip out. Even though you know you should have breakfast in the morning to switch off Fat-Maker Switch #6, it's easy to get into the habit of skipping. And you may feel as if you just don't have the appetite for breakfast.

There's a good chance that's because you've learned to override your morning body clock. Once you re-establish your normal, healthy metabolic rate, you'll begin to feel hungry when you get up in the morning.

In addition, "you will be hungry at appropriate times throughout the day and will lose the urge to binge in the evenings," observes C. Wayne Callaway, M.D., obesity specialist, clinical professor at George Washington University in Washington, D.C., and former director of the Nutrition and Lipid Clinic at the Mayo Clinic in Rochester, Minnesota.

If you've long avoided morning meals, you might simply begin with a piece of just-ripe fruit—an apple, a banana, an orange or half a grapefruit, for example. Then have some 100% whole-grain toast or a bagel with nonfat cream cheese on it and a cup of tea or coffee. On some mornings you may enjoy mixing whole-grain cereal with a four-ounce serving of nonfat or low-fat yogurt. You'll reap the benefits all day long.

Go for the classics—plus. One of the best combinations for breakfast is the classic "health food special"—a bowl of old-fashioned oatmeal with low-fat or skim milk and a piece of fruit. Another classic is my personal favorite, Bircher-Benner Muesli (see the easy recipe in "The 'Master Breakfast' from Switzerland" on page 77).

The food you get in the morning should provide both protein and carbohydrate, in part because of the overnight activity of your liver. "In the morning your liver will be about 75 percent depleted of glycogen," notes Lawrence E. Lamb, M.D., medical consultant to the President's Council on Physical Fitness and Sports and author of *Stay Youthful and Fit* and *The Weighting Game: The Truth about Weight Control.*

As I've noted, glycogen is the energy fuel that the liver makes out of blood sugar, or glucose. "If you want to protect your body protein, you had better provide some carbohydrate food early in

Switchbreak
SKILLPOWER
--▶ NOT
WILLPOWER

If you're in the habit of skipping a low-fat breakfast because you don't have enough time in the morning, reset your alarm clock right now.

Set it 5 or 10 minutes earlier. Or 15. Or even 20, if necessary—whatever it takes to allow yourself enough time for breakfast.

Don't want to give up those additional minutes of sleep?

Well, breakfast will give you a far greater payoff than the extra bit of sleep you might gain—especially if staying in bed longer means that you have to ditch your morning meal. Ten minutes is all it takes for a glass of juice and some whole-grain rye bread or crackers or a bowl of cereal.

the morning to replace that glucose," adds Dr. Lamb. "Your brain will function better, too, as it needs that glucose to maintain its ability to do all the complex tasks required of it."

But there's another reason to get protein and carbohydrate in this first meal of the day, and it has to do with the processes in your autonomic nervous system. That's the network that activates body parts that you never have to consciously think about, such as the lungs, heart, liver, intestines and brain. When you feed this system an early-morning start-up breakfast of carbohydrate, protein and fiber, you tend to automatically rev up hormones and neurotransmitters that prime you for an active day. So the right kind of low-fat breakfast actually helps set the fat-burning rate for the whole day.

Protein and carbohydrate are easy to get in this first meal. The protein can come from low-fat dairy products such as skim milk, low-fat cottage cheese, nonfat yogurt or nonfat cream cheese. Since fiber-rich complex carbohydrates are found in any whole-grain food, be sure to have whole-grain bread, a whole-grain boxed cereal or old-fashioned oatmeal.

Though I prefer old-fashioned cooked oatmeal or Bircher-Benner Muesli, your supermarket probably has a good selection of boxed cereals. Just be sure to go for whole-grain products. Among them are Walnut Acres Nonfat Whole Oat Granola, Nature's Path Heartage, Hidden Valley Amaranth, Kellogg's Extra Fiber All-Bran, General Mills' Fiber One, Kellogg's Fiberwise and Kellogg's Heartwise.

Eat on the drive in. If you drive any distance to work, you've got more than enough time for breakfast.

True, a bowl of cereal is a bit difficult to handle when

The "Master Breakfast" from Switzerland

One of the world's best known natural-healing medical clinics and hospitals is the Bircher-Benner Clinic in Zurich, Switzerland. And a pillar of the clinic's health-building regimen is a unique breakfast cereal long favored by European mountain people.

Bircher-Benner Muesli, as it's called, is easy to make and very satisfying. Instead of cooking old-fashioned oats, you mix them with water the evening before, then soak them overnight. You can serve the muesli with just-ripe fruit and yogurt. Here's how to make a single serving.

½ cup slow-cooking oats, uncooked
    Just-ripe fruit (apple, banana, orange, berries) or canned
        unsweetened fruit such as peaches
    Nonfat or 1% low-fat plain yogurt
1 teaspoon brown sugar (optional)
    Cinnamon, vanilla or other natural flavorings

Place the oats in a bowl and add enough pure water to cover. Cover the bowl and place it in the refrigerator overnight.

In the morning, slice the fruit. Add it with the yogurt, brown sugar (if using) and flavoring to taste to the oatmeal and stir.

---

you're obliged to steer, shift and change lanes. But a number of low-fat breakfasts may lend themselves to the morning commute.

Before you leave home, add some frozen berries and a handful of nonfat whole-oats granola to a cup of nonfat plain yogurt. Mix it all together in a pint container with a screw-on lid, and you're ready to go.

Another idea: Slice a whole-grain, rye or pumpernickel bagel in two and spread it with nonfat cream cheese. Put the halves together and slip the bagel into a sandwich bag; you can have your breakfast break anywhere along the morning route.

Meet to eat. Make the first meal of the day more fun and interesting. Begin a breakfast partnership with your spouse, your child, a friend or a co-worker.

If you eat with someone at home, take turns making the low-fat breakfast for each other. When you're meeting with a friend or co-worker, remember that you don't have to go to the local diner or gourmet-muffin breakfast shop, especially in good weather. Instead meet in a nearby park, where you can combine breakfast with a walk and a bit of sunlight. You can also meet a few minutes early at work or drop by a fellow commuter's house first thing in the morning and share a low-fat breakfast before starting out.

Steer clear of country specials. Stay away from the kinds of food that Ma and Pa Kettle used to have before hitching up Nelly and working in the fields. A high-fat breakfast of scrambled eggs and sausage is an invitation for fat to come right in and make itself at home—in your cells, that is.

Don't think you have to go to a greasy spoon to get more than your share of morning fat. You're also getting an overload of fat if you microwave some instant oatmeal, cover it with whole milk and butter up a couple of slices of toasted white bread.

With any kind of high-fat breakfast, your blood sugar rises fast. Fat with breakfast sends your blood sugar up at twice the rate of lunchtime fat. And the fat-forming processes after breakfast may be double what they are after lunch.

Chapter Five

Fat-Burner Switch #2

Eat Low-Fat, High-Fiber Snacks

I know it may be hard to believe, but it's true: Eating healthful, low-fat between-meal snacks increases your energy and metabolism, triggering an energizing process that produces heat and burns calories. Eating these snacks also reduces the urge to overeat, especially at night.

During the day when you go for four or five hours at a stretch without eating, your blood sugar levels drop and your energy wanes. It may take a strong dose of willpower just to get out of your chair, let alone do some daily exercise. So instead of stuffing yourself at two or three meals a day, it makes far more sense to eat less at each meal and eat more often, according to research published in the *New England Journal of Medicine* and the *American Journal of Clinical Nutrition*.

The studies show that moderate-size meals plus small between-meal snacks may help lower blood cholesterol levels, reduce body fat, enhance digestion, lessen the risk of heart disease and increase metabolism. In one study researchers found that people who ate more frequently had lower cholesterol levels than those who ate just a few big meals. Furthermore, cholesterol levels went down even though the more frequent eaters consumed more food during the day.

Planning That Pays Off

There are many good scientific reasons why it's time for most of us to change not only what but also when and how much we eat.

The large, traditional American meals that stimulate excessive insulin production essentially build up the body's strongest pro-fat hormone. A burger and french fries—or any high-fat variations on this theme—promote fat storage. Such meals also speed the conversion of sugar to body fat.

In contrast, moderate meals and between-meal snacks (as illustrated in "The Low-Fat Living 3-plus-4 Eating Plan" on page 83) promote a steadier production of sustained energy. This eating plan also promotes fat-burning and tends to produce a smaller, healthier insulin response.

It's important to note that the 3-plus-4 Eating Plan still allows for the normal and necessary storage of some body fat, which is vital to health. Yet the plan is targeted to prevent the storage of needless, excess body fat.

The plan changes that by altering not just when and how much you eat but also what you eat. If you follow this plan—keeping your calorie intake in the range shown for each snack and meal—you'll satisfy your appetite while stoking your energy system at just the right intervals.

Feeling Snackish?

There are many other good reasons for snacking. Since ancient times, people have instinctively and traditionally taken a pause several times a day to make tea and consume a favored serving of food. Then, while enjoying each sip and every bite, they look out at the horizon or share a warm conversation or reflect on the path just traveled. It is through these simple actions that the day—and life—remains in a bit better perspective, and one of the simplest and healthiest of human pleasures is not forgotten. Few choices provide greater rewards, no matter how fast the world seems to be moving.

So here are some guidelines for taking low-fat snack breaks—yes, even in the rush of twenty-first-century life.

Scatter your snack attacks. Snacking on low-fat foods throughout the day has considerable weight-loss advantages, observes Dean Ornish, M.D., founder and president of the Preventive Medicine Research Institute in Sausalito, California, and assistant clinical professor of medicine at the University of California, San Francisco, School of Medicine. By eating low-fat snacks in midmorning and midafternoon, you're less likely to stuff yourself at main meals or lapse into stress-related eating binges in the evening.

Keep favorite snacks nearby. Adults make an average of 20 to 30 food decisions a day, according to

Don't Snatch Sat-Fat Snacks

When you're scanning the supermarket shelves for low-fat snacks, you not only want to avoid saturated fats from animal sources, you also need to be particularly wary of snacks and other packaged foods that list "pure vegetable oil" as an ingredient. Often this oil is coconut, palm-kernel or palm oil—which are comprised of 86 percent, 81 percent and 49 percent saturated fat, respectively. Coconut and palm-kernel oils are even more saturated than beef fat and lard!

Even if the food label says "cholesterol-free," read the tiny print listing nutrients. It's true these three vegetable oils don't contain cholesterol, but they do raise cholesterol in the blood.

George L. Blackburn, M.D., Ph.D., associate professor of surgery at Harvard Medical School and chief of the Nutrition Metabolism Laboratory at Deaconess Hospital in Boston. Therefore, it's critically important to have low-fat snacks readily available to make your between-meal food choices as easy as possible.

If the only food on hand is a monster soda and a bag of chips or a huge candy bar, you may end up consuming 50 or 60 grams of fat or 1,000 calories all at once, just because you grabbed what was convenient. Be sure to look at the low-fat snacks I recommend in this chapter, then shop for those, so they'll be on hand the next time you reach for one.

Make teatime your snack time. "Many, if not most, people are better off with low-fat snacks at midmorning and

Switchbreak
SKILLPOWER
---▶NOT
WILLPOWER

Things have changed a lot since Adam and Eve's day, and fortunately, fresh fruit is no longer forbidden. The same goes for fresh vegetables. The trick—if there is one—is to keep these temptations within reach.

If you find yourself getting hungry around midmorning or midafternoon every day, what's available? Packaged crackers? A bag of chips? A turbocharged candy bar or a bag of peanuts?

Right now, think about one place you can put an apple, a banana, an orange or a bag of carrots, celery or radishes where it will be ready for a snack break tomorrow.

It sounds like a simple change, but just having a fresh snack in your desk drawer or in your glove compartment actually changes your environment.

And "it's when you make changes in your environment that it's easier to succeed" at low-fat living, according to Diane Hanson, Ph.D., lifestyle specialist at the Pritikin Longevity Center in Santa Monica, California.

especially at midafternoon," says Richard N. Podell, M.D., director of the Overlook Center for Weight Management in New York City.

As the day wears on, what and when you eat take on increased significance, because metabolism gradually starts falling off. An afternoon snack helps to boost the glucose supply that you need for energy, according to Dr. Podell. "Eating at this time helps you handle the midafternoon blood sugar dip," he notes. "Also, an afternoon snack helps keep your blood sugar levels steady, so you won't become ravenous by the time you eat dinner."

In mid- to late afternoon the brain has a strong tendency to crave high-fat, high-sugar foods. It's important to head off the pattern of having a late-afternoon snack that's high in fat or a high-fat dinner. That too-hearty dinner, especially, sets off signals that prime you to consume far more fat late at night.

Turn the fat down low. Generally, the snacks that you want have less than five grams of fat per serving—and an even better target may be three grams per serving. And if you're eating a packaged low-fat food, be sure to read the label carefully to find out exactly what is meant by a "serving." Remember, if you overeat snacks—even fat-free ones—you may turn on Fat-Maker Switch #2 and end up converting existing calories into body fat.

Pare the calories. Though fat comes first, you need to keep an eye on calories as well. Even if you're eating nonfat food, the calories can increase quickly if

The Low-Fat Living 3-plus-4 Eating Plan

"Eat three square meals a day" was the old advice—but it came from another era. Today you're much better off eating three low-fat meals and three or four low-fat snacks every day. Research now points to the conclusion that this pattern—not the three-square plan—will help you turn off your Fat-Maker Switches and turn on the fat-burners, keeping your body fat to a comfortable minimum.

The chart below shows how the plan works. All meals are less than 500 calories, with a maximum of 20 to 25 percent of those calories from fat. But in addition to the three meals, you should treat yourself to at least two—and up to four—snacks during the day, at approximately the two- to three-hour intervals shown in the chart. All snacks should be lower in calories—and therefore lower in fat—than the meals. If you space your meals and snacks as shown and stick to the recommended calorie levels, you'll help keep the calories stored as excess fat to an absolute minimum.

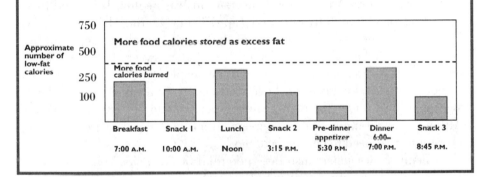

you eat fast or go back for a second or third serving. All the snacks listed in "A Quality Cornucopia: The Best Energy-Boosting, Fat-Fighting Snacks" on page 88, for instance, are under 300 calories in the amounts shown. But if you eat two or three servings at each snacktime, you can quickly exceed your daily calorie limit. And that means that instead of turning on a Fat-Burner Switch, you're turning on a Fat-Maker Switch by mistake.

Dole out the dried fruit . . . slowly. The problem with dried fruit is that it's so tasty! This food is so easy to munch—and leaves you eager for more. Not only that, it seems so healthy. Just fruit that's been dried—what could be more naturally delicious?

Eat Low-Fat, High-Fiber Snacks

Don't Trust "Diet Foods"

Under normal conditions, the body knows when to stop eating—that is, when its nutrient needs are met. But artificial sweeteners block the natural cues to the brain and body. Thus, after you've had an artificially sweetened food or beverage, you'll probably find yourself craving another food.

Experiments indicate that the taste of sweets can increase general appetite and prompt us to eat far more than we need, sometimes to the point of obesity.

Whether it's an artificial sweetener with no calories or a caloric sweetener such as sucrose or fructose, the body responds in a similar way. This may be due in part to the liver's increasing hunger: As it gobbles up excess glucose, it lowers blood sugar and helps turn the ingested fuel into fat.

"Studies conducted on the effects of artificial sweeteners have shown no evidence that they contribute to an overall reduction in calories or to weight loss," says C. Wayne Callaway, M.D., obesity specialist, clinical professor at George Washington University in Washington, D.C., and former director of the Nutrition and Lipid Clinic at the Mayo Clinic in Rochester, Minnesota. "It appears that the calories simply get replaced by other foods. It has also been demonstrated that sweets (even artificial ones) stimulate an appetite for fats in some people."

Some studies, for instance, have shown that aspartame (the artificial sweetener sold under the name NutraSweet) actually increases appetite. Although not all findings are in agreement on this subject, there are other objections that need to be weighed, too.

"Chemical sweeteners also pose potential health risks," observes Neil Barnard, M.D., faculty member at George Washington University School of Medicine, president of the Physicians Committee for Responsible Medicine and author of *Food for Life*. "People struggling with weight problems get no miracle cure from artificial sweeteners."

Well, here's the surprise: If you munch about 20 pieces of dried fruit—which is easy to do—you may consume as many as 500 to 1,000 high-sugar calories. Even though the sweeteners in the fruit are "natural," those handfuls of fruit can shift your fat-forming processes into overdrive.

"Fruit sugar causes significant increases in blood fats (triglycerides) in some people," explains internist John A. McDougall, M.D., founder and director of the McDougall Program at St. Helena Hospital in Santa Rosa, California. "These fats are the very ones stored in fat tissues. Fruit also stimulates insulin production, which stuffs these fats into fat cells."

Even fruit juice can be a problem when you consume lots of it. "Processing fruit into sauce or juice disrupts and/or removes fiber, increasing the speed of absorption and the amount of carbohydrate absorbed by the bloodstream," says Dr. Mc-Dougall. "Fruit puree, such as applesauce, raises insulin more than whole fruit."

Guard against generation of new fat cells by avoiding large intakes of food at one time. Space smaller meals throughout the day. This tactic reduces the hormonal signal that causes fat cells to divide and multiply.

—*Peter D. Vash, M.D., eating disorders specialist at UCLA Medical Center*

Spurn the sly sweets. Studies suggest that synthetic sweeteners may reinforce your taste for sweet foods. "Artificial sweeteners may impede weight loss by increasing hunger," warns Dr. McDougall.

It's thought that in large quantities the fake sweeteners may decrease the level of serotonin, which is one of the chemicals that signal the brain "I'm full! Don't eat any more!" At the same time, the sweeteners may increase insulin, with the usual result of reducing fat-burning.

Avoiding sweeteners, however, does not mean you have to ban them completely. On occasion, you may want to have an artificially sweetened food or drink or use very small amounts of sucrose or table sugar. Many of the recipes in part 4 taste sweet and delicious even though added sweeteners are kept to a minimum.

Dodge the fake fats. Substitutes for fat are being tested all the time, and there's no telling when the next breakthrough will come.

But if you're following a Low-Fat Living Program, you don't need them—and you probably don't want them. Any imitation fat is likely to increase your appetite for fat-rich, even greasy foods.

"Fake fats may be a shot in the arm for manufacturers," warns Neil Barnard, M.D., faculty member at George Washington University School of Medicine in Washington, D.C., president of the Physicians Committee for Responsible Medicine

Snacks to Rein In

Many snacks that are labeled "healthy" by food producers really are healthy—but only up to a point.

The trouble is, even if they're completely free of fat, some foods trigger an unusually strong insulin response if they're eaten in large quantities. And when the insulin response kicks in, that triggers fat-making in the body.

What this may mean, especially for anyone who struggles with being overweight, is that it's all right to eat one serving of food that's labeled "healthy," but reconsider before you go any farther than that.

Polishing off an entire bag of fat-free rice cakes or nonfat potato chips, for instance, may actually slow down fat-burning and rev up fat-forming processes.

To avoid the potential insulin response produced by any of the foods in the list below, I recommend you choose them less frequently than those in "A Quality Cornucopia: The Best Energy-Boosting, Fat-Fighting Snacks" on page 88. And if you do have these low-fat treats now and then, be sure to eat them in carefully limited amounts, as I've specified here.

- Fat-free rice cakes—no more than three
- Air-popped popcorn—less than one cup
- French bread and other white breads—a maximum of two ½-inch slices
- Fat-free potato chips—one handful
- Fat-free corn chips—one cup (which may be eaten with salsa)
- Refined wheat-flour crackers—no more than three
- Sugar-coated, white-flour nonfat devil's food cookies (and other nonfat cookies)—no more than three
- Fresh carrot juice—one small glass (eight ounces)
- Dried fruit—no more than two ounces

and author of *Food for Life*, "but they are no answer to America's weight problems. Not only is their safety in doubt, but these additives reinforce the taste for fatty foods rather than help you break the habit."

Snack for sharpness. Eating smaller, nutritious meals and snacks helps to stabilize blood sugar levels, which in turn optimizes memory, learning and performance, according to psychologist and chronobiology researcher Ernest Lawrence Rossi, Ph.D.

The Best of Leftovers

Some of my all-time favorite snacks are leftovers from delicious low-fat meals.

If you're at home, these tantalizing day-after specials are right in the fridge, just waiting to be served. If you're taking them to work, all you need are some small plastic containers and a spoon or fork.

Like the woodchopper who gets warmed twice—first from chopping the wood and then from burning it in the stove—you get a double benefit from a low-fat meal that stores well as leftovers. (The recipes are all from part 4.) Although your own tastes will guide you, here are the ones I like best as leftovers.

- Roasted Chestnut and Wild Rice Soup (page 292)
- Four-Bean Salad with Balsamic Vinaigrette (page 290)
- Tex-Mex Pasta Salad (page 294)
- Gingerbread Muffins (page 298) and other whole-grain muffins
- Lentil Spread in Pita Pockets (page 305)
- Thick and Zesty Gazpacho (page 268)
- Green Chili and Cheddar Buttermilk Biscuits (page 270)
- Thick and Hearty Vegetable Chili (page 302) or Southwestern Chicken Chili (page 303)
- Old-Fashioned Cornbread (page 304)
- A slice of Linguine Frittata with Broccoli (page 271)
- Chicken Salad with Peaches and Pecans (page 277) or Chicken and Wheat Berry Salad (page 278) on a slice of Cracked-Wheat Quick Bread (page 280)
- Greek Pasta Salad (page 286)
- Raspberry-Currant Scones (page 360)
- Perfect Pumpkin Pudding (page 377)
- Apple Crisp (page 375)
- A slice of whole-grain bread with Cucumber and Yogurt Spread (tzatziki) (page 381)

By taking a break to snack, you allow your mind and body to resynchronize, Dr. Rossi notes. "Oxidative waste products and free radical molecules that have built up in the tissues during preceding periods of high performance and stress are 'cleared out' of the cells. The stores of messenger molecules so vital to

(continued on page 90)

Eat Low-Fat, High-Fiber Snacks

A Quality Cornucopia: The Best Energy-Boosting, Fat-Fighting Snacks

One of the lucky things about the 3-plus-4 Eating Plan is that so many low-fat snacks are included. At first you might have to change your shopping patterns somewhat—and even visit a few new food stores—to gather an interesting range of tempting low-fat snacks. But there are many to choose from.

Here are some suggestions to help make up your list—and these are just for starters. Step into the fresh fruit and vegetable section when you're looking for snack food, and you'll find specials that change with the seasons.

The quantities given here are for one good, solid low-fat snack. For fresh fruits and vegetables, however, I don't give any particular quantities, since it's almost impossible to go overboard with those foods.

But remember, even before you snack, have a look at the other Fat-Burner Switches. You may actually be thirsty (Switch #3), or your body needs light and exercise (Switch #4).

If you do decide to have a snack, just be sure to eat the moderate sizes shown here, timing them according to the 3-plus-4 Eating Plan. As long as you're eating the amounts shown, you can be sure that Fat-Burner Switch #2 is turned on.

◾ One thick piece of 100 percent whole-grain bread topped with nonfat cream cheese and 100 percent all-fruit preserves. Some favorite breads include Ezekiel Sprouted Grain Bread, Shiloh Farms 100, Shiloh Farms Sprouted Wheat Bread, Vermont Bread Company's 100% Whole-Grain Bread and Wild's Whole-Grain Bread. Also be sure to try any locally made whole-grain breads carried by supermarkets, farmers markets and health food stores.

◾ A whole-rye cracker or bagel with nonfat cream cheese or nonfat cream cheese and a piece of fresh fruit.

◾ A whole-wheat English muffin with all-fruit preserves and nonfat cream cheese.

◾ A whole-wheat English muffin with nonfat mayo and a thin slice of part-skim cheese such as Jarlsberg light Swiss.

◾ A Health Valley Fat-Free Whole-Grain Muffin or Snack Bar.

◾ A low-fat whole-oats granola bar.

◾ One to three pieces of RyKrisp, Wasa Crispbread, Scandinavian-style bran crispbread or another whole-rye cracker with all-fruit preserves and/or nonfat cream cheese.

◾ A whole-grain bagel with one teaspoon of Dijon mustard, one teaspoon of nonfat mayo and two slices of turkey breast.

■ A whole-grain bagel with one teaspoon of Dijon mustard, one teaspoon of nonfat mayo and two thin slices of part-skim cheese such as Jarlsberg light Swiss.

■ A Nature's Choice Whole-Grain Fat-Free or Low-Fat Snack Bar.

■ One to three whole-grain cookies such as Health Valley Fat-Free Cookies.

■ One to three fat-free rye or other 100 percent whole-grain crackers spread with fat-free bean dip.

■ One cup of nonfat plain yogurt with fruit—fresh or unsweetened canned or frozen.

■ A half-cup of nonfat old-fashioned whole-oats granola with skim milk or yogurt.

■ One cup of low-fat or nonfat yogurt sweetened with fruit juice.

■ One cup of tomato soup, made with skim milk, and two whole-rye crackers.

■ One cup of noninstant oatmeal with skim milk and one teaspoon of brown sugar.

■ A quarter-cup of nonfat ricotta cheese topped with a handful of nonfat whole-oats granola.

■ Four ounces of nonfat frozen yogurt.

■ A half-cup of 1 percent or nonfat cottage cheese with fresh or unsweetened frozen or canned fruit.

■ Eight ounces of tapioca pudding, made with skim milk.

■ One cup of nonfat or low-fat bean, lentil or vegetable soup, such as Progresso, Pritikin or Healthy Choice products.

■ A variety of fresh-cut raw vegetable and fruit pieces with three whole-grain crackers, served with a nonfat dip or dressing.

■ One piece of angel food cake with unsweetened fresh berries. (For the cake recipe, see page 366.)

■ One piece of whole-rye or whole-grain bread with one teaspoon of nonfat mayo and two ounces of water-packed albacore tuna.

■ Eight ounces of unsweetened orange juice with a small low-fat whole-grain muffin. (If it's store-bought, read the label to make sure it's low-fat.)

■ One celery stalk stuffed with one tablespoon of nonfat cream cheese or cottage cheese.

■ One apple or other fresh fruit with three whole-grain crackers.

■ Sliced fruit and berries mixed into a half-cup of nonfat plain yogurt or nonfat cottage cheese.

mind/body communication are replenished, and energy reserves are restored."

Treat yourself on occasion. One of the great tastes to emerge from the new generation of light, lighter and lightest foods is low-fat or nonfat chocolate. Since it's available, why not have some once in a while?

On a cold winter's afternoon, make a cup of fat-free hot cocoa with skim milk—or for a summertime treat, add fat-free chocolate syrup to ice-cold skim milk. For true chocolate lovers, one or two chewy chocolate fat-free whole-grain brownies or cookies can be just as good as the real thing (among my favorites are the ones made by Auburn Farms and Health Valley.)

If your taste buds whine for chocolate ice cream, you might occasionally choose a fat-free frozen chocolate fudge bar, which delivers the flavor but not the fat of chocolate. (For more low-fat chocolate dessert ideas, check the delicious recipes created by my wife, Leslie, in chapter 20.)

Savor it all. The bottom line: If you want to "burn off" excess body fat and think, feel and perform at your best all day long and well into the evening, make it a priority to take a low-fat snack break at midmorning, midafternoon and mid-evening.

Use these minutes to stop what you're doing and step off the fast track. Look out the window, walk outside and find a quiet spot to lift your vantage point and savor some food and drink that you love.

As simple as it sounds, few of us make this choice in the 1990s. And we pay the price for it every day—not just in lessened fat-burning power but in our personal effectiveness, relationships, mental outlook and life satisfaction.

Chapter Six

Fat-Burner Switch #3

Drink Water and Other Fat-Fighting Beverages

For years, physicians have been advising us to drink eight eight-ounce glasses of water every day for best health. And it makes good sense, since our everyday environments seem custom-designed to leave us parched.

Homes and offices have radiant or forced-air heating in the winter and low-humidity air-conditioning in the summer. Cars and public transportation have temperature-controlled air that's usually a lot drier than it needs to be for comfort. All the time we're sitting in our living rooms, offices and cars, we're usually drinking much less water than we're losing.

It takes surprisingly little fluid loss—only 1 to 2 percent of the body's total water content—to cause dehydration. Each day the average person loses at least two cups of water through breathing, another two cups through invisible perspiration and six cups through urination and bowel movements. That's ten cups a day.

There are other factors that contribute to water loss. Drinking caffeinated beverages and others that act as diuretics causes you to lose invisible perspiration and to empty your bladder more often, and additional moisture evaporates as you sweat during exercise or hard physical labor.

On the intake side, you do have some easy sources, even when you're not thinking much about it. Many foods contain a large amount of water; you'll get approximately 3½ cups of fluid from what you eat during a typical day. And the body itself does a modest amount of water recycling. As you burn energy, one of the by-products of your metabolic processes is water—about ½ cup every day.

Since you lose ten cups of water a day and get only four from food and metabolism, it seems obvious that you need to drink at least six cups just to stay on an even keel. And if you can drink eight as recommended, you're even better off.

Tap In

Of course, the eight cups' worth can come in many forms. You might keep an eight-ounce glass nearby and top it with water every couple of hours or so. Or drink the equivalent amount of other liquids, such as skim milk, unsweetened juices or a variety of other noncaffeinated beverages.

Heat, humidity, exercise and diet can all make a difference in how much you actually need. Stroll around Tucson in August, and you'll require a lot more than eight glasses of water to keep yourself hydrated. And the person who munches dry tortilla chips at snacktime needs more fluids than the person who eats a couple of oranges as a snack. But while exact needs may change depending on the environment and the type of food you eat, the point is that you nearly always need extra fluids.

But getting your fill of liquids is more than an energy preserver: It's also a fat-burner. Hidden dehydration, as we saw, is the culprit that turns *on* Fat-Maker Switch #7. When you get your fill of thirst-ending beverages, you turn *off* that switch and turn *on* a brand-new fat-burner—because drinking water and other fat-fighting beverages not only speeds up fat-burning but also fights tension and tiredness.

Have a Hunger Quencher

Many of us mistakenly perceive our thirst drive as hunger and eat high-fat snacks when we're really thirsty, not hungry.

A good way to distinguish between the two is to drink a glass of ice-cold water when you feel hungry and then wait for a few minutes. You might find that you're no longer hungry at all. If you are, then go ahead and eat a light snack. The important thing is that you feed your body's real thirst and hunger and feed them appropriately, drinking water when you're really thirsty and eating food when you're actually hungry.

"Drinking generous amounts of water is overwhelmingly the number one way to head off food cravings and reduce appetite," says George L. Blackburn, M.D., Ph.D., associate professor of surgery at Harvard Medical School and chief of the Nutrition Metabolism Laboratory at Deaconess Hospital in Boston. When you drink plenty of water throughout the day, it takes up room in your stomach, helping you feel full and reducing your desire to eat. Research by Wayne Miller, Ph.D., director of the Weight Loss Clinic at the University of Indiana in Bloomington, and his colleagues indicates that high daily water consumption is related to successful, lasting weight loss.

And some studies indicate that as part of an active lifestyle, increased water intake may actually help reduce fat deposits. When the body is fully hydrated, the bloodstream has all the fluid it needs to transport lipids, or fatty acids, from place to place. Drinking water also enhances the physiological processes that release fat cells' fatty acids into the bloodstream for delivery to the muscles for burning.

There's also some evidence to suggest that the chillier the beverage, the greater its fat-burning power. You can "maximize calorie burn by keeping the water ice-cold," says Ellington Darden, Ph.D., exercise scientist and director of research for Nautilus Sports/Medical Industries. "A gallon of ice-cold water requires over 200 calories of heat energy to warm it to core body temperature." Even if you consume only a glass or two, Dr. Darden notes that it takes heat energy to warm up water to body temperature—and that might use up a few calories now and then. You're simply putting some of your body energy into that internal water-heating process.

Studies on the fat-burning benefits of drinking ice water

have thus far been conducted only on three groups of 100 women, ages 20 to 65, yet the principle being studied does seem to make biological sense. And according to observations by the research team conducting these studies, the findings would seem to apply to both men and women.

Whatever the water temperature, however, it's certain that drinking more water is a sound choice for lifelong good health and weight control. "Water may be the simplest, most powerful key to fat loss," suggests Dr. Darden.

Add-Ons for Variety

In addition to its fat-burning bonuses, water pours other benefits into your body systems. Although it may seem obvious, it's important to point out that water counters dehydration and by doing so counteracts some of the body-damaging side effects (besides fat-making) that can result from dehydration.

"If you don't drink enough water, your body's reaction is to retain the water it does have," says Dr. Darden. "This in turn hampers kidney function, and waste products accumulate. Your liver is then called on to flush out impurities. As a result, one of your liver's main functions—metabolizing stored fat into usable energy—is minimized."

Feeding your internal reservoir is also essential for staying alert and contributing to energy storage. "Because a deficiency of water can alter the concentration of electrolytes such as sodium, potassium and chloride, water has a profound effect on brain function and energy level," says neurosurgeon Vernon H. Mark, M.D., author of *Brain Power*.

There are sports medicine researchers who confirm this observation. "Even a slightly dehydrated body can produce a small but critical shrinkage of the brain, thereby impairing neuromuscular coordination, concentration and thinking," says Robert Goldman, D.O., president of the National Academy of Sports Medicine. Because you're preventing dehydration when you drink plenty of water, you're helping to decrease fatigue.

More Revs in Your Bevs?

What about caffeinated beverages? It's probably just fine to have an occasional cup of coffee or black tea or a caffeinated soft drink. Yet it's important to know that caffeine-containing beverages such as coffee, tea and some sodas act as diuretics, increasing urine production and prompting loss of fluids.

In addition, according to a study published in the *New England Journal of Medicine*, even moderate amounts of caffeine consumed on the job during the week can leave you feeling out of sorts on weekends if you suddenly withdraw from the caffeine on Saturday and Sunday.

The long-term health effects of caffeine are unclear. Data from a study at the University of Geneva in Switzerland suggest that for some adults, a moderate intake of caffeine may increase metabolism. In other individuals, however, caffeine may increase symptoms of stress, and it can either increase or decrease appetite.

In general, claims that caffeine revs up your metabolism may be overstated. "Caffeine stimulates in a negative way, because it provokes insulin release and may in fact enhance the storage of what is eaten as fat," says Judith Rodin, Ph.D., former professor of psychology and psychiatry at Yale University and now president of the University of Pennsylvania in Philadelphia. "Countless women drink caffeinated diet sodas to help them through their days of (diet) fasting or eating very little. This practice may lead them to feel even more hungry, and it prepares their bodies for maximally storing (as body fat) whatever food they eat." And if you do drink coffee or tea, make sure you stay away from the cream, high-fat milk and any nondairy creamers that are high in fat.

Pour It In

Look at the nearest table. Is there a full glass or water bottle on it right now?

If the answer is no, you probably need to develop some everyday habits and patterns to turn on Fat-Burner Switch #3. Here are some tips that will help you flick on this important switch for low-fat living.

Sniff out dryness. Breathe in through your nose and pay attention to the sensation. Do you feel a slight tightening in the nasal passages?

If you begin to pay attention to such body signals, you'll have a ready reminder that it's time for a drink. Another sign is

Switchbreak
SKILLPOWER
---▶ NOT
WILLPOWER

If you're keeping a water bottle with you during the day, how do you keep track of your refills? Here's a quick trick to make sure you're taking an adequate number of water breaks: Put some rubber bands around the container in the morning, then take one off every time you refill it.

If you have a 16-ounce container, for instance, you know you need to refill it four times to get your recommended daily dose of water. Start the morning with four rubber bands around the container and remove one band each time you refill.

By about 10:00 A.M., the first band should be gone, and by noon the second. Sometime in the afternoon and evening, you should refill the container twice more, removing the last of the rubber bands by the time you go to bed.

Next morning, of course, it's the brand new start of a brand new day. Put all the rubber bands back on and start over.

dryness of the mouth or eyes. These are vital signs that you're starting to become dehydrated.

You might be in the habit of reaching for candy or a cough drop when your mouth is dry, putting in eyedrops when your eyes feel dry and itchy or using a saline nasal spray to soothe dry nasal passages. Next time, before you try any of these methods, have a good tall glass of water—or one of the other beverages that help fend off dehydration. Chances are just the extra liquid in your body will help soothe dry eyes, mouth or nose, without any other remedy.

Put zing in your water. Plain, pure, energizing, fat-burning water is fine, of course, but there are lots of ways to dress it up. You can add zest to it with just a drop of natural, unsweetened lemon, lime, orange or berry flavoring. Water with a dash of pure peppermint flavoring is also delicious.

Don't sweeten it. Either real or synthetic sweeteners may push your appetite and metabolism in the wrong direction. If you're reaching for soda, punch, fruit juice or even a sports drink, read the label. The sweeteners to avoid in excess are both artificial (aspartame or saccharine, for example) and natural (such as fructose, which is usually corn syrup, or sucrose, which is table sugar). Drinking large quantities of beverages high in refined sugars is just one habit that can contribute to obesity.

Go for the fizz. Pure carbonated mineral water is just as thirst-quenching as regular water, but many people prefer the extra fizz. All the citrus, berry and peppermint flavorings that taste good in plain water are even more tongue-tingling in carbonated water, creating a great natural soda without any sweeteners.

Try tea for you. If an iced tea break sounds good to you, I can recommend plenty of variations. One of the best is green tea (my preference is Republic of Tea Brand), unsweetened or served with one teaspoon of sugar, maximum, per eight-ounce glass.

Also check your supermarket shelves for some of the naturally flavored decaffeinated black teas that appeal to the tastes of connoisseurs. Tantalizing flavors include Republic of Tea Brand Mango Ceylon, Ginger Peach, Cinnamon Plum, Blackberry Sage, Orange Ginger Mint, Lemon Winter Mint, Carob Cocoa Mint and Cardamom Cinnamon. Celestial Seasonings offers many varieties as well. They are all delicious unsweetened and iced. Or if you prefer some sweetness, you can add just a teaspoon of sugar per eight-ounce glass. If you like the traditional flavors, have iced decaffeinated black tea such as Lipton or Nestea.

Despite the power of tradition, you can have your iced tea in winter as well as summer. And you may get the same potential fat-fighting benefits as you would from ice water.

Decaf your café. Iced decaffeinated coffee tastes great with skim milk and a teaspoon or less of sugar. Now that America has entered the era of gourmet coffees, you have your choice of flavors and varieties to suit your taste.

Chapter Seven

Fat-Burner Switch #4

Enjoy Do-It-Anywhere Active Minutes and Low-Intensity Aerobics

I know. You're too busy. Or too out of shape. Or your knees, back, arms, hips or feet hurt. And as you get older, you have a more crowded lifestyle.

If you have responsibilities for taking care of children or parents, if you're moving upward in a profession where you have loads of job demands, if you have chores and projects at home, along with obligations to your friends and community, it all adds up to little time for exercise.

But are these the things that really get in the way of exercise—or is it more likely to be what's happening on TV?

A good prescription for the 30 to 50 million mostly sedentary and unfit Americans is "turn off the television, get up off your fanny, go out the door and move around a bit," says Steven N. Blair, P.E.D., president of the American College of Sports Medicine and director of epidemiology at the Cooper Institute for Aerobics Research in Dallas. Research has shown

Join the Long-Life Group

The best reason to turn on Fat-Burner Switch #4 is for enjoyment. By getting the active minutes that you need every day, you'll not only burn fat, you'll also feel better in nearly every way.

But just in case you're wondering whether those active minutes have some life-lengthening benefits, have a look at the graphs below, which are based on a large-scale study published in the *Journal of the American Medical Association*.

To present a picture for each sex, researchers reviewed the statistics on death rates for three fitness groups—those who engaged in low, moderate or high rates of regular exercise. The "low" exercisers were almost sedentary; they did lots of sitting and not much else. The "moderate" group got about 200 minutes of light physical activity every week—a little less than a half-hour a day. Those in the "high" group exercised much more: They went reg-

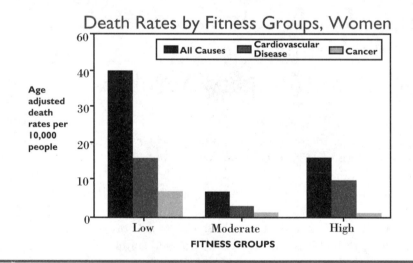

Death Rates by Fitness Groups, Women

All Causes · Cardiovascular Disease · Cancer

Age adjusted death rates per 10,000 people

FITNESS GROUPS — Low · Moderate · High

that all forms of exercise help improve your health and burn calories. "Any activity that increases your metabolic rate and burns more calories provides benefits," according to Dr. Blair.

Exercise, Not Punishment

Most of us still view exercise as an all-or-nothing issue, believing that something must be unpleasant to be good for us.

ularly to aerobics classes or ran or played a sport almost every day.

For researchers looking at these three distinct exercise groups, the first question was: How do the death rates compare? But the researchers also looked at specific causes of death, especially cardiovascular disease and cancer, to see how the groups compared in those areas as well. The graphs show the age-adjusted death rates for each 10,000 people.

Among women, for example, the age-adjusted death rate from all causes was nearly 40 per 10,000 for those who got low amounts of exercise. Just contrast this to the death rate for women who got moderate daily exercise. In that group, the death rate from all causes was less than 5 per 10,000.

The men's graph shows a similar pattern in the death rates of low and moderate fitness groups—proof that moderate exercise can make a dramatic difference in your life expectancy.

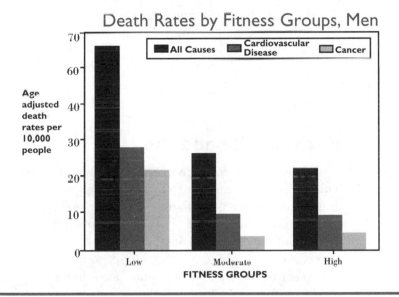

Death Rates by Fitness Groups, Men

"Exercise is loathsome," said Mark Twain. And based on some exhausting experiences, many people might agree with him.

The good news is that you don't need to have an iron will in order to get enough exercise.

That's right: You don't have to get out there every day and do a carefully orchestrated workout. And it's lucky you don't, because a full-scale workout can easily eat up a couple of hours a day, especially if you have to get to and from a health club.

Can't even find a full hour today? Well then, skip it. But you can probably find some shorter time slots here and there, and that's almost as good.

If you just add a few "active minutes" here and there, you'll also be taking giant strides toward controlling your dietary fat intake. Actions as simple as taking the stairs instead of the elevator or walking an extra block or two can help you neutralize natural cravings for high-fat foods.

"Research is even showing that exercise may enhance your preference for fruits and vegetables," explains Diane Hanson, Ph.D., a lifestyle specialist at the Pritikin Longevity Center in Santa Monica, California.

Moreover, when you find some do-it-anywhere active minutes throughout the day, you automatically turn on Fat-Burner Switch #4. With each active minute, you slowly, steadily begin to burn off excess body fat and improve your health. You help reduce the risk of obesity, as well as heart disease and high blood pressure.

Mix the Mild and the Hot

By combining do-it-anywhere active minutes (some days) with low-intensity aerobics (other days), studies show, you may dramatically lower your chances of having osteoporosis, breast cancer and colon cancer. Even small amounts of exercise throughout the day may help alleviate depression, anxiety and distress.

"Inactivity is an unnatural state for human beings," says psychologist Keith Johnsgard, Ph.D., author of *Exercise Prescription for Depression and Anxiety*. "Without (exercise), we gain weight, our muscles atrophy, our cardiovascular systems suffer, and to make matters worse, we feel depressed and anxious."

What happens if you don't get regular physical activity in your life? Well, for one thing—and this may be a hard pill to swallow—you actually lower your expectations of having a long and healthful life.

"A staggering quarter of a million deaths each year can be attributed to physical inactivity," reports a panel of experts convened by the Centers for Disease Control and Prevention in Atlanta and the American College of Sports Medicine. Regular physical activity and exercise can produce body fat losses even if you don't restrict your calorie intake.

Some studies show that regular exercise may be the single most important factor in maintaining weight-loss success. In a study at the Department of Social and Administration Health Sciences of the School of Public Health at the University of California, Berkeley, 90 percent of the individuals who reached and maintained goal weights reported exercising regularly, compared with only 34 percent of the relapsers—those who went back to higher, undesired weights after dieting.

Exercise may also help you reduce dietary fat intake by offsetting your natural cravings for high-fat food. Studies indicate that lipoprotein lipase, a key fat-storing enzyme, is restricted by exercise. And the reduction in lipoprotein lipase helps reduce excess body fat.

"For people who are very sedentary, a little extra physical activity can reduce the risk of disease as much as quitting smoking," says Dr. Blair, one of the experts on the panel. Even if they become physically active late in life, people who get their fat-burning exercise tend to outlive inactive people.

Breaking It Up

Even though preventive medicine groups have long been urging Americans to exercise regularly, reports show that little progress is being made. In fact, less than one in ten Americans meets standards for regular exercise, and 70 percent of those who begin exercise programs quit during the first year. After age 40, the typical American becomes less active with each passing year.

But if you break up your exercise into simple, small units, it's easier to do. Also, you should reward yourself after every set of active minutes.

Besides the direct fat-fighting benefits, small, brief interludes of exercise also give you some stress relief, which, as we'll see, brings up some reinforcements in the fight against fat. Just five or ten minutes of activity has a direct effect on your ability

Middle-age Americans who are overweight move their bodies for an average of only 50 minutes a week, and they need to move them for 200 minutes a week.

—George L. Blackburn, M.D., Ph.D., associate professor of surgery at Harvard Medical School and chief of the Nutrition Metabolism Laboratory at Deaconess Hospital in Boston

to handle everyday stress. And when stress diminishes, so does your body's tendency to store more fat.

In general, studies have found that people who are physically active have fewer psychological and physiological overreactions to stressful situations and daily hassles. In other words, when you build active minutes into your day, it is less likely that you'll become emotionally upset or that you'll start pumping out anxiety- and tension-producing hormones that can also prompt abdominal fat-storing.

Research at Harvard Medical School's Institute for Circadian Physiology has shown that every time you use muscular activity, even briefly, you increase your energy and alertness. So even if you're taking just a few active minutes here and a few there, you're still getting a solid metabolic boost.

Sneak Attacks on Time

For on-the-go people who are determined to fit active minutes into their daily lives, there are hundreds of ways to flick on Fat-Burner Switch #4. Here are some of the tactics that you can use to fit exercise into your Low-Fat Living Program.

Walk on by. You can begin by taking several short walks every day to build your enjoyment of a more active lifestyle. If it seems like there's no good time to walk, consider some of the prime-time opportunities.

■ Before or after a meal
■ After a long meeting—when you're taking a break anyway
■ At the end of the workday
■ A couple of hours after dinner, when it's still too early to go to bed

Try some fancy footwork. If you naturally sink into a comfortable chair every time you answer the phone, set a new pace next time it rings. While you're talking, stroll around, look out the window, do some knee bends. Sitting still is unnecessary when you have a long cord or—better yet—a cordless phone. If you use this time to good purpose, even a ho-hum phone conversation can turn into a fat-burning pastime.

Relish your chores. Many people regret that they don't have time to get to the health club or swimming pool because there are so many household chores to be done. Well, honor those chores—they're great fat-burners.

You can lose a pound of fat a week just by ratcheting up your activity level a notch or two, according to Janet Walberg-Rankin, Ph.D., associate professor of exercise physiology at Virginia Polytechnic Institute and State University in Blacksburg. Among the activities she includes on her list are mowing the lawn, chopping wood and cleaning the basement.

If you hardly have time to get through your daily to-do list—including brisk vacuuming, mopping or leaf-raking—consider these minutes as part of your daily "active living" total. True, some fitness routines can incinerate calories faster, but anything that gets your body moving helps you fight fat.

Extend your range. "It's not the intensity of physical activity that leads to better health," says John Duncan, Ph.D., exercise physiologist at the Cooper Institute. "It's the total number of minutes you spend each week exercising."

If your goal is 30 minutes a day of exercise, you don't need to be sweating out those minutes on a resistance-training machine. "We used to believe that you had to walk briskly enough to improve your VO_2 max (aerobic capacity) before you would gain any health benefits," Dr. Duncan observes. "But now we know that metabolic changes occur at very moderate exercise in-

---

Switchbreak
SKILLPOWER NOT ◄-- WILLPOWER

Standing burns more calories than sitting. So—stand up!

Right now?

Sure.

There's no reason why you have to sit down while you're reading a book. On the contrary, evidence shows that you're likely to be more alert and energized when you're doing some kind of activity, no matter how inconsequential it may seem. Standing while you're reading is just one way to get your body in motion.

The next step: When you have to write a letter or even work at the computer, rearrange your work area so that you can easily stand for a while and sit for a while. Even this small amount of exercise, multiplied throughout the day, can make a difference.

---

tensities. Those metabolic changes confer health benefits, even if there is little measurable cardiovascular improvement."

Put more spring in your offspring. Even if you don't want to be more active for your own sake, perhaps you'll want to do it for your children or grandchildren. When both parents are active, children are nearly six times more likely to be active than children of two inactive parents, according to research presented at the annual National Institutes of Health Conference on Physical Activity and Obesity.

Finding Time for Playtime

Discovering time to exercise is like trying to get more laughter in your life: It's usually easier said than done. To master the tricks, you need to be part escape artist and part strategist, but most of all an opportunist. The moments that you can grab for activities come suddenly and pass swiftly, and if you don't take advantage of them, every cell of your body pays a certain price.

Here are some ideas to help plan your playtime.

Take up stairing. Whenever you have a choice, climb the stairs instead of getting on an escalator, a moving walkway or an elevator. You burn ten times more calories climbing the stairs than you do sitting still. If this means you need to allow yourself a few more minutes to get to your office or to make your way through an airport, so be it. Just allow time, even if you have to leave for your office, your appointment or your plane flight a little earlier.

Keep your distance. Parking at the mall? Shopping at the supermarket? Instead of cruising the lot to find the closest space, go for those vast empty spots on the far side of Nowheresville. It won't take you that much longer to get to the store (no, you won't miss the sale), and the long-distance walking boosts your metabolism and burns calories.

Pull up short. When you're taking a cab, allow some extra time and have the driver drop you off a few blocks from your destination. If you're taking a bus, get off a stop or two before you need to, then cover the distance with some fat-burning strides.

Make every minute count. When you're standing in line, for example, you can tighten and relax your gluteal muscles (that is, your rear end). When you're on the phone and someone has put you on hold, you have a good opportunity to do a few repetitions of abdominal breathing techniques like the abdominal vacuum exercise on page 162 and the transpyramid breathing exercise on page 163. "These little motions aren't going to replace really good training, but they help strengthen muscles in a surprisingly easy manner," observes Charles Kuntzleman, Ed.D., national program director for Fitness Finders, a physical fitness and wellness consulting firm in Spring Arbor, Michigan.

Waste some moves. For a fat-fighting aficionado, TV commercials aren't for snack-fetching—they're for stretching. Get up, stretch, move around. If you're upstairs and there's a quick chore to be done downstairs, or vice versa, seize the commercial break as an opportunity to get it done. Or hang a jump rope near the TV and skip to the jingle. Even that small amount of activity will help you break out of the fat-making mold.

Meet and flex. Make active dates with friends and do some physical activities together. If you're accustomed to meeting for lunch or drinks, figure out some other meeting arrangement and make sure it involves exercise. Maybe your lunch partner has been wanting to take up tennis again—and so have you. Maybe you can get some people interested in a pickup game of Frisbee, table tennis, basketball, soccer or volleyball. Even if your lunch hour is literally that, no more than an hour, you and a friend can plan on a short lunch together, followed by a long walk.

Try a clean sweep. Often, chores are more pleasant if you do them in mini-doses rather than as cellar-to-rafters whole-house overhauls. When the weather's good, step outside and sweep your sidewalk, patio, driveway, balcony or deck for a few minutes. Raking leaves and pulling a few weeds are other outdoor chores that can fill a few minutes—with multiple benefits for your mood and metabolism.

Make the night moves. It's usually easy to get away for a few minutes in the late evening to stroll under the stars. Invite your partner or child or a friend along; you'll get a chance to catch up on the day. Or put on some of your favorite music this evening and move your feet. (Even tapping your feet burns more calories than sitting still.)

Get on a good cycle. Whether you're pedaling a moving bike or a stationary one, you'll pleasantly wheel off the calories.

Switchbreak
SKILLPOWER
--→ **NOT**
WILLPOWER

All around America, tucked away in dusty basements, stored in attics and stuffed in cobwebby closets, are tons of unused exercise equipment—the promising tools of a lower-fat future.

If your home is a storage unit for such riches, take this opportunity to dust off the rowing machine or walking machine and bring it out of hiding.

No question about it: The active minutes strategy works best when you keep your home fitness equipment where it can be used. When you want to get to a rowing machine or stationary bike for a few minutes of steady pulling or pedaling, you don't want to waste extra time pulling it out of a hidden nook.

Right now, move the fitness equipment to the "action area" of your home. Doesn't fit the decor? Well, just give it a designer name—*nouveau vie*, for instance, which means "new life," because that's really what it represents. If that equipment is available for your active minutes, you can pedal, ski, walk or pull your way to better health in the comfort of your own home. You can even do it with the TV on.

Go to the dogs. If you're the proud owner of a sprightly canine, you know your pup is eager to go out anytime. Instead of resisting the eager pleading in those friendly eyes, give in! The more you can walk your pet, the less fat you have to lose.

Or if you don't have a dog but neighbor Wilson does, astonish him by offering to perambulate with his pet twice a day. Not a bad combination: Make your neighbor a friend for life while you lengthen your life with more exercise.

Lunch at length. Walk someplace at least five minutes from your work area to eat your lunch. Then, after eating, return by a roundabout route, so you enjoy a ten-minute return walk.

End the weight. Are you waiting for the washer to finish its last cycle or for the bathtub to fill? Use that time to go up and down the stairs. If you have a rowing machine, sit down and do some smooth strokes. If a walking machine is available, get on it and move out. The pace doesn't have to be fast or the interval long. Any rhythmic exercise is a boon to your body.

Make motion your dessert. If there is no muscular activity to burn off the carbohydrate consumed in low-fat meals or low-fat or nonfat snacks, neurochemicals in your brain and body respond by quickly converting the carbohydrate directly into body fat for storage. And studies suggest you may get up to twice the usual calorie-burning benefits for each active minute of exercise you spend if you begin your activities within 15 to 30 minutes after eating a snack or full meal.

Research indicates that your body's metabolic rate goes up by about 10 percent after a meal or snack as a result of the chemical processes that are activated to get that food digested. There's evidence that this 10 percent can be increased—and in some cases may be doubled—if you do 5 to 20 minutes of moderate physical activity such as walking while these initial digestive processes are still going on.

By "pulling oxygen into the body within a half-hour of eating, food can be made to burn hotter, in a sense, with fewer calories being available for fat storage," explains Bryant A. Stamford, Ph.D., exercise scientist and director of the Health Promotion and Wellness Program at the University of Louisville in Kentucky.

Also, research shows that a single ten-minute walk may trigger a two hour boost in your sense of well-being by raising energy levels and lowering tension.

Taking On Airs

While short activity breaks are all to the good, for Switch #4 to burn the most fat, you also need a second element: low-intensity aerobics.

The most effective exercise program for good health—including building up your defenses against aging—is to exercise several times a week the "lower-intensity way," according to preventive medicine specialist Kenneth H. Cooper, M.D., founder and chairman of the Cooper Institute. According to Dr. Cooper, you need to maintain that comfortable level of exercise "for at least 30 minutes three times a week, or for 20 continuous minutes four times a week."

One of the first noticeable signs of improved aerobic fitness is a lowered resting heart rate, because your normal heartbeat slows as your fitness improves. While many nonathletes have heartbeats in the range of 75 to 80 beats per minute, elite athletes in endurance sports can become so well-conditioned that they have resting heart rates between 30 and 45 beats per minute. That change occurs because the heart that's been strengthened through regular aerobic exercise becomes more powerful and efficient.

Shake a Leg

"But I'm just too busy to exercise," you may be saying.

And that's probably close to the truth—if what you mean by exercise is driving to the health club, putting on sweats, working out for an hour, showering, dressing, driving home and then getting back to the million things you have to do.

But you're not too busy to try the Four Fives and a Ten Plan. In fact, here's your chance to stop, look ahead to tomorrow and plan your breaks.

■ You'll need five minutes of easy physical activity in the morning. Are you going to get up earlier to do that or do it after breakfast?

■ Plan on taking a five-minute walk before you have lunch. Decide when you'll actually need to break for lunch in order to get that additional walking time.

■ You'll want at least a five-minute walk after lunch. Count on it.

■ Plan on doing five minutes of easy stretches or muscle-toning (see Fat-Burner Switch #7 on page 155) when you get home.

■ Ask your partner, a family member or a friend whether anyone would like to take an after-meal walk at a fairly brisk pace for ten minutes.

That's all there is to it. Within a week or so your energy and stamina may increase to the point where you feel like you've gained more productive hours in a day. The active minutes won't cost you time; they'll save you time by upping your effectiveness and improving your mental focus.

People who have developed good cardiovascular fitness from regular aerobic exercise will generally have hearts that beat 45 to 50 times a minute when at rest, according to Dr. Cooper. Their hearts are pumping at least the same amount of blood as an unconditioned person's heart that beats up to 80 times a minute when resting. Result: Over the course of a day, the unconditioned person's heart must beat 50,000 times more than a conditioned person's heart. In a year, that's a workload of more than 18 million extra beats that an unfit person's heart must provide!

What Is Aerobics?

In the 1960s, when I first began studying exercise science, the kind of workout we favored was for "cardiovascular fitness." A few years went by, and the name changed to "cardiorespiratory exercise." Today it's "cardiovascular endurance" or—best known of all—"aerobics."

So what does this ever-changing term actually mean? Have we all been talking about the same thing for the past 30 years, though under different names?

Actually, cardiovascular endurance is somewhat different from aerobics, though the benefits are similar. As you build cardiovascular endurance, you're essentially training your heart, lungs and blood to perform at their optimum or peak levels. Aerobics, on the other hand, means that oxygen intake, transport and utilization are improved with regular training.

Many people began discovering aerobics when the term was popularized by Dr. Cooper. Under the supervision of his research team, more than 1.25 million exercise hours, with nearly 52,000 participants, have been recorded and assessed over a 20-year period.

Aerobic exercises are those that safely and comfortably increase your breathing and heart rate for an extended period of time—usually at least 20 minutes—without disturbing the balance between your intake and use of oxygen. In other words, you pick up the pace of your activities until you're breathing hard and your heart is pumping fast, but because you build up to that pace, the concentration of oxygen in the blood remains virtually the same.

In contrast, activities that require sudden, excessive bursts of energy—like sprinting—are anaerobic. With anaerobic activities you're "giving your all" for a short time, which actually depletes the oxygen in your blood. So your nerves and muscles suffer short-term oxygen deprivation until that explosion of super-effort is over.

Dr. Cooper has promoted aerobic exercise as a fundamental of good health precisely because it helps develop your body's ability to sustain exercise, build muscle tissue and burn fat. According to Dr. Cooper, aerobic exercise increases the amount of blood in your system and increases the amount of oxygen-carrying hemoglobin in your blood.

Your blood becomes, in a word, richer: It can carry more oxygen to each cell and take away more carbon dioxide and other wastes than it could before you started regular aerobic exercise. Also, your muscle cells improve their ability to process the oxygen and eliminate wastes more efficiently.

The Heart of Aerobics

To treat your heart better as well as burn fat, you need to shoot for the target set by Dr. Cooper—getting aerobic exercise for at least a half-hour three times a week or for 20 minutes four times a week.

On some days, you can move toward that goal simply by extending your 10-minute walk into 20 or 30 minutes. Or perhaps you can pinpoint some other exercises that you'd like to do, nonstop, for 20 or 30 minutes several times a week. Here's where it pays to take advantage of low-intensity aerobics.

In my household, we go through a relaxed, low-intensity aerobic exercise session three times a week for a half-hour each session, right after our evening meal. On evenings when the weather is good, the session is nothing more complicated than brisk walking.

How can you spare the time if you have a growing family?

I can speak only from our own experience. We have two daughters, ages five and two, who love the playground equipment in a nearby park. So they're in the playground while my wife, Leslie, and I walk around the perimeter of the park, keeping them in sight. Sometimes the five-year-old will tag along with us. Even the two-year-old occasionally starts out with us and later hitches a ride on my shoulders. (Now there's a workout.)

When our 16-year-old son is at home, he often heads out the door with us. He enjoys going for a run or shooting baskets while we walk.

Two or three evenings, after our brief aerobic walk, we go through 15 to 20 minutes of muscle-toning exercises, like those shown in Fat-Burner Switch #7, beginning on page 155. Sometimes we do these exercises with the television on in the family room while the children watch a videotape of *Sesame Street* or play games.

We're fortunate to have an array of exercise equipment to use, and I'd definitely recommend getting whatever equipment you can afford. A stationary cycle, treadmill, cross-country ski machine or stair-climber is easy and efficient to use, and I've gotten many energizing, fat-burning hours of enjoyment from exercising in the same room with the rest of the family.

Whatever exercise we're doing, our goal is always to make

Reaping Aerobic Benefits

When you're doing aerobic exercise, you take in more air and get rid of more carbon dioxide with each breath. In addition to strengthening your heart and making blood flow more efficient, this process provides some other benefits, according to preventive medicine specialist Kenneth H. Cooper, M.D., founder and chairman of the Cooper Institute for Aerobics Research in Dallas. Among the other pluses of aerobic exercise:

■ Your blood vessels become more flexible, so they're less likely to get fatty deposits from the blood that passes through. That means there's less resistance in the blood vessels and less work for your heart.

■ The number of capillaries, the tiny blood vessels that form a network throughout the cells of your body, increases. Perhaps triggered by increased circulation or as the result of a chemical trigger, your body spontaneously creates new capillaries when you increase aerobic activities.

■ Lung capacity increases. Some studies have associated this rise in "vital capacity" with greater longevity.

■ The heart muscle grows stronger and is better supplied with blood. With each beat, the heart can pump more blood, increasing what doctors call the stroke volume.

■ Your blood acquires more HDL, which is the good cholesterol. At the same time, the ratio of total cholesterol to HDL decreases, which is a clear sign that your overall cholesterol level has improved.

■ Because of the improvement in the cholesterol picture, you reduce your risk of developing atherosclerosis.

this time fun. Often that means planning the indoor activities so that our girls and teenager all enjoy themselves, and we have a chance to spend some laughter-filled time together.

Not that we do this seven days a week. In fact, we usually take several evenings off. But at least three times a week we go for a full half-hour of this aerobic exercise, with or without some of the muscle-toning exercises. The other evenings, we always try to spend some active time after dinner, even if it's just ten minutes playing "chase" or other get-up-and-go games with the girls.

Since that exercise after mealtime helps prevent cravings for high-fat foods, we're less likely to gravitate to the kitchen, wondering why we're still hungry long after the meal is over.

Relishing Your Active Time

There are several reasons why any kind of aerobics or muscle-toning is so valuable. First, as I've mentioned, aerobic exercise within 30 minutes of the evening meal revs up fat-burning before bedtime, just about the time your metabolism begins to fall. While you always get some immediate, thermic (heat-producing), metabolic boost from physical activity, your body usually returns to a near-resting level an hour or so later. But studies show that you get an enhanced metabolic lift from the one-two combination of eating and exercise when they take place within a half-hour of each other. In some cases, your body continues to burn calories at a higher-than-normal rate for more than ten hours.

Leslie and I have both noticed that the evening active time really does help bring our family closer together. Having this active time together has also improved our love life, perhaps by helping to align wavelike "ultradian" biological rhythms. And the additional activity produces another benefit that links up with Fat-Burner Switch #10—helping everyone in the family to measurably deepen each night's sleep.

Guidelines for Go-Getters

What if you happen to work evenings, or morning exercise is more enjoyable or more convenient for you?

Answer: You might not be able to gather the family for a comfortable activity time. But for your own sake, you should definitely include these periods. You'll get significant benefits no matter when you choose to be more active and to exercise.

Whenever you do your low-intensity aerobic workout, it should always be enjoyable—not only while you're doing it but also in the glow that comes afterward, when you're feeling refreshed and alert. To get the most out of your low-intensity aerobics, however, it's essential to build up gradually, avoiding overexertion and possible injury.

Here are some guidelines to help your aerobic workouts work for you.

Start slowly. Precede each session with at least five minutes of gentle warm-up that mimics your upcoming aerobic activity or sport, moving at an easy pace. If you stretch, do it

Are You Fit to Pump Air?

Many experts will recommend that you get a medical examination before you begin an exercise program. And some doctors may tell you that you should have an exercise tolerance test (ETT) or a maximal graded exercise test (MaxGXT).

Do you absolutely need such exams?

The answer, in the view of many medical authorities, is that it all depends.

The National Heart, Lung and Blood Institute in Bethesda, Maryland, advises that if a person is at low risk for heart disease and has no symptoms, he does not need to see a physician before starting a moderate exercise routine.

The American Heart Association has simply stated that "older sedentary individuals may . . . wish to seek medical advice."

But turn to other authorities, and the answers become somewhat more complicated. The American College of Sports Medicine (ACSM) says you can begin exercise programs without undergoing an ETT or a MaxGXT if you've been healthy and you're under the age of 45 with no major coronary risk factors. But the list of risk factors is long.

The ACSM says you should have the exercise tests if you have a family history of high blood pressure, heart attack or cardiovascular disease prior to age 50, a history of high blood pressure that measures above 145/95 or an elevated total cholesterol/HDL cholesterol ratio (above 5 for males or 4.5 for females). The organization recommends exercise exams if you have an abnormal electrocardiogram, smoke cigarettes or have diabetes. Also, the ACSM says that individuals at higher risk (above age 35 with one or more coronary risk factors) and individuals at any age with symptoms suggestive of metabolic, pulmonary or coronary heart disease should undergo a physician-supervised exercise tolerance test.

And even if you're not at risk because of these factors, you should begin the exercise program slowly and proceed gradually. "Be alert to the development of unusual signs or symptoms," the ACSM advises.

gently, without bouncing movements, after your muscles are warmed up. Otherwise you may cause injuries to your joints.

Feel the rhythm. Exercise at a rhythmic, comfortable pace using major muscles, such as the thighs. Begin gradually. Listen to your body. Stop at any sign of pain.

How to Calculate Your Target Heart Rate Zone

The predicted maximal heart rate (PMHR) is the maximum number of heartbeats that you should have when you're exercising. As we age, our hearts become a little less powerful and resilient even if we're in the best of health. So the PMHR goes down as your age goes up.

The method for calculating PMHR is simple. Just subtract your age from 220. If you're 45 years old, for instance, your PMHR is 220 minus 45, or 175. Your heart shouldn't pump any faster than that, even when you're going all-out.

The lower and upper limits of your target heart rate zone are 60 and 75 percent, respectively, of your PMHR. You can calculate those limits by multiplying the PMHR by 0.60 and 0.75. The target zone is in the middle. For the 45-year-old whose PMHR is 175, the lower limit of the heart rate zone is 105, while the upper limit is 131. If the pulse rate is anywhere between 105 and 131 while exercising, the 45-year-old is safely within the limit of the target heart rate.

Take the talk test—and find your target. Choose an exercise intensity that allows you to work steadily while still being able to talk without gasping for breath. This is known as the talk test.

Many physicians recommend, in addition, that you find out your target heart rate zone and then stay within that zone during aerobic exercise. That is, as long as your heart is beating at a certain rate per minute, you can be sure you're gaining solid benefits in a safe exercise range.

To find your target heart rate zone, you first need to know your predicted maximal heart rate (PMHR), which can be determined with a simple math calculation (see "How to Calculate Your Target Heart Rate Zone"). The target heart rate, determined from that, is a sensible aerobic intensity level that's usually 60 to 75 percent of the PMHR.

To maximize this Fat-Burner Switch, some authorities suggest exercising near the lower end of this range. That's based on the theory that when you drive your heart rate toward the top of the target heart rate zone and your muscles are pushed to high-intensity levels, you use more blood glucose for energy rather than stimulating your system to metabolize stored fat and burn that when you exercise.

To measure your heartbeat, you should take your pulse three times: shortly after beginning to exercise, again at a midway point in the aerobic session and once more when cooling down. Gently touch the inside of a wrist or the pulse point on your neck (just under the curve of your jaw) with your fingertips and feel for the pulse.

To make a quick estimate of your pulse, count the number of beats you feel in 15 seconds (call the first beat zero, not one). Multiply by four to get the beats per minute.

Better yet, you can use an electronic heart rate monitor that does it all for you, measuring your pulse and providing you with instant feedback. A state-of-the-art heart rate monitor is the kind that you strap to your chest. An electronic wristband provides a visual readout, along with some sound signals. This monitor can give you a continuous reading of your heart's responsiveness to various physiological variables such as stress, intensity of exercise and tension levels. Taken together, these are keys to regulating the intensity and quality of aerobic fitness.

The advantage of a heart rate monitor is that you don't have to stop during exercise to measure your pulse, which interrupts the exercise and interferes with concentration. Once you've set it, the monitor automatically guides you into the optimal zone with visible numbers and a series of distinctive tones.

Buy some time. When it fits your schedule, plan to do 20 to 30 minutes of low-intensity aerobics three or four times a week. But remember, on days when you just can't find that amount of time to spend on aerobic exercise, substitute a few 5- to 10-minute mini-walks, or climb several flights of nearby stairs in the morning and again after lunch.

Don't try to go harder and faster. Here's a finding that may come as a surprise: Competitive thoughts during exercise can increase harmful stress. According to a study at Shippensburg University in Pennsylvania, levels of stress hormones such as norepinephrine, which normally increase by moderate amounts during strenuous activities, rise dramatically when you mentally drive yourself with words like *harder* and *faster*.

People should "abandon competitive thinking during workouts," says Kenneth France, Ph.D., the psychologist at Shippensburg University who studied the effects of thoughts on norepinephrine levels. His study included athletes from a wide variety of disciplines who did identical workouts. The athletes were given alternate sets of mental cues, beginning with words like *calm*, *relaxed* and *steady*, followed by more competitive words like *faster*, *harder* and *better*. Dr. France found that both types of mental signals produced equal pulse rate

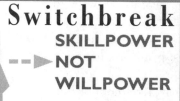

Switchbreak
SKILLPOWER
- - ► NOT
WILLPOWER

Do you have a small electric fan stored away—maybe an old one that you use only in the summertime?

Get it out right now and put it near your exercise area or exercise equipment. When you're doing indoor activities, turn it on.

According to researchers, mental boredom can be partly heat-related. With a cool breeze blowing, you're more likely to feel invigorated and alert while you're using an exercise machine or doing low-intensity aerobics.

If you don't own a small fan, you can find a variety of them at most hardware, discount or household goods stores. The clip-on fans that attach to the edge of a desk or window frame are especially convenient and easily adjustable.

changes, but the aggressive words caused norepinephrine levels in the urine to more than double. "Performance may even improve when you take pressure off yourself," he concluded.

In short, keep things fun—a word seldom heard in rigorous exercise circles. Begin thinking of exercise as time for something special for yourself, and include friends in your fitness sessions if that's enjoyable for you.

Add easy speed-ups. As your fitness improves, consider speeding up the pace—not instantly, but gradually.

According to Dr. Stamford, you may want to try aerobic exercise at two paces if you want to burn off even more fat.

First, it must begin with enough vigor to trigger a substantial adrenaline release. "One of the jobs of adrenaline is to increase the free fatty acids in the bloodstream, so the body can use them as fuel for activity," observes Dr. Stamford. "A prime location for that to occur is the stores of fat in the abdominal area." (It may be that those fat cells are particularly sensitive to adrenaline.) You can probably get this effect from brisk walking. "Just step up the pace or even jog a bit now and then to boost adrenaline output," advises Dr. Stamford.

This level of activity, however, must then be followed by prolonged, less intense aerobic exercise that will burn up the liberated fat molecules. Walking or any steady, enjoyable means of movement can be effective.

With other common activities like gardening, the same principle applies. You might start out hoeing or digging and then move to some other, more sustained aerobic activity such as steady raking.

Wind down. At the end of each aerobic session, keep moving until your heart rate gradually returns to normal. This cooldown period, however brief, is critical from a health and safety standpoint because it allows the body to return gradually to its pre-exercise state.

Never stop exercising suddenly. After some heat-generating exercise, you might be tempted to come to a standstill, sit down or start talking to a friend. But don't let anything distract you from a sensible cooldown period of up to five minutes. If you are not hooked up to a heart monitor but are taking your own pulse by touch, learn to check it while moving rather than standing motionless.

Chapter Eight

Fat-Burner Switch #5

Have a Fat-Fighting Lunch

L unch is the crossroads of your day, the time when morning ends and your afternoon takes off—with either a healthy dose of mind/body invigoration or, for many people, the beginning signs of an afternoon decline.

In America and many other parts of the industrialized world, speed has become the midday theme: Grab a quick bite. Eat on the run. Gotta hurry back to work.

With lunch, these days, chances are you barely notice it, hate it, scarf it down or skip it altogether.

But this approach punches a hole in the middle of a Low-Fat Living Program. Studies point to the conclusion that you need a good lunch "for both health and work efficiency," says Etienne Grandjean, M.D., director of the Department of Ergonomics at the Swiss Federal Institute of Technology in Zurich and an expert on work productivity.

If you look at the way your metabolism reacts to skipping one meal, you realize that bypassing lunch can be a costly mistake. It leads to a ravenous appetite late in the day and heightened cravings for high-fat foods, according to C. Wayne Callaway, M.D., obesity specialist, clinical professor at George Washington University in Washington, D.C., and former director of the Nutrition and Lipid Clinic at the Mayo Clinic in Rochester, Minnesota. "People who skip breakfast or lunch tend to binge in the evening, instead of eating moderately," Dr. Callaway observes.

Eating Well—The Best Revenge

For low-fat living it's essential that you not only have lunch but also make a habit of avoiding high-fat and fat-forming foods at that time. Most lunchtime problems arise from the fact that what you think is a good choice at first glance could be loaded with hidden fat. And beyond the obvious weight-gain problems, one of the main reasons to avoid high-fat lunches is that they cause fatigue.

"Fat seems to slow other processes, like thought or movement," says Judith J. Wurtman, Ph.D., a nutritional researcher in the brain and cognitive sciences department at the Massachusetts Institute of Technology in Cambridge. "It makes people very lethargic. During the long digestive process that follows a high-fat meal, more blood is diverted to the stomach and intestines and away from the brain."

Women, as I've noted, need to be careful about consuming animal fats because these extra fat calories may increase production of the pro-fat hormone estrogen. And both men and women need to avoid simple carbohydrates and include more fresh vegetables, legumes and whole grains at lunchtime.

All in Good Taste

The lunchtime challenge is to eat foods that have vivid, distinct, tongue-tingling flavors but are low in fat and relatively high in energizing protein.

Nutritional scientists have realized that most people will not trade taste for health. If you're offered an incredibly healthful, nutrition-rich, high-fiber veggie burger that tastes like straw, you might eat it once or twice because you know it's good for you. But soon, studies show, you'll go back to the good old burger.

That won't happen, however, if the veggie burger offers a range of flavors and textures that you've never experienced before. As soon as you get to like it better than the fat-filled alternatives, you'll forget about turning back to the relics of a former dining style.

So the single most important factor in enjoying lower-fat lunches—and all other meals and snacks—is taste. To an astonishing extent, "the brain is more interested in what's happening on the tongue than in the body," explains Harvey Weingarten, Ph.D., chairman of the psychology department at McMaster University in Hamilton, Ontario.

Which brings us to the tasty low-fat lunches I love best— as does the rest of the family (even our picky 16-year-old). You'll find some of these favorites in chapter 18. And they're all designed to turn on Fat-Burner Switch #5.

We've created these lunches with the goal of putting great taste into eating, with less fat and none of the guilt. "There's the idea that either you lead a sensual, rich life and die young or you avoid life and eat boring food," says Dean Ornish, M.D., founder and president of the Preventive Medicine Research Institute in Sausalito, California, and assistant clinical professor of medicine at the University of California, San Francisco, School of Medicine, whose program of exercise, stress reduction and a very low fat diet has been shown to reverse heart disease. "That isn't the choice at all." The fact is, you never have to eat a boring lunch!

The formula is quite simple: You have to make sure you're not depriving your taste buds of the excitement and interest of good flavor. Eating well is a sensual experience that most of us anticipate with good feelings. If you're looking forward to just bland taste and deprivation, it's almost guaranteed that you won't stick to low-fat eating long.

15 Ways to Zap the Fat from Your Lunch

But what if you're not home at lunchtime—or you don't have time in the morning to prepare one of the Low-Fat Living Program lunches?

Any time you take a lunch break, you can make a good, satisfying choice and turn on your Fat-Burner Switch. All

Lunch Launchers

What do you want your lunch to do for you? Depending on what you eat, you can get a charge of high energy—or you can end up feeling calmer and more focused.

One key to high energy may be having a lunch that is not only low in fat but also relatively high in protein. High-protein foods may help promote faster thinking, greater energy, increased attention to detail and quicker reaction speed. Among your choices are baked or broiled skinless chicken breast, turkey breast or fish; a bean or lentil salad, soup or casserole; low-fat or nonfat yogurt or cottage cheese with fruit; or a glass of skim milk with a piece of fruit. Then balance the menu with some complex carbohydrates from fruit, vegetables, whole-grain bread, rye crackers or a side dish of beans or lentils.

If you want to shift your energy toward calmness rather than high energy, emphasize the complex carbohydrates. Research suggests that meals and snacks that are low in fat and protein but high in complex carbohydrates may produce a calm, focused state of mind and may help relax you. You're likely to get this effect from low-fat pasta salad served with fruit, vegetables or 100 percent whole-grain bread, a muffin or rye crackers topped with your favorite all-fruit preserves. Very small amounts of these carbohydrate-rich foods—1 to 1½ ounces for many people—are usually enough for a calming, focusing effect. (There are exceptions, however. You're more likely to need between 2 and 2½ ounces of carbohydrate-rich foods for lunch if you're 20 percent or more overweight. And women in the days just preceding menstruation also need this higher amount.)

Note: A few people have biological cravings for carbohydrates and, rather than being calmed by them, find them energizing. For this small group of individuals, the "sugar buzz" is real. But contrary to popular belief, carbohydrates do not generally cause hyperactivity or increased energy or aggressiveness in normal, healthy people.

Just-ripe fruits and vegetables (except potatoes, corn and popcorn) appear to be mind-mood neutral, say researchers. That is, these foods don't directly affect alertness or calmness and therefore can generally be eaten with either protein-rich or carbohydrate-rich foods.

around you are opportunities to squeeze out the fat and calories but keep the taste.

It's easier than you think—especially if you don't let fast foods fool you. Even if you're on the run today, here are a few

Strengthen Your Strategies

In general, steer clear of the fat/sugar duo.

"It's typically American," observes Bryant Stamford, Ph.D., exercise scientist and director of the Health Promotion and Wellness Program at the University of Louisville in Kentucky. "We like to combine simple sugars and fats at the same meal—a hamburger, french fries and a cola, for example."

But when your body gets the jolt of simple sugars from a soda (a 12-ounce serving has an average of ten teaspoons of sugar), it releases a surge of insulin in response.

Dr. Stamford describes insulin as "a pro-fat hormone that 'opens up' the fat cells, making them ready to store fat." Once you have a high-sugar soda or fruit drink that raises the glucose level in your blood, the insulin just pours into your system to control the blood sugar. "Then here comes the fat from the hamburger and fries, and bingo—the arrow is pointing toward storage," says Dr. Stamford.

It's not just sweet sodas that can produce this effect. Any high-glycemic foods, including spoonfuls of ordinary table sugar, may produce an insulin response that results in rapid fat storage.

insights and tips that can help you out of high-fat patterns and get you into low-fat gear.

1. Go for mineral water. "I'll have a diet (whatever)" has become the clarion call of a weight-loss-focused society. But a monster-size Diet Coke, Pepsi or ginger ale or any other soft drink is not your best option at lunch. All that sweetness, in whatever form, stimulates your appetite, while the drink itself may do little to quench your thirst.

And what does it do to taste? You can be sure that any chef worth his garnish would be horrified to see someone drinking an overwhelmingly sweet-tasting soda and drowning out the subtle and fascinating flavors of a well-prepared meal with an ultra-dose of syrupy sweetness.

For your lunchtime beverage, seize other options. Ask for ice water or sparkling water and then add a squeeze of fresh lemon. Or if you like the taste of milk, you might consider having skim milk with your meal. Your system craves that additional calcium to help stop the bone loss of osteoporosis. (Women, take note: You're especially prone to osteoporosis, and every glass of skim milk is a low-calorie, high-calcium dose of prevention!)

These are only two options, and you have many more. Be sure to check Fat-Burner Switch #3 on page 91.

2. Don't picnic on chips. For some people, lunch without chips is like love without kisses. One of the biggest self-deceptions is to think that you can "eat just a few." If you're eating at a restaurant and some unidentified chips come with your meal, skip them. They're sure to be high-fat, and even if they aren't, you don't need them during your midday meal.

If you're eating at home or taking your lunch to work, have some crunchy rye crackers or other low-fat whole-grain crackers instead. On occasion, you might have a serving of fat-free tortilla chips.

3. Be a fat-dip skipper. Say no to mystery dips and traditional high-fat soft cheeses, especially the mysterious orange concoction that dresses up nachos in so many fast-food outlets. Making your own lunch? Get some delicious fat-free bean dip, nonfat sour cream dip or ultra-low-fat Cheddar cheese. They're delicious on rye crackers or fat-free whole-grain tortilla chips.

4. Watch out for soup fat. "Soup's on!" is a dinner call that can subvert your fat cravings and slash total calories. In fact, soup is the best of nourishing, appetite-quenching appetizers, according to weight-loss researcher Barbara Rolls, Ph.D., at Johns Hopkins University in Baltimore. But obviously, they aren't applauding chicken gumbo in a fatty broth or double-thick clam chowder made with whole cream.

To get the fat-fighting, appetite-suppressing benefits of soup, you have to lean toward soups made with light broth or vegetable stock. A good example: tomato soup made with 1 percent or nonfat milk. Or for variety, try fresh gazpacho.

Luckily, many soup producers have responded to the cry for low-fat products, and you now have your pick of brightly labeled low-fat soups at the supermarkets. Just avoid any soups that are still beef-, pork- or cream-based.

5. Get fresh. If you're headed for the salad bar, pile on the fresh salad. A well-stocked salad bar these days will have a wide array of fresh greens and garden-grown fixings—Bibb lettuce, Boston lettuce, red-leaf lettuce, romaine. In addition, you may find shallots, spinach, alfalfa and bean sprouts, arugula, Chinese cabbage (bok choy), red cabbage and cucumbers.

Some restaurants and fresh-food markets also have mesclun greens—a wonderful taste explosion of mixed greens.

If you go for only the greens you recognize and steer clear of the unknown, you may be depriving yourself of some brand-new, wonderful flavors. Have you had fresh chard, kale, radicchio, endive, kohlrabi or escarole? (Not all salad bars have these varieties, of course, but some do.) And before you start to pour on dressing, add zero-fat flavors with zesty herbs that add so much interest to a salad—cilantro, cress and watercress, fresh dill, fresh parsley, fennel or garlic. For a spark of onion flavor and naturally hot spices, add red onions, regular onions, green onions (scallions), radishes or hot peppers.

Mushrooms can look less than appetizing at the salad bar if they've been sitting out too long, but add them if they're fresh. With tomatoes you run the same risk. They may be pale and limp if they were sliced too early and have sat too long, but the fresh ones give a burst of good taste.

Fresh peppers hold their flavor well, so be sure to sprinkle your salad with green peppers, red peppers, yellow peppers and pimentos (roasted red peppers).

6. Don't dress with fat. A garden salad can be part of a great lunch, but when you pour on regular salad dressing, you add a whopping 25 or more grams of fat!

High-fat salad dressing is now the number one source of fat in the diets of American women ages 19 to 50. It accounts for almost 10 percent of their fat intakes, according to the National Cancer Institute in Bethesda, Maryland, and the U.S. Department of Agriculture Human Nutrition Information Service. (The culprits next in line are margarine, cheese and ground beef.)

Many full-service restaurants now offer zero-fat salad dressings, as do fast-food restaurants like McDonald's. If you're shopping for bottled dressings, you'll soon get an affinity for low-fat flavors you especially like. Mine include Pritikin Italian, Pritikin French Style, Pritikin Garlic and Herb, Kraft Free Italian, Newman's Own Light and Wish-Bone Fat-Free Italian.

Or you can skip the dressing entirely and just squeeze on lemon juice or lime juice. Try it a few times: You'll discover that the zesty sprinkling of sharp citrus adds its own tangy freshness, especially if you already have fresh herbs, peppers and other garden treats livening up your salad.

Have a Fat-Fighting Lunch

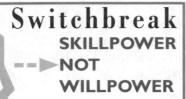

Switchbreak
SKILLPOWER
---▶ NOT
WILLPOWER

What warms you up can help slim you down.

As you look ahead toward your next lunch, stop now to figure out how you can get some spicy heat in it. In addition to planning a low-fat menu, you'll help switch on your fat-burner if you can add at least one hot or super-hot food.

For instance, you can add a dab of hot mustard or a dash of chili powder to soups or sandwiches. Or if you like the flavor of Tabasco, shake it on until your palate sings "Olé!"

Now plan where you'll eat out next time. Instead of a traditional American restaurant, plan on a Mexican, Thai, Indian or Chinese restaurant where the cook is bold with the curry, hot peppers and other sizzling ingredients.

These spices may help increase your after-meal metabolic rate, according to some Canadian medical studies. Also, if you eat that hot stuff, you'll be less likely to stuff yourself. The flavors are so intense that the meal itself signals "All full!"

7. Be very dairy careful. Many dairy foods have far more fat than anyone needs. Just say no to regular (full-fat) milk, regular cream cheese and cottage cheese as well as other high-fat cheeses. There are many alternatives: low-fat or nonfat cheeses (I like Jarlsberg light Swiss), nonfat cream cheese, nonfat cottage cheese or skim milk.

8. Spread it thin. Use all-zest, no-fat sandwich spreads such as mustard, hot sauce or fat-free salad dressing instead of butter or margarine. If you love mayo, make it fat-free to save a whopping 11 grams of fat per tablespoon!

9. Please pass the pasta. You can please your palate with fresh pasta, one of the great low-fat foods. The trick with pasta, however, is to choose your sauce cautiously. Pick tomato or wine-based pasta sauce instead of cream or oil or cheese sauce. And if you're making a cold pasta salad, go "lite" with the ingredients: Choose fat-free dressing, skip the olives and opt for low-fat cheese.

10. Don't sink with subs. Submarine sandwiches and other deli-made, hoagie-style mammoths can be low in fat, but you have to choose the ingredients carefully. First of all, try to get whole-grain bread instead of a regular roll. (And especially stay away from a croissant, which may have 12 grams of fat as opposed to the 1.4 grams in two slices of 100 percent whole-grain bread.) If the deli doesn't have a whole-grain bun, ask for something that's better yet—old-world whole-grain rye or pumpernickel bread.

Now for the fixings: Order your sub or sandwich with sliced turkey breast instead of ham, bologna or sausage. Hold the mayo, unless you have the option of fat-free. Nix the olives, cheese and oil. And above all, watch out for any premixed chicken or tuna salad that happens to be sitting in the deli's serving tray. Just to give you a sample of the danger: A six-inch tuna-salad sub made with regular mayo contains a staggering 36 grams of fat!

Whether you're getting your sandwich from the deli or making it yourself, pile on any quantity of lettuce, tomato and other fresh veggies to add crunchiness, flavor and fiber. Some other favorite fat-free extras include green peppers, jalapeño peppers, sprouts, pickles and onions. Instead of high-fat spreads, add a dash of spicy mustard and a splash of vinegar.

11. Subtract fat, and add pizzazz, to pizza. Pizza makes a quick and lovable lean lunch if you don't order extra-fat toppings and if you go very light on the cheese. Olives are almost pure fat, and most pizza meat toppings—including sausage, pepperoni, ham and ground beef—are excessively high. If you do want toppings, add extra veggies and a dash of fresh pepper.

12. Invest your pesos in low-fat fare. If you're eating Mexican, choose nonfat bean burritos or nonfat bean soft-shell tacos, light on the cheese, with extra veggies and plenty of salsa. Watch out for the many fat-packed favorites that can sabotage your low-fat living faster than a bear trap. Nachos and taco salads are two of the worst fat-slingers: A single taco salad can contain 55 grams of fat and 800 calories!

13. Beef up on burger evasion. If you find yourself craving a burger, hunt as hard as you can for alternatives. You'll cut way back on fat if you choose a grilled chicken breast or ground turkey-breast burger, for instance. But they need to be grilled, not fat-fried, and free of high-fat toppings. For added flavor, season either of these with a spicy meat or poultry sauce.

If the burger dream just won't go away, find a restaurant that has the American classic in a new and kinder low-fat form. The Garden Burger, developed by Wholesome and Hearty Foods of Portland, Oregon, is now available at T.G.I. Friday's, Hard Rock Cafe and many other restaurants. It's low in fat and served with nonfat mayo or mustard. The cheese-burger version is served with very little cheese.

But when you're looking for a way around burgers, be sure

to say no to anything that's fried or batter-fried, even if there's a kernel of chicken, fish or vegetables at the core of that breading. Think of that pale batter as a sponge that soaks up the fat and grease, raising the total fat grams sky-high.

As for eating bacon with or in anything—or by its own fat-packed self—it's like eating a crispy strip of butter.

14. Despise french fries. Many restaurants are now claiming that their french fries are less likely to pack on the fat because they may be fried in "healthier" vegetable oils. True, those oils have less saturated fat, but they may be high in triglycerides, which have been shown to raise the risk of high cholesterol and other heart-related problems.

Best policy: Scratch the fries, no matter what oil they're fried in. Substitute some whole-grain breadsticks or a low-fat bean salad.

15. Get your just desserts. When your sweet tooth speaks up, go ahead with a bite or two of dessert. But make sensible choices.

You're fine with a nonfat whole-grain brownie or several cookies. (I especially like the ones made by Health Valley.) Other choices include a nonfat granola bar and nonfat pound cake. Or have a small cup of nonfat plain yogurt, sweetened with fresh or canned fruit. Another good treat is a single chocolate mint.

Chew these bites of your dessert very slowly, savoring the taste. Then immediately brush your teeth (which helps end the craving for more sweets) before you head into your afternoon work.

Or try this alternate dessert that may completely satisfy your yen for an after-dinner sweet. After your meal, just pop in some mint gum. Chew slowly, then ditch it when the flavor disappears. By then, you'll be into the heart of the afternoon, and your twinge of dessert longing will be faded or gone.

Chapter Nine

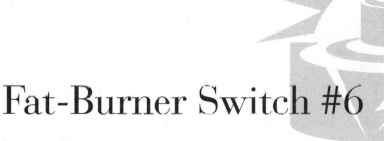

Fat-Burner Switch #6

Use On-the-Spot Distress Blockers

It's always something. Bills. Slow drivers. Traffic. Waiting in line. Just a few of the minor irritations that turn into major bugbears when you're feeling stressed.

I've already discussed how stress can become a fat maker (it's Fat-Maker Switch #10; see page 63) and how you can reduce fat-making processes in the body by identifying your own stress "hot spots" and seeking ways to keep distress at bay whenever possible. These actions are a good start.

Now, when you turn on Fat-Burner Switch #6, you're taking the next step. Here you'll learn a series of on-the-spot distress-dissolving techniques that let you rise above daily hassles and defuse tension and anger, thereby enabling your mind and body to sustain a higher energy level. And along with that higher energy comes correspondingly higher-efficiency fat-burning and a greater likelihood that you'll be alert to turning on other fat-burners all day long.

Burning Fat, Not Burning Out

According to research presented at the 1994 International Conference on Obesity, the less distress you hold on to, the greater your metabolic power may be. That's because anxious, angry or hostile people tend to metabolize fats more slowly than others.

Those who seethe with anger are slowest at getting rid of dietary fat, says psychologist Catherine Stoney, Ph.D., of Brown University in Providence, Rhode Island. "Sitting on high anger levels just doesn't work," she notes.

People with the slowest rates of metabolism often seem to be hostile and anxious, studies show. These people report higher daily stress and sometimes suppress their anger.

Whenever you're hit with increased pressures, your body responds by secreting adrenaline, the fast-acting hormone that stimulates the release of fat from cells throughout the body. In the moments following that surge of adrenaline, though, you lapse into a period of being tense or upset.

"During a stressful situation, adrenaline causes fat cells from all over the body to squirt their contents into the bloodstream," says Redford Williams, M.D., director of the Behavioral Medicine Research Center at Duke University Medical Center in Durham, North Carolina. "Once in circulation, those free-floating molecules can provide the body with the extra energy it needs to meet the physical demands of whatever situation you're in."

Does Your Cup Boileth Over?

Back in our Neanderthal yesteryear, this response to danger and stress poured energy into our hairy bodies, so we could hurl stones at wild beasts and dash away from woolly mammoths running amok. This reaction was probably very appropriate for prehistoric people who needed to flee from danger or charge into battle. But in the modern world, during most daily situations these fat molecules remain unused—except when the stress hormone cortisol enters the picture.

As described earlier, cortisol is released whenever you enter a tense phase. Following biological pathways that have helped preserve humankind throughout the eons, cortisol dampens

Testing the Currents:
Your Response to Foods

Research suggests that the foods you eat can influence production of brain messenger chemicals called neurotransmitters. These chemicals in turn affect your mental energy, concentration, attitude, mood, behavior and performance, according to researchers who conducted studies at Harvard University, Massachusetts Institute of Technology in Cambridge and the National Institutes of Health in Bethesda, Maryland.

While choosing the right foods and combinations of foods can help you manage your emotions and mind, these responses are different for each person. Therefore, you need to carefully observe your body's responses.

One way to do this is to keep a food journal. Over the next few weeks, take notes on your state of mind and your mood 10 to 15 minutes before meals and snacks. Do you feel alert and motivated? Calm and focused? Tense and irritable? Note these observations in your journal.

Then, one hour after eating, reassess your state of mind and emotions and quickly write down your honest observations.

After two weeks, review your appraisals to create a list of the food choices that seem best for you. Use that list as a helpful tool in monitoring your day-to-day eating patterns. Continue the journal for a third and fourth week, reviewing it at intervals to find out whether your observations are consistent. At the end of a month, you should have a clear idea of the foods that give you the responses you want—in terms of both energy and your overall sense of well-being.

fat-burning processes. Fat gets tucked away for storage (emergency use) while the cortisol stimulates carbohydrate-burning to meet the body's cry for more fuel.

Research at Yale University indicates that overweight men and women who carry most of their fat in the abdominal region produce more cortisol than those with less fat there. In one study at Wake Forest University in Winston-Salem, North Carolina, stressed male monkeys—both those who exercised and those who were sedentary—had more intra-abdominal fat than their nonstressed counterparts. The researchers say this suggests that a chronic stress-induced arousal syndrome plays a role in abdominal fat distribution.

During times when we're often tense and stressed (but not

facing life-or-death physical situations), a significant portion of the spare fat harbored in the bloodstream goes wandering off to your abdomen for storage. Thus, whenever you experience some lasting feelings of distress, there are many measurable effects on the brain and body, including slower fat-burning.

Fortunately, there's preliminary evidence that breathing techniques, meditation and other stress reduction methods may help keep cortisol levels down. And that could make a big difference in how your body handles fat when stress stalks.

Bank on Small Changes

Identifying simple, practical new ways to stay on top of the stresses in your life can make a direct difference in your energy level and fat-burning power and make it easier for you to turn on all your other Fat-Burner Switches throughout the day. Best of all, research shows it's the small stress management choices that can lead to major, lasting changes.

"There are rapid, simple strategies that anyone can follow," say stress management authorities Ronald G. Nathan, Ph.D., Thomas E. Staats, Ph.D., and Paul J. Rosch, M.D., authors of *The Doctors' Guide to Instant Stress Relief*. "Are they truly 'instant'? We believe they are."

In other words, strategies can be played out immediately, at the moment of stress, to combat its effects. "The stress response starts in seconds," the researchers have noted. "Instant stress relief is important because it can keep stress—and distress—from accumulating and overwhelming you."

You're the Switch Master

It makes sense to expand your arsenal of do-it-anywhere stress reduction techniques. "Whether it's meditation, biofeedback, yoga or whatever, all relaxation techniques lead to a common set of changes in the body, one of which is to dampen the stress-induced production of cortisol," says Herbert Benson, M.D., associate professor of medicine at Harvard Medical School and president of the Mind/Body Medical Institute at Deaconess Hospital in Boston.

These changes come under the heading of behavior modification. The American Medical Association, the California Dietetic Association and the International Congress on Obesity have all concluded that behavior modification is necessary for successful, lasting weight loss and good lifelong health.

Top 30-Second Stress Neutralizers

Here are some of the fastest scientifically based stress management techniques that we've tested. They're all quick, taking less than 30 seconds to implement—but if you use them, you can get some deep and long-lasting benefits.

Breathe Away Stress

Surprisingly, many of us halt our breathing for several seconds or more at the start of a stressful situation. This reduces oxygen to the brain and pushes you toward distress and feelings of anxiety, anger, frustration and panic. While all this is going on, you may have faulty reactions while feeling a general loss of control.

So whenever you feel yourself getting hit with increased stress—as evidenced by muscle tension, irregular breathing, cool hands or nervous sweating—one of the best ways to regain calm is to change the way you breathe.

The action step here is simple: Continue breathing smoothly, deeply and evenly. When the cue of fear, threat or stress first captures your attention, you could be anywhere in the inhalation or exhalation cycle, so the first thing you need to do is concentrate on finishing that cycle. And at the same instant, say to yourself "Alert mind, calm body."

"It is the inner breathing of the (100 trillion) cells in your body that enables you to produce biological energy," observes Sheldon Saul Hendler, M.D., Ph.D., assistant clinical professor of medicine at the University of California, San Diego, and author of *The Doctor's Vitamin and Mineral Encyclopedia*.

What produces this biological energy? Dr. Hendler points to a specific complex chemical, adenosine triphosphate (ATP), which he calls "the basic currency of life." ATP is like a coiled spring that "springs" open to release energy when it's combined with a cellular fuel like glucose. In other words, to convert fuel into energy, your body desperately needs an adequate supply of the chemical that does the conversion—and that key chemical is ATP.

"Without ATP there is no energy, no life," says Dr. Hendler. "It is ATP that we utilize to act." The body and brain are extremely sensitive to even very small reductions in ATP production, Dr. Hendler has observed. "This sensitivity is expressed in terms of fearfulness, anxiety, aches and pains, confusion and intermittent fatigue." The production of ATP, Dr. Hendler says, is directly influenced by the "inner breathing" of your cells. "Breathing is unquestionably the most important thing you do in your life. And breathing well is unquestionably the most important thing you can do to improve your life."

We each breathe about 20,000 times every day. With that much air going in, it seems natural to assume that we take in plenty of oxygen. But the fact is that most of us breathe just deeply enough to keep from becoming unconscious. Neuroscientists have reported that although we technically remain "alive," we don't supply our brains with optimal levels of oxygen.

According to experts, vital lung capacity decreases about 5 percent with every decade of life, mostly as a result of lost elasticity of lung tissue. Research at the Baltimore Gerontology Research Center of the National Institute on Aging shows that it's common to find a huge drop in the amount of oxygen taken in by the lungs as we age. Most—perhaps nearly all—of this loss can be prevented with proper breathing habits, good posture and regular aerobic exercise.

Studies by the National Institute on Aging indicate that the circulating blood of a 20-year-old man takes up an average of nearly 4 liters of oxygen per minute. In contrast, because of his shallow breathing and loss of lung elasticity, the blood of a 75-year-old man takes up only 1½ liters of oxygen a minute. This is typical, but it isn't inevitable. Research suggests that a fit 75-year-old can take in as much oxygen as a fit 20-year-old.

But many of us get into the habit of shallow breathing throughout our lives. That means we're taking in much less breath—and giving our cells much less oxygen—than people who regularly do diaphragmatic breathing.

In diaphragmatic breathing, the diaphragm muscle moves downward, creating a natural pressure vacuum that draws air into the lower lungs. This is quickly followed by a slight expansion of the abdomen and lower ribs. Finally, as the inhalation cycle is completed, the chest expands and the upper lung areas are filled with air.

Upper chest breathing automatically leaves you underoxygenated and interferes with fat-burning and other forms of energy production in the body. Diaphragmatic breathing, on the other hand, fills your lungs almost to capacity. And that's an important distinction, because the more parts of your lungs the air gets to, the more oxygen you can get into your bloodstream.

When it's traveling from the heart to pick up oxygen, blood flows to different areas of your lungs at variable rates of speed. It's estimated that blood flows to the top areas of your lungs at the rate of about one tablespoon per minute, to the middle areas at the rate of a pint a minute and to the bottom areas at the rate of about one quart a minute.

When you first try it, diaphragmatic breathing may seem like more work than shallow breathing, but that's really just because you have to concentrate to change your shallow-breathing habits. In actuality, smooth diaphragmatic breathing requires only about 1 percent of the body's ongoing energy consumption to bring air in and out, tests have shown. In comparison, typical shallow chest breathing takes at least twice as much energy to accomplish the same work.

So training yourself to use diaphragmatic breathing is tremendously important in mastering stress and staying healthy. Plus, you get an added benefit from using your diaphragm: As it contracts, this muscular hollow gently pushes the internal

Switchbreak
SKILLPOWER NOT ◄-- WILLPOWER

How can you switch on diaphragmatic breathing so that it becomes the way you breathe all the time?

Practice, at first—and then it will become a habit. But you have to begin with awareness. Focus on each step of the process.

1. Sit or stand with your shoulders back and relaxed, your neck comfortably stretched and your head erect.

2. Place your hands right over your belly, below your rib cage.

3. Slowly inhale through your nose. As your abdomen expands slightly downward and forward (with your lower back staying flat), feel your lower ribs move out to the sides. Then, as you complete the inhalation, feel your chest expand comfortably.

4. Exhale slowly through your mouth, feeling a wave of relaxation flood your abdomen, chest, throat and face.

Be sure to place your hands over your diaphragm. Touching the outside of your lower ribs improves the results.

As you repeat the exercise, you will become increasingly aware of the exact sensation of breathing correctly.

Switchbreak
SKILLPOWER
--▶NOT
WILLPOWER

You can practice, right now, to develop the strength of a cue word. Once you have the word planted in your subconscious, you can use it anytime, anywhere to help beat fat-building stress.

1. Sit in a relaxed, comfortable place, breathing slowly and deeply. Permit yourself to let go of all anxious or work-related thoughts for a few minutes.

2. Direct your attention to your breathing, focusing on the air as it gently passes into and out of your nostrils and chest. Begin to feel the sensations of your body—the air or clothing on your skin, the weight of your shoulders and arms, the texture and support of the surface you're sitting on.

3. Vividly imagine thinking, feeling, looking, sounding and performing at your relaxed best in a specific past place and circumstance. Focus on a time when you felt safe, loved, respected and at your best.

4. When this image feels strongest and most calming, vividly picture the word (or words) in your mind that suggests or describes this place. That word becomes your cue.

organs down, massaging them and, some researchers suggest, improving circulation and digestive elimination functions.

Use an Instant Mind-Escape Word

For an instant leap from stress and tension into a state of greater calm, behavioral scientists recommend a cue word.

The cue word can be a command to yourself, like "Relax" or "Take time out." But other word cues with specific personal meaning are usually more effective, like "beach" or "mountain" or "summer vacation." Personalize these associations by substituting the names of your own favorite getaway places.

When you practice using your cue word, try to develop every aspect of the mental image that goes with it. Here's a checklist to help you make sure you've used all your senses to conjure up the stress-soothing sights, sounds, tastes, feelings, temperatures and emotions that the word should suggest. If anything's missing, go back to that place and reimagine it, filling out the details until your cue word becomes a total sensual, emotional and mental experience.

■ How deeply were you relaxed?

■ Did you feel a sense of ease or compassion or joy or discovery or wonder?

■ What did it feel like to have this inner balance—to be in touch with your spirit?

■ Were you indoors or out? In sunlight or shade, clear air, rain or snow?

■ What was the temperature? Did you notice air currents?

■ What were you wearing and how did it feel on your skin?

■ What could you see in all directions from the surface where you sat, stood or lay?

■ Was there a sweet taste in your mouth? Forest or floral scents in the air?

■ How did the muscles in your body feel?

■ What was the rhythm of your breathing?

■ What were the sounds around you and off in the distance?

■ Where was your mind focused? In what specific ways did you feel connected to nature and the universe around you?

Each time you use your cue, the instant-recall power of the word becomes stronger. It becomes an automatic tool. When stress rises here and there throughout the day, you can think—and perhaps say aloud—this cue word and recapture the feelings of relaxation and inner control.

If you've been harried by phone calls all day long, for example, the next time the phone rings you might pause before answering and say your cue word aloud. The word becomes your "instant tranquilizer." In a single moment you can find yourself more calm and confident, and when you do pick up the phone, that calmness will be conveyed in your voice.

Relax Your Face and Hands with a Wave of Relaxation

Certain areas of the body have large corresponding "maps" in the brain and are keys to staying calm, alert and ready to respond rapidly and appropriately to whatever situation arises. Two of these "signal" muscle areas are the face and hands.

The action here is to flash a mental "wave of relaxation," beginning with the muscles in your face and around your eyes. Then let this wave pass through your neck, shoulders and whole body, right out through your fingertips and toes.

To see how this works, stand with your shoulders loose and your arms hanging freely at your sides. Close your eyes and imagine that a warm waterfall is washing through you,

Streamlining Your Stress-Stoppers

Sometimes all it takes to put the brakes on stress is a rapid switch-over to another activity—or a complete break from whatever's causing the stress to build. Here are some tactics you can employ on the spot. Though they seem simple, you'll be surprised at how effective they are.

■ Stand up and do some gentle stretching exercises.

■ Escape from the telephone. The next time it rings, let your answering machine handle the call. If you don't have an answering machine, unplug the phone or turn the ringer all the way down. If it's really urgent, you can be sure the person will call back.

■ See your blessings. Just close your eyes and take a few seconds to visualize the people, possessions or memories that you value or love.

■ Sip a glass of iced herbal tea and think only of its flavor.

■ Sit down and list five things you've enjoyed in the past week or month.

■ Remember your most perfect romantic moment.

■ Take off your shoes, rotate your feet and wiggle your toes.

first through your face, then through your neck, shoulders, arms and hands and on down until it flows out through your toes. And as it flows along, this waterfall clears away all tension.

Shift Your Attention

"Changing your thoughts can give you immediate new control over how you respond to stress," notes Frank Ghinassi, Ph.D., instructor in psychiatry at Harvard Medical School. What you do with your mind and directed energy in the initial moments of a stressful situation will help determine the outcome.

When you shift your attention away from the situation, you're prompting the brain into a state of relaxed alertness. And that gets you away from the more typical reactions to stress—anger or paralysis.

To put this in perspective, recall a time when someone's safety (maybe your own) was threatened and you overreacted to the pressure. You'll realize that if you had remained calmer and more flexible—if you'd been able to think more clearly during the first moments of the situation—you could have chosen a more effective response.

That's the key to rapid stress relief: Learn to insert a gap that's filled with calm alertness at the very start of each stressful or fearful scene. With practice you can enlarge this gap between stimulus and response and use your creative imagination to seek out new solutions. Here are some techniques to help you arrive at those solutions.

■ Focus on what you can control rather than on what you can't.

■ Divert your mind from the situation, so you don't get knotted up again and again in worries or imaginary fears.

■ Listen for just one extra moment, keeping an open mind, instead of instantly talking back.

■ Ask yourself "Will my reaction harm the other person?"

When you're skilled at protecting yourself from blind reactions, you not only help avoid creating a stressful situation fraught with tension, you also avoid hurting yourself.

Deflect Distress with Physical Activity

Research at the University of Pennsylvania School of Medicine in Philadelphia has shown that exercise has a direct effect on how well you handle everyday stress. In particular, if you are physically active, it is likely you will not become as distressed or emotionally upset when faced with stressful events.

When you do some physical activity during high-pressure times, you're more likely to recover more quickly, both physically and emotionally.

So the next time you're stressed, why not get up and move around? Chances are you'll reduce the negative effects of stress and capture a quick-surge boost of mental and physical energy.

"Exercise has a powerful impact on the way we view ourselves," says Robert Motta, Ph.D., director of the doctoral program in school community psychology at Hofstra University in Hempstead, New York. A number of studies support Dr. Motta's view and further show that regular exercise enhances mood and improves stress control.

In a study at Stanford University, researchers examined the psychological effects of physical activity on 357 adults ages 50 to 65 over a one-year period. Researchers compared groups of people who participated in exercise classes of various types and those who exercised at home. The study showed that all the exercisers, regardless of how they went about their exercise, had reduced levels of stress and anxiety compared with nonexercisers. And those who exercised most regularly had greater reductions in symptoms of anxiety and depression.

According to health psychologist Richard Dienstbier, Ph.D., of the University of Nebraska in Omaha, studies show that a vital attribute in stress management is "mental resilience and toughness." These qualities are strongly influenced by a set of physiological changes in the pituitary/adrenal/cortical "arousal system." The changes accompany or result from a program of regular physical exercise, especially aerobics.

"Once the physiological pattern called toughness is achieved through regular exercise and other health-building means," says Dr. Dienstbier, "the tough individual takes the increased energy level and reduced feelings of anxiety and depression into account in judging potential success and failure in new situations. Knowing energy levels will be sufficient to accomplish most tasks, the tough individual predicts success rather than failure. That very prediction leads, in the short term, to hormonal changes associated with energy. On the other hand, the individual who is not tough, burdened by feelings of anxiety more than energy, is likely to predict failure and, as a direct result of that prediction, to produce higher levels of cortisol."

Since cortisol is a powerful body-produced chemical that can induce fat storage, you're turning off a Fat-Maker Switch every time you use exercise to combat stress.

Use Your Pause!

As you take a calming breath at the beginning of each stressful situation, wait for a moment before speaking, especially if you feel the first flash of anger. This one strategy can make a big difference in your relationships with others, especially a spouse, close friend or relative who is likely to be hurt by your anger.

"Our research has shown that it takes only one put-down to undo hours of kindness you give to your partner," say Clifford Notarius, Ph.D., professor of psychology at the University of Denver and director of the Center for Marriage and Family Studies, and Howard Markman, Ph.D., professor of psychology at Catholic University in Washington, D.C., authors of *We Can Work It Out*. They point to the small changes in behavior that can turn the tide in your favor.

"Listening to your partner rather than walking away or yelling just once in the heat of an argument can produce substantial changes in stress relief and marital happiness," they observe.

Shift Your Point of View

Whenever you find yourself feeling a surge of anger or hostility, shift your attention. Ask yourself "Is this really a deliberate affront?" Try to reframe the provocation and see things from the other person's view.

■ There's no need to get upset about this.

■ Maybe he is angry about something else and is letting off steam.

■ If this turns into a difficult situation, stay calm.

Finally, be sure you cope with any effects of antagonism. Relax tense muscles. Slow your breathing. Whenever possible, use humor.

"But the situation's not funny!" you say. Well, maybe it can be, if you imagine the ridiculous. If you're in heavy traffic, for instance, and the person ahead of you has cut into your lane without signaling, you could replace anger by thinking to yourself "What a clown!" Then envision a huge disembodied clown face, with red lips and nose pressed to the wheel. When you've got the image of Bozo the Clown trying to steer his way down the road, you're more likely to chuckle than to stew in outrage.

For a variation, I like the suggestion of Martin E. P. Seligman, Ph.D., professor of psychology at the University of Pennsylvania. Say to yourself "What an ass!"—and then go ahead and visualize a pair of buttocks steering the car that just cut you off. Decorate them with some feathers or glitter paint. Imagine what it will be like when a cop stops the driver for reckless driving and discovers there's nothing but a pair of buttocks behind the wheel.

Anger gone yet?

If it lingers despite your attempts to see the ridiculousness of the situation, you might visualize yourself as a bomb disposer. Your job is to slowly and coolly defuse the bomb of anger, then move ahead with some kind of action without attacking. In conversations, for instance, you might rely on a short list of "defusing words" tailored to reduce anger on the part of your spouse, children, boss, difficult co-workers or irritating neighbors.

Of course, it's tougher if you're on the receiving end of anger, and many people feel that the only good defense is a spirited offense. But before you strike back, pause and find the humor.

What if your spouse comes home after a rough day at work and takes out frustrations by yelling at you or the kids? Instead of becoming angry and emotionally off-balance, try a dose of fun. You might imagine your spouse as a grouchy, irritable yet cuddly teddy bear in need of a hug, a kiss or a kind word.

You can take the grumpiness less seriously because you're not the target of that anger, even though you're obviously getting the negative fallout. What your partner really needs is your support and care, rather than a confrontation and a ruined evening or weekend.

In response to grumbling grunts and grouchy comments, take a deep breath and say, in as warm a tone as you can muster, "I can tell you've had a really rough day." And then you might add, reaching out to give a reassuring pat on the back or squeeze on the arm, "I'm happy you're home now, here with us." The outcome—and the mood of your entire evening—will be very different than it would be if you snapped "If you think you had a rough day . . . !"

If grouchiness is a chronic behavior, then other strategies may be called for. But if it happens only occasionally, your willingness to be compassionate and have fun can be contagious. Humor and well-timed jokes, backed with kind words, give your partner a chance to cool off.

Hide Your Bathroom Scale

I know. It may seem hard to believe that the bathroom scale can be your enemy in low-fat living. But if you're accustomed to a morning weigh-in that leaves you feeling guilty, angry, discouraged or demoralized, then it's worse than your enemy—it's a skilled saboteur that stands ready to undercut your fat-fighting work.

Think about what happens when you step on that accusatory scale. Most of the time, it just delivers the bad news— that you haven't lost weight or, worse, you've gained weight. Sure, the numbers are accurate, but the tale they tell is not the whole story.

"Those numbers on your scale typically tell half-truths," says Wayne L. Westcott, Ph.D., consultant to the National YMCA, the American Council on Exercise and the National Academy of Sports Medicine. "Your scale may tell you that you've gained ten pounds in the past decade, when in truth you may have lost 5 pounds of muscle and gained 15 pounds of fat." If that's happened, the scales give you the illusion that you're only 10 pounds overweight, when in fact you need to shake off 15 pounds of fat.

On the other hand, the news might be better than the scale says. If you've been on the Low-Fat Living Program, for instance, your scale may say you've lost only 7 pounds after three months. But in fact you may have gained 5 pounds of muscle and lost 12 pounds of fat, giving you a net improvement in body composition that's much more impressive than the scale is telling you. Or the scale may show you gaining weight when that weight is all muscle, which actually weighs more than fat.

Not only are the scales indifferent to the balance between muscle and fat, they cannot distinguish between water weight and fat weight, either. An added pound or two may be just water and may vanish in a day or so.

Among the reported 70 percent of all dieters who regularly weigh themselves, most forget that their body weight reflects an intricate combination of water, muscle, fat, bone and related tissues. The balance among those factors can vary from hour to hour, day to day, even when there's no fat loss occurring.

What this means, then, is that there's no reason to weigh yourself every day, or even every week. When you're on the track with low-fat living, in fact, you may actually gain weight (as measured by the scale) while losing fat, changing body proportions, getting healthier and increasing your energy.

"The focus should be on healthy lifestyle change. The more you focus on the scale, the worse the outcome," says John Foreyt, Ph.D., a faculty member at the Baylor College of Medicine in Houston and co-author of *Living without Dieting*.

If you're a stickler for mathematical progress checks, there's still some measuring you can do if you want to, and it's far more useful than referring to the scale. Measure your waist, hips, thighs and arms; they'll all start to change as you lose excess fat. Then check these measurements every month or two for a simple indication of your progress.

The fit of your clothing is another valid sign of improvement. You may want to try on a tight pair of jeans now, then put them away for future comparison.

Just keep the bathroom scale out of sight and out of reach. You have enough stress in your daily life without a morning dose of guilt, doubt and Monday-morning quarterbacking.

Use On-the-Spot Distress Blockers

Before You Eat under Stress—Question Yourself!

"Eighty-five percent of my patients have psychological reasons for overeating and eating high-fat foods," says Maria Simonson, Sc.D., Ph.D., director of the Health, Weight and Stress Clinic at Johns Hopkins Medical Institutions in Baltimore. "And one of the major reasons is stress. Stress makes you eat more quickly than anything else.

"Some people who are stressed out go for soft, creamy, comfort foods, like mashed potatoes with plenty of butter," Dr. Simonson observes. Another typical comfort combo is the old late-night standby—milk and cookies. If you find yourself turning to food in response to bad feelings or fatigue, it's vital to have on-the-spot nonfood strategies to feel better.

"Before you eat," advises Dr. Simonson, "ask yourself 'How am I feeling about myself right now? What's happened to upset me? Am I eating this because I'm hungry or because I'm upset?' "

Tune Out the TV Blues

Watching television for long periods—more than two hours at a stretch—generally leaves people in worse moods than before they began to watch, concluded a study supported by the National Institute of Mental Health in Rockville, Maryland. As they observed more than 1,200 subjects over 13 years, researchers gained a better understanding of what happens to people when they watch TV as an escape from stress or as an attempt to feel better.

In many cases, the strategy backfires. Their moods sink. And generally, the worse mood you're in, the harder it is to handle stress. That lost-in-a-fog look in people's eyes after hours of TV gazing isn't entirely due to eyestrain.

The tube has a measurable effect on metabolism as well. In another study, researchers at Memphis State University monitored young girls watching an episode of *The Wonder Years* and found that their metabolic rates dropped as much as 16 percent below resting levels. In other words, they burned fewer calories watching TV than they did just sitting still with the TV off.

Though further research is still under way to determine the exact effect of TV inertia on adults, the basic message seems clear: To counter the metabolism-lowering, mood-depressing, stress-inducing effects of television, you need some form of relief from its influence or a counterbalance to its effects.

The best way to find relief? Turn on your Fat-Burner Switch by staying more active in the evening. If you're in the habit of logging in early and continuing until you can barely see the commercials through drooping eyelids, your first goal is simply to cut back on television time. Or mix some energy into your media experience as I've suggested, by pedaling an exercise bike or striding along on a ski machine while you watch.

Knitting, mending, ironing and folding laundry are other things you can do while you watch TV, and any of these metabolism-raising activities will help counteract the mood- and energy-lowering effects of the tube.

Reconnect with a Loved One or Friend

When the pressures in your life increase, remember to stay in close touch with the people you care most about. Pull back from pressure and take a few moments to jot a quick note to a friend. If you have access to a computer network system, send an e-mail across the wires. Or pick up the phone and say a kind word to your loved ones. All these relationship strengtheners can help protect you against lasting distress.

"If you look at the factors that predict successful, permanent weight loss, social support ranks near the top of the list," says Dr. Foreyt. "I'd go so far as to say it is absolutely critical."

Say a Kind Word—To Yourself

It's amazing to realize that high metabolism may be as much a reflection of mental outlook as of physical condition.

Does that mean we can think ourselves thin? Probably not. But when it comes to coping with distress, your thought processes can have both direct and indirect effects on your energy and fat-burning power.

Let's take several examples: Many of us have been led to believe that we can find solutions to emotional distress if we think or talk about it enough. But thinking or talking about our difficulties and inadequacies—excess body fat or looking and feeling older, for example—may inadvertently keep the feelings of distress alive.

Self-suggestion, or self-talk, can magnify distress if we're directing negative comments or criticisms against ourselves.

Neutralizing Your Saboteurs

Take an extra few minutes about once a month to use a well-proven method for identifying and changing self-talk habits. It's called the double column technique.

1. Divide a piece of paper down the middle. Label the left column "Saboteur" or "Negative Self-Talk," the right column "Coach" or "Voice of Truth."

2. In the left column record negative self-statements you've noted over the past several hours or so. Pay special attention to self-talk that includes "shoulds" and "shouldn'ts." Also list anything that sounds like a put-down.

3. Across from these negative statements, in the right-hand column, write down positive statements. These are the statements that you can use to "coach" yourself out of negative thought patterns and into a new frame of mind.

To get started, list entries under a few general categories. One category, for instance, might be weight loss.

Under "Saboteur," you might put the statement: "I shouldn't have overeaten those high-fat foods again." Your "Coach" column would respond with: "It's perfectly all right to occasionally eat some high-fat foods. That's because most of the time I'm eating the lower-fat, high-taste foods I'm coming to enjoy."

Or your "saboteur" might say: "I've got so far to go, and I've tried and failed so many times before, why should things be any different now?" And your "coach" replies: "Maybe the things I tried before weren't effective—or maybe they just weren't right for me. This time there's more to it than simply losing fat. I'm building up my health and fitness one small choice at a time."

As you review this list, make the "Coach" remarks part of your thinking and feeling, internalizing them to the point where you find you're truly thinking and feeling more positive in every way about every facet of your life.

We live with this inner mind chatter all day, every day. It's a natural human tendency, and unfortunately, most of us have learned to emphasize self-defeating messages.

We often have trouble being as compassionate or rational with ourselves as we would be with a friend or loved one. Perhaps this is because critical parents, teachers, bosses and peers have inadvertently led us to believe many negative things about ourselves.

According to several surveys of conversations between parents and children, researchers have found that most parents give their children a dozen criticisms for every single compliment or positive comment. In the average secondary school classroom, the ratio of criticisms to compliments made by teachers to students is 18 to 1. As for business situations, a survey at Stanford University showed that the negative comments from bosses outnumber the positive by ratios that range from 4 to 1 to as much as 8 to 1.

Nagging, critical voices are sure to be echoed by your subconscious mind. They can hold considerable harming power, especially when they keep you trapped in old, self-sabotaging behavior patterns.

"If you find that your self-talk—that little, nagging voice in the back of your mind—is highly critical and judgmental, or self-discounting, or self-indulgent, or emotionally upsetting, you need to retrain the way you are thinking," says Joyce D. Nash, Ph.D., a clinical psychologist in the San Francisco Bay area and author of *Now That You've Lost It: How to Maintain Your Best Weight*. "You need to teach your little voice to be more objective and supportive, like a coach for a team. When you allow your self-talk to be negative, you allow it to sabotage you, to rob you of motivation, to enmesh you in painful emotions."

Time and again people say "When I feel bad, I get all tensed up, stop exercising and can't sleep"; "When I'm upset, I yell at other people and then feel terrible about myself"; "When I'm angry at myself, I punish myself by sitting around in front of the TV and begin eating nonstop."

Psychologists have discovered that when people feel distressed about something and react by stuffing themselves with food, the resulting feeling of failure is usually not based on reality. That is, most people aren't even aware of how many extra calories or excess grams of fat they've eaten. Instead, the feeling of failure is generated almost completely by the notion that they've lapsed or cheated.

A sense of failure can prompt many forms of emotional distress, from a feeling of unattractiveness to a collapse of self-esteem, suggests Marcia Germaine Hutchinson, Ed.D., adjunct professor of counseling psychology at Lesley College in Cambridge, Massachusetts. As a result, she says, each time we feel distressed it can lead to "poor posture—rounded shoulders,

Switchbreak
SKILLPOWER
--- ► NOT
WILLPOWER

As you read this, are you starting to think about what you shouldn't have eaten for dessert last night or the high-fat snack you shouldn't have had today?

If so, you could be playing into the hands of a fat-maker called guilt. Just a small dose of it may raise your stress level—and the irony is that stress, rather than a high-fat indulgence, could be the bigger fat-contributing culprit.

Instead of worrying about a slip-up or two, turn things around right away. Be kinder to yourself.

Yes, on occasion you'll eat small amounts of "forbidden" foods. If you do happen to overeat and don't automatically yell at yourself, you'll likely eat less, recover more quickly and keep your Fat-Burner Switches turned on. So:

■ Forgive yourself for not being perfect; remember, everybody has ups and downs.

■ Become more active. Head out the door for a five-minute "mini-walk."

■ Continue with your regular meals and snacks. If you try to eat less to compensate for overeating, you'll simply confuse your body's metabolism.

drooping head—which is not only unattractive but unhealthy and interferes with our ability to breathe properly and keep our energy and metabolism high."

One of the simplest ways to shake off this negative mind-set and start being constructive and self-supporting is by choosing a variety of quick, practical daily habit changes. By turning off the Fat-Maker Switches and turning on the Fat-Burner Switches, for instance, you take immediate, active steps to rev up your energy and your calorie-burning power. There's good scientific evidence that in addition, your mood will tend to stay more positive when you control those switches.

A few moments is all it takes to shift your thinking and give yourself a dose of emotional support—and these steps pay off. Be sure to guard against the "if onlys" that tend to tie us in knots. Many people who have been up and down on various diets live in a tightening web of "if only" statements such as "If only I could lose those 15 pounds" or "If only I had more willpower, I could change."

Often when we say "If only I were thin," what we're really saying is "I hate myself the way I am."

To move forward, you first need to forgive yourself, today, for not looking the way society has coerced you into thinking you should look. It's hard enough to be overweight in our thinness-driven culture without adding to the problem by being hard on yourself.

It's also essential to distinguish between having a body and being that body. Remind yourself that the best of who you are, as a human being, is in your head and heart. The fact that you have a body to live in is something to be thankful for. But while being thankful for it, don't be lured into thinking you are your body—or you may end up with the distorted and negative feeling that you're made up of chunky thighs or a protruding abdomen!

Keep Looking on the Lighter Side

There are powerful scientific reasons that explain why people who are quick to laugh—especially at themselves—are generally more active, more energetic, healthier and better able to bounce back from stressful situations. And medical research has shown that people with this kind of humor are less likely to experience stress-triggered binge eating and to avoid exercise.

"In order to laugh at yourself, you have to forgive yourself for not being perfect," says Mark Therrien, the director of Innerplay, an organization based in Lakewood, Wisconsin, that promotes the therapeutic use of humor and play. In presentations he has made to the American Dietetic Association and other organizations, Therrien explains how humor comes into play in a weight-loss program: "The forgiving attitude allows you to look at your mistakes, learn from them . . . and

Switchbreak
SKILLPOWER NOT ◄-- WILLPOWER

One of the simplest and most important steps you can take toward a different life is to recognize and guide your self-talk.

Here are two steps you can take right now to change the critical voices to complimentary ones.

1. When you notice self-talk turning negative—and putting you down—make it a point to pause and say something more helpful to yourself.

2. Follow that statement with some action step to bring out inner strength and self-pride.

Negative self-talk is often triggered by a critical comment from a friend about your appearance or a glimpse of your physique in a mirror. If you're focused on losing weight or changing your appearance, you're likely to feel a swelling of self-doubt or impatience when you don't get the "final results" you'd hoped for or when you have a sudden urge to eat high-fat foods.

Right now, try to detect the sound of any negative self-talk that may be in your head. The next step: Contradict it. Then choose one Fat-Maker Switch to turn *off* and a Fat-Burner to turn *on*.

There—you have the upper hand again.

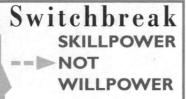

Switchbreak
SKILLPOWER
--▶ NOT
WILLPOWER

Having trouble getting perspective on your anger, stress and day-to-day problems?

Ask yourself "Is it worth dying for?" suggests Robert S. Eliot, M.D., cardiologist, stress researcher and author of *From Stress to Strength*.

When you chronically let stress get the better of you, you risk not only losing your cool but also shortening your life. Researchers know that mismanaged anger and hostility can contribute to high blood pressure and the risk of an unexpected fatal heart attack. And there may be a link between anger or helplessness and certain forms of cancer. And your stress can eventually destroy relationships.

So what throws your frustration into high gear? Waiting for someone who always shows up late? Long lines? Slow-poke drivers? Bank machines that refuse to cooperate? Rude kids? Go on—list them all.

Reframing your priorities with the Big Question should make it easier to "go with the flow" and let go of needless anger and tension.

laugh at them. Besides, laughing burns calories."

In truth, humor has very little to do with telling jokes. It's about perceiving the absurdities of everyday life and then chuckling at them, even through hassles, heartaches and hard times. It means taking yourself more lightly even when you're doing serious work. And it's about laughing—harder and more often than most of us usually do.

The body and brain are extremely sensitive to even very small escapes into "mirthful laughter." A sense of the absurd, and the laughter that goes with it, works its wonders by initially arousing and distracting the mind and then leaving us feeling more relaxed.

Scientists theorize that laughter stimulates the production of neurotransmitters and hormones that affect hormonal levels in the body. These body chemicals are related to feelings of joy, an easing of pain and strengthened immune response.

Want to lighten up? Here are two ideas suggested by humor experts and psychologists.

Cultivate cosmic humor. Spontaneous mirth is something you allow to happen naturally through a sense of relaxation and fun. Start looking for more ridiculous, incongruous events that go on around you all the time. Point them out to others. Make up short stories about the funniest things you see or hear and use them to spice up family discussions at the end of the day.

Start a family humor library. What makes you laugh?

Whether it's cartoons, letters from friends, posters, biographies, old or new comedy movies, joke encyclopedias or humorous stories, expand your collection. And don't forget audiotapes with live comedy or humorous stories that can give you a quick shot of delight at the beginning or end of the day. Pay attention to whatever harmless humor tickles your funny bone—and make it a point to surround yourself with more of it.

Use On-the-Spot Distress Blockers

Fat-Burner Switch #7

Count on Fast Firm-Ups: Quick and Easy Muscle-Toning

Reach up and press the fingertips of your left hand to the upper muscles of your right arm. Tense those arm muscles. Now place your fingertips against your abdomen and tighten your abdominal muscles.

What did you feel when you tensed these areas? Did the muscles feel firm? Or did they feel a little bit loose, even though you tightened them as hard as you could?

You have more than 400 muscles in your body that you use every day. You don't have much direct power over some of the involuntary muscles, such as the fistful of fibers that makes up most of your heart or the nimble intestinal group that urges food and waste through your digestive system. But many of the voluntary muscles that control posture and movement, like those in your shoulders, upper arms, chest, back, waist, thighs and calves, are under your control.

All these voluntary muscles have one thing in common.

They need to be strengthened and balanced in relationship to each other—and kept that way. And that part is up to you. If you don't keep up the balancing and alignment part of your body maintenance, it's almost guaranteed that your muscles will start to wither away, actually losing the ability to do whatever they were designed to do. And one of the prices you pay for this gradual atrophy of the muscles is reduced metabolism.

The Warranty on Your Body

One of the most important fitness discoveries in the past decade has been that well-toned muscles serve a vital role in fat distribution. They act as fat-burning furnaces 24 hours a day, providing a remarkable metabolic boost.

"To wage war effectively against body fat, you need to be a good calorie-burning machine 24 hours a day, and having adequate muscle tissue is the only way to do that," observes Bryant A. Stamford, Ph.D., exercise scientist and director of the Health Promotion and Wellness Program at the University of Louisville in Kentucky.

Many of us seem to have accepted the "fact" that we have to fight a battle against waistline flab—and too often we view this single battlefield as the Waterloo of our campaign. To remain slim and fit, however, you have to look past your abdomen to all the other major muscles in your body.

Here's why: Your body comes with a built-in warranty. If you consistently use all your muscle groups in adulthood, those muscles will remain firm, flexible and well-balanced throughout your life.

Muscle loss begins in the midtwenties. If you're sedentary, you have been losing muscle at the rate of about a pound a year since age 25 or so. And even if you have exercised regularly for many years, doing aerobic activities such as walking, jogging or cycling, you have lost some muscle since that time.

This muscle is called lean mass, as distinguished from fat tissue, which has no muscle at all. If your lean mass steadily decreases, so does your resting metabolism. As a result, your body needs fewer and fewer calories to function, and the excess calories are more easily stored as body fat.

Getting Tuned with Toning

By toning your muscles you actually raise your metabolic rate, so you burn more fat, even when you're resting. And different kinds of exercises tone the muscles in different ways.

Taking the prize in most categories are the exercises involved in resistance training. This is any kind of training that involves lifting weights, even if they weigh just a few pounds. (A big distinction: I'm not talking here about Arnold Schwarzenegger–style muscle-building.)

According to the latest guidelines from the American College of Sports Medicine, all it takes for solid, progressive strength-training results is a total of 15 minutes of strengthening exercises three or four times a week, using free weights, supported weight machines or body-weight calisthenic exercises.

Muscle-making resistance exercise may be the single most effective weapon you can employ if you're over 40 and gaining weight, according to William Evans, Ph.D., director of the Noll Physiological Research Center at Pennsylvania State University in University Park. Strong, well-toned muscles keep your circulation high, draw in more oxygen, rev up calorie-burning and increase your overall metabolism, helping you to "burn off" stubborn layers of excess body fat.

The maintenance deal on your body never runs out. Scientists say it's never too late to get stronger—and stay stronger. "There's a myth that we lose the ability to respond to exercise as we age, that we can't get stronger or make muscles bigger," observes Dr. Evans, former director of the Human Physiology Laboratory at the Jean Mayer USDA Human Nutrition Research Center on Aging at Tufts University in Boston. "That's not true."

According to Dr. Evans, the right kind of muscle-toning can make people 65 and over stronger than they've ever been in their lives. "We can triple muscle strength in old people. We can make a 90-year-old stronger than a 50-year-old," Dr. Evans says. "Our oldest exerciser is 100 years old."

> *Of all the calories burned in the body, 50 to 90 percent are burned by your muscles—even when you sleep.*
>
> —Covert Bailey, author of
> The New Fit or Fat

The Calorie-Gobbler and Muscle-Builder

Aerobic exercise, as we've seen, burns calories whenever you're doing it, and that's why you need Fat-Burner Switch #4. But beyond aerobics, when you develop and maintain lean muscle mass through resistance exercise, the new active muscle fibers consume calories 24 hours a day, just to maintain themselves.

Doctors have compared the effectiveness of aerobics in building lean muscle mass with that of resistance training and concluded that you're best off with both. To make a comparison of the two, an eight-week study of 72 men and women was conducted by Wayne L. Westcott, Ph.D., consultant to the National YMCA, the American Council on Exercise and the National Academy of Sports Medicine. In the study, Dr. Westcott had one group that did only aerobics for eight weeks. In that group, people lost an average of 3 pounds of fat and ½ pound of muscle. A second group combined brief strength-training sessions and aerobics. They lost an average of 10 pounds of fat and gained 2 pounds of muscle! Several follow-up studies reported similar results.

Muscle-strengthening exercises are just as vital for women as they are for men, says Barbara Drinkwater, Ph.D., past president of the American College of Sports Medicine. "It's healthy that women are now accepting muscles as part of a normal human body."

Strength training confers other benefits on women, too, according to a study published in the *Archives of Internal Medicine*. Researchers reported that strength-training exercises for premenopausal women were associated with decreases in levels of "bad" LDL cholesterol.

Overcoming Resistance

The basic principles of strength training are simple: If you stress your muscles by making them work against resistance, they'll get stronger to meet the challenge. Because muscles respond immediately to the resistance they're facing, toning begins at once and continues as long as you continue training. So each of us has the lifelong capacity to develop more strength and tone with resistance training.

I want to emphasize again—since it's such a common misperception—that strength training doesn't mean that you'll develop huge muscles. And it doesn't mean that you have to spend dozens of hours in the gym on the weight machines. You can begin with whatever types of strengthening exercises interest you. Then, once you've selected some basic exercises, listen to your body, maintain good posture and begin with light resistance and smooth, well-controlled movements. You'll quickly feel and see the results.

All the muscle-toning exercises in this chapter will help turn on Fat-Burner Switch #7. Of course, if you do a complete routine that includes the various exercises with the recommended number of repetitions, you'll maximize the efficiency and effectiveness of this program. For that reason, I've summarized a comprehensive program, with my recommendations, in "A Sample Weekly Fast-Firm-Up Schedule" on page 179.

But remember, any of these exercises, in any combination or amount, will help tone your muscles and burn excess calories. Each of them is based on the fundamentals. All that's required for some are a pair of hand weights or ankle weights and a chair—and some require no props at all. There's no need for special exercise clothes. No requirement to go to a fitness club or gym. No call for expensive equipment. If they're done in sequence, you'll be working nearly all the important muscle groups in your body.

Getting started is simple. You don't need a long warm-up, though you might want to take a five-minute walk beforehand. Best of all, you can begin in the privacy of your own living room, den or office. Simply select whatever body area you want, first and foremost, to shape and strengthen. Here are the parts I'll be covering in the sections ahead.

- Abdomen
- Lower back
- Chest, shoulders and upper back
- Upper arms
- Thighs and buttocks
- Lower legs

Your Rule Model

If you haven't done muscle-toning exercises before, it's easy to get into the swing of the routines. But there are some general rules that it's helpful to know beforehand. These are important to help prevent injury and to get the maximum muscle-toning, fat-burning benefit out of each routine.

1. Precede every strength-building session with some smooth, comfortable warming-up motions to increase blood flow and loosen up your muscles and joints.

2. If you're using weights, you should know your one-repetition maximum (1RM) for each exercise and use weights that are 80 percent of that. One RM is the most weight you can lift with a single movement or muscle contraction. It's a weight so heavy that you cannot lift it again without resting for a while.

The amount of this weight varies from person to person, and it also varies as you become accustomed to the exercises. Once you know your 1RM, be sure to keep checking it every two to four weeks.

Experts recommend that you choose a resistance level that is 80 percent of your 1RM in order to build strength without injury or muscle strain. When you check your 1RM after two to four weeks and find that it's higher, be sure to recalculate the 80 percent level, so you can make upward adjustments in the weight you're using.

3. Listen to your body. If you feel any pain during a particular movement, stop immediately. Continue if the pain subsides, but only after reducing the amount of weight you're lifting.

You may have a mild burning sensation while you're exercising, and slight soreness the next day is common when beginning to exercise. But if you feel actual pain, or if the discomfort continues in any area, you should consult your doctor before continuing.

4. During each strengthening exercise, use good posture and smooth, controlled movements, and keep your breathing as even and steady as possible.

To maintain balanced posture throughout every movement, don't arch your back or use any twisting or turning motions that are not part of the exercise.

Smooth movements are essential. Each exercise has a concentric (lifting) portion and an eccentric (return) portion.

"Without the eccentric component in an exercise, you don't get much muscle growth," says Maria Fiatarone, M.D., professor of medicine at Harvard Medical School. Other experts concur. "Slow, controlled movement is the best for building muscle and for burning fat," says Dr. Westcott. Therefore, be sure to go through each exercise slowly and smoothly from start to finish. This also helps prevent injuries.

Never hold your breath while exercising, since that could cause an unhealthy rise in blood pressure.

5. Once you've worked up to it, go through two sets of five to ten repetitions (a repetition, or rep, is the complete motion of an exercise) of each exercise. The exercises take a total of about five minutes for each body part.

For example, using 80 percent of your 1RM resistance level for a given exercise, go through a first set of five to ten reps. It may be helpful to rest a few seconds between repetitions.

When you're using weights, you'll know the resistance level is correct when, after five to ten reps, your muscles are too tired to continue without resting. At the end of the first set, rest for a full minute or two to let your muscles recover. Then go through a second set of five to ten reps and rest again. And then, if you have the ability, the desire and an extra few minutes, add a third set.

6. Cool down for at least several minutes after the exercise session. Don't stop suddenly or sit still after exercising. Keep moving as you ease back into your normal routine and let your heart rate and blood flow return gradually to their pre-exercise levels.

Ab Solutions: How to Flatten Your Stomach

Okay, let's get to the waistline first.

Without a doubt, a slim, toned abdomen is the most sought-after symbol of low-fat living success. When the abdominal muscles are strong and balanced, they flatten your waist and help hold your internal organs in place.

But you might not realize how much good it does your back to have well-toned abdominal muscles, or abs, as they're more often called. Strengthening the abs helps the back at a

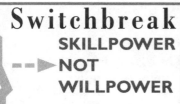

Switchbreak
SKILLPOWER
--->NOT
WILLPOWER

You can start toning your midsection before every meal, and it's literally as easy as breathing if you use the following technique.

The abdominal vacuum exercise is a simple breathing technique that has been used for years by fitness experts to firm and slenderize their midsections. Try it right now.

1. Breathe in and out normally a few times. Then, on the final breath, force every last ounce of air from your lungs.

2. With that final exhalation, allow your lower abdomen to come in and up as much as possible.

3. Hold that forced-exhalation position for about five seconds, then inhale.

4. Repeat once or twice more.

There are two key muscles in your lower abdomen: the transversalis and pyrimidalis. These move in and up when you exhale forcibly.

Do a few of these exercises before every meal, and you'll begin to feel those muscles gathering strength and control as you continue to tone them. It won't happen all at once, but as you get in the habit of doing this exercise, the two muscles will "wake up" and start working again.

strategic point—the lumbosacral angle of the pelvis. Lower back pain often gets started or aggravated in this area, so the firming exercises that help burn calories may also help prevent future back trouble.

What's the best way to flatten your stomach? I'm sure many people think of traditional sit-ups and leg-lifts, which are still America's two most popular abdominal exercises. Well, the problem is that they don't slim the waistline, no matter how many times you do them. That's right: You could do 5,000 a month without making a whit of difference in your waistline.

In fact, these traditional favorites often cause or aggravate lower back pain by pulling on the front of the lower spine, which causes pelvic tilt. When this happens, your back is swayed inward and your lower abdomen pushes out. The posture you end up with only spotlights a potbelly appearance.

In a way, it's good news that sit-ups and leg-lifts aren't effective when it comes to tightening your waistline and toning your abs. That means you don't have to do them!

The following abdominal exercises, along with the abdominal vacuum technique described in the Switchbreak, are the ones I've found to be most effective. And as you'll see, a number of them can be done with variations. Whether you do all of them every day or repeat just a few is entirely your choice. But I recommend that you try each of them at first to find out which ones you prefer and to get a feel for the ones that seem to benefit you the most.

Transpyramid Breathing Exercise

This exercise, a more complete version of the abdominal vaccuum technique, will help you build a toned, fit lower abdomen. It's called the transpyramid breathing exercise because of the two muscles it targets—the transversalis and pyramidalis. Sometimes called voluntary contractions by exercise experts, these are "the most important exercises to flatten your abdomen," according to Lawrence E. Lamb, M.D., medical consultant to the President's Council on Physical Fitness and Sports and author of *Stay Youthful and Fit* and *The Weighting Game: The Truth about Weight Control*.

1. Lie on your back with your shoulders relaxed and your knees bent just enough that your feet rest comfortably on the floor. Place your hands on each side of your hips, with your fingers spread across your abdomen. The index finger of each hand should point to your belly button, but without touching it.

2. Take a deep breath and then exhale. As you breathe out, notice which way your lower abdomen moves. At the end of the exhalation you should feel your lower abdomen moving inward, toward your spine. This motion tells you that the transversalis and pyramidalis muscles of the lower abdomen are getting their workout.

3. Now inhale. Notice how your belly tends to "pop" outward against your fingers.

4. When you repeat, exaggerate to make a very clear distinction between these two motions—pulling your abdomen in

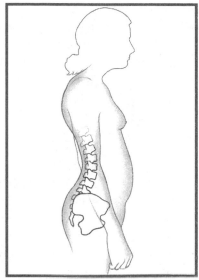

When you do sit-ups and leg-lifts, the abdominal muscles may pull on the front of the lower spine, pushing out the lower abdomen.

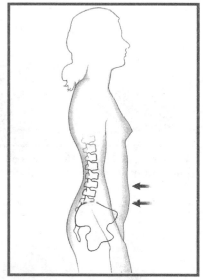

By doing the exercises in this chapter, you'll pull in your abdomen, flattening your belly.

and up during the exhalation, then popping your abdomen outward on the inhalation. (For muscle-toning, the key half of the movement is the exhalation phase.)

5. At the end of each exhalation, tighten the lower abdominal muscles to press that area inward even more. Then, on the next inhalation, consciously release the abdomen out against your fingers.

It's a good idea to learn this movement while lying on the floor in a comfortable position. Once you've got the exercise motion mastered, however, you can do it sitting or standing.

Variation: When you're seated and doing this exercise, you should be in an upright, straight-backed chair. Slowly exhale, and as you reach the place where you normally finish breathing out, smoothly and forcefully breathe out more, using the power of your lower abdominal muscles. At first you might use your hands to gently push up on the lower abdomen during the exhalation part of the exercise.

Repetitions: Work up to doing ten repetitions of this exercise each day. But they don't have to be done all at once. Fit them in wherever you can—one or two in bed before rising in the morning, several right before each meal or even at traffic lights when you're running errands or driving home from work. Since they can also be done while standing, you can pause for an exercise break as you're stepping up to the kitchen counter or just before you sit down at your desk.

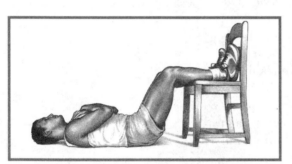

At the start of the abdominal roll-up, your upper body should be relaxed, with your arms crossed on your chest.

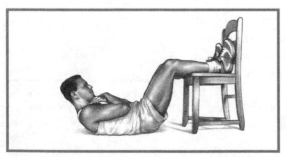

As you lift your head and shoulders, you'll feel the pull on your abdominal muscles.

Abdominal Roll-Ups

Also called crunches or curls, abdominal roll-ups are among the easiest and most effective exercises for toning your upper abdominal area. Here's how they're done.

1. Lie on your back with

your knees bent, your calves resting comfortably on the seat of a chair and your feet free, as shown. (If you find that the chair seat isn't a comfortable height for supporting your lower legs, you can just bend your knees a little and place your feet flat on the floor.) Cross your arms on your chest.

2. With your middle and lower back still flat, slowly raise your head and shoulders off the floor about 30 to 45 degrees. During this movement, keep your lower abdomen flat. Make sure it doesn't pouch out during the upward movement.

3. Pause for a second at the top of the motion and then slowly lower yourself to the starting position.

When you're doing this exercise, make sure your legs and feet stay free. You might be tempted to secure your feet or legs under the edge of a sofa, but I strongly advise against it. If your feet are held down, you're not doing the abdominal muscles much good. Instead, the hip flexor muscles take over the movement, and that can seriously stress your lower back.

Also be sure to keep your arms crossed in the position shown when you lift yourself. If they whip upward, the sudden motion may cause injury to the neck.

Repetitions: When you begin doing abdominal roll-ups, start very gradually. Do just a few repetitions, then take a break and see how you feel. As long as there's no serious discomfort or pain, over a period of weeks you can work your way up to 25 or more repetitions.

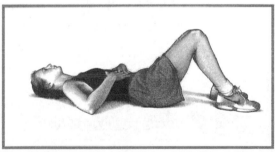

To get into position for the exhalation roll-up, lie on your back in a relaxed position, breathing normally.

Exhalation Roll-Ups

This exercise combines the abdominal roll-up and the transpyramid breathing exercise in a single abdominal-strengthening move. Have a look at the illustrations and then follow these guidelines.

1. Lie on your back with your knees bent and your feet

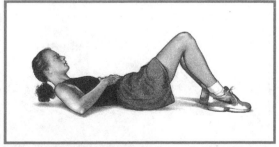

When you exhale and lift your neck and shoulders, the tension puts pressure on the abdominal muscles.

flat on the floor. Your fingers should be on your lower abdomen with your index fingers pointing toward your belly button.

2. Do a roll-up exercise as shown, lifting only your shoulders and upper back from the floor.

3. At the top of the motion, gently force out an exhalation.

4. Pause for a two-second count before slowly returning to the starting position.

Repetitions: Work up to five or six repetitions.

Twisting Exhalation Roll-Ups

This exercise and the next one—reverse trunk rotations—are great firm-ups for the sides of the waistline. Here's how to do twisting exhalation roll-ups.

1. Lie on your back with your knees bent and your feet on the floor, with your head gently cradled in your hands.

2. Now imagine your abdomen "sinking" into your lower back. Try to hold on to this feeling throughout the roll-up.

3. Begin with a regular abdominal roll-up, but as you bring your head and shoulders off the floor, make sure the lower part of your shoulder blades remains in contact with the floor.

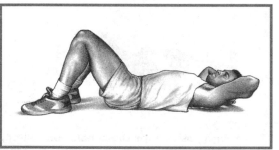

For the twisting exhalation roll-up, begin in position for the transpyramid exercise.

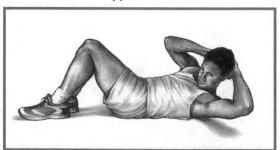

Raise one elbow and bring it toward the opposite knee—exhaling and relaxing your back muscles.

4. Go through a transpyramid exercise, exhaling to flex your abdominal muscles as you slowly bring one elbow and shoulder toward the opposite knee, as shown. While you're doing this, keep your elbow and back relaxed to ensure that the twist is gentle and comes from your waist, not your arm or neck.

5. Return to the starting position.

6. Repeat, bringing the other elbow and shoulder toward the opposite knee and turning your rib cage in the same direction.

Repetitions: Work up to

doing five left and five right repetitions. But even when you add more repetitions, make sure the motions are always slow and steady.

Reverse Trunk Rotations

Here's another proven exercise for abdominal fitness and good posture. This movement involves the external and internal obliques, a set of midsection rotation muscles that help keep your abdomen slim and toned.

When you do reverse trunk rotations, you'll also strengthen the deep spinal muscles (multifidus and rotatores), the posterior spinal surface muscles (erector spinae) and an important lower back muscle, the quadratus lumborum. The full range of motion of this exercise builds both flexibility and strength in the waist and lower back, an ideal combination for helping to prevent injuries and back pain.

1. Lie on your back with your arms extended to the sides, as shown. Your arms should be perpendicular to your torso so that if viewed from above, your body forms the letter T.

2. Bend your knees at a sharp angle, pulling your heels toward your buttocks with your knees together.

3. Maintaining the same angle at your knees, slowly lower your legs to one side until the outside of your lower leg lies flat on the floor.

4. Smoothly raise your legs to the starting position. Your arms and shoulders should remain in contact with the floor throughout the exercise to stretch and strengthen the internal and external obliques.

5. Repeat the movement, lowering your legs to the other side.

Variations: If your shoul-

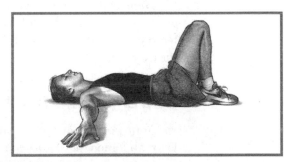

When you first try reverse trunk rotations, your heels should be as close to your buttocks as possible.

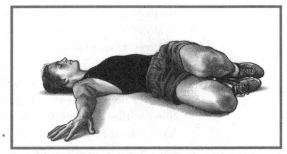

For the most benefit, try to maintain the same knee angle as you lower your knees to the floor.

ders come off the floor as you lower your legs to the side, you may wish to have a friend gently hold them down as you do the exercise. If you still find the exercise difficult, use less knee bend. Or you might begin by having a partner support your knees as you gently lower them. With your partner helping, test both sides to assess your current strength and flexibility levels.

One rehabilitative medicine authority suggests another slight variation that could also make this exercise easier. As you gently lower your legs toward the floor, let your knees come up toward your shoulders, suggests Rene Cailliet, M.D., chairman of the Department of Rehabilitative Medicine at the University of Southern California School of Medicine in Los Angeles.

As you get in great shape, you can pull in your heels more and more to raise your knees higher. The exercise becomes more difficult as your knees go higher, approaching a 90-degree angle to the floor.

Repetitions: Begin with very few repetitions and then gradually, over a period of weeks, work your way up to six to ten reps. Over time, gradually bend your knees more as you do the exercise.

Lower Back Muscle-Toning

Your posture and back strength can influence how much your abdomen protrudes and also whether or not you can safely, enjoyably perform other exercises without injury or tension-related fatigue. Here are several simple exercises, each recommended by at least one medical specialist on back care, that can gently stretch and strengthen your back. If possible, perform these exercises on the days when you also do abdominal-toning exercises.

A word of caution: It's best to do lower back muscle-toning only after you've warmed up with a brief walk or another form of low-intensity aerobics from Fat-Burner Switch #4. Start with only one or two repetitions of each exercise. If you have a history of back problems or are currently experiencing back pain, consult your physician before doing these or any other exercises.

Single Knee-to-Chest Lifts

This easy-does-it exercise helps stretch the muscles and connective tissues of your back and hips.

1. Lie on your back with both knees bent and your feet flat on the floor.

2. Lift one leg and raise the knee until you can grasp your thigh just below the knee with both hands.

3. Gently pull your knee toward your chest for a slow count of five. Relax.

4. Release your leg and slowly return it to the starting position.

5. Repeat with the other leg.

Repetitions: Six to ten with each leg.

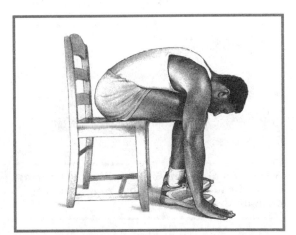

When you do knee-to-chest lifts, you should feel the stretch along your back and hip.

Seated Lower Back Stretches

The advantage of these stretches is that you can do them almost anywhere—at home, in the office or even while you're waiting somewhere. Just don't try to do them too fast, wherever you are, since they really do stretch the lower back muscles to the max, and sudden movements can pull or strain those muscles.

1. Sit in a firm-seated chair with your feet flat on the floor and your knees apart.

2. Slowly and gently bend forward, reaching down to place the palms of your hands on the floor.

3. Hold the down position for a five-second count.

Repetitions: Six to ten.

If you can't reach the floor with the palms of your hands, just stretch as far as you can—but don't bounce.

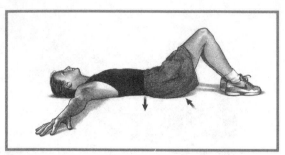

By pressing the small of your back to the floor, you shift the position of your pelvis, which helps to align your back.

Pelvic Tilt Movements

This simple, relaxing exercise helps strengthen some of the front spine structures and stretch the back.

1. Lie on your back with your arms extended to the sides, your knees bent and your feet flat on the floor, as shown.

2. Gently press your lower back flat against the floor.

3. Hold for a few seconds. *Repetitions:* Six to ten.

Chest, Shoulder and Upper Back Muscle-Toning

The muscles in your upper back and shoulder area are so closely interconnected that it makes sense to work all of them in the same session. Three specific exercises—modified push-ups, chest and shoulder raises and chest crosses—are targeted to help strengthen and tone all the muscle groups. For best results, when you do one exercise for this area of your body, do them all.

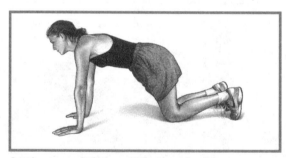

At the top of the modified push-up, your arms should be fully extended, but your knees remain on the floor.

Modified Push-Ups

This revision of a classic exercise strengthens muscles in your arms, chest, shoulders and back. Even if you can't lift your knees off the floor at first, you may be able to work up to regular push-ups gradually.

1. Lie facedown on the floor with your knees together.

2. Place the palms of your

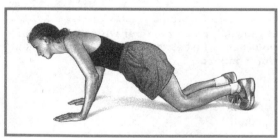

Lower your upper body slowly, feeling the stretch in your shoulders and upper back.

hands flat on the floor on either side of your chest, near the fronts of your shoulders.

3. Support the weight of your upper body on your arms and keep your knees in contact with the floor as you slowly raise your body. During this movement, keep your back as flat as you can.

4. Smoothly return to the starting position.

Variations: To increase the strengthening effect on your upper arms and back, move your hands directly underneath your shoulders for the push-ups. If you want to increase the strengthening effect on your chest, move your hands slightly outward so that they're positioned just a little wider than your shoulders.

Repetitions: 6 to 25.

Chest and Shoulder Raises

For these exercises you'll need a small handheld weight. Adjustable dumbbells come with small round plates that are weighted in two-, five- and ten-pound increments. But if you don't have dumbbells, you can start out by lifting a book instead. Another alternative is to pour water into a plastic milk

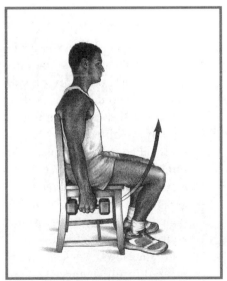

As you begin chest and shoulder raises, your arm should be relaxed and hanging straight at your side.

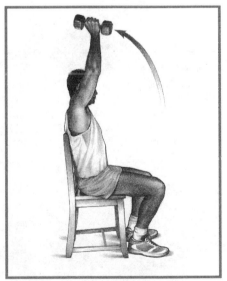

Keep your arm fully extended as you slowly lift the weight, using the muscles in your shoulder and upper arm.

or juice container that has a sturdy handle. Fill the container until it's the correct weight, then securely fasten the lid.

1. Sit upright in a chair with one arm at your side and the weight in your hand.

2. Keeping your elbow straight, slowly raise your arm forward and up.

3. Pause when your arm is fully extended almost above your head, but not quite perpendicular.

4. Slowly return to the starting position.

5. After you finish the repetitions on one side, do the same number with the weight in the other hand.

Repetitions: Six to ten. If you can't perform six correct repetitions without getting too tired to lift the weight, then it's too heavy and you should reduce it. If you can easily perform ten repetitions or more, however, you should gradually increase the weight.

Chest Crosses

Here's another exercise with weights that will give the muscles of the front part of your chest and shoulders an excellent workout. You can use a pair of equally weighted books or partially filled milk or juice containers if you don't have regulation adjustable weights.

1. Lie on your back on the floor with your knees bent and your feet in a comfortable position. Your lower back should be pressed firmly against the floor. Hold a weight in each hand as shown, with your elbows bent at 90-degree angles.

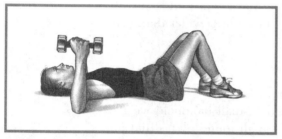

At the start of the chest cross, your forearms should be straight up and down, perpendicular to the floor.

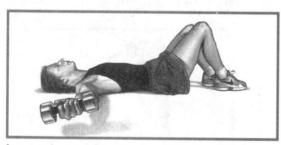

Lower the weights slowly to the floor, keeping the tension in your chest and shoulders.

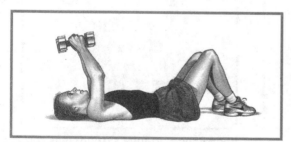

Lift your arms very slowly as you raise the weights, maintaining tension on your shoulder and chest muscles.

2. Extend your arms straight out, level with your shoulders, holding the weights in your hands with the palms up.

3. Keeping your elbows slightly bent, raise your arms very slowly and move them in an arc toward each other until the weights gently touch above the center of your chest.

4. Slowly move the weights apart and reverse the motion to bring them to the starting position.

Repetitions: Six to ten.

Upper Arm Muscle-Toning

The two toning exercises included here will help you work on both the front and back of your upper arm. For both you'll need weighted objects or dumbbells. The arm curls, however, can also be done with stretchy resistance cables, available in many sporting goods stores. As in other exercises that require weights, you'll need to experiment to find your ideal starting weight, then adjust upward as you get more proficient.

Arm Curls

This is a popular, easy exercise to strengthen the biceps muscle in the front of your upper arm and to help tone your forearms.

1. Sit on an armless chair or a bench.

2. Holding a weight in one hand, bring your forearm straight up toward your shoulder, keeping your elbow bent. At the finish of the motion, your palm should be facing your shoulder, as shown on page 174.

3. Slowly return to the starting position.

4. After finishing the repetitions on one side, move the weight to the other hand and do an equal number of repetitions.

Variations: In this exercise you can either lift both arms at once or alternate left and right. And you can vary the exercise by doing it with your palms down.

There's also an isometric variation, which means pushing against an immovable object instead of lifting weights. The variation, which is easy to do at your desk, is recommended by Dr. Stamford. Sitting in a normal position, just push up against the underside or lip of the desk and exert pressure for six sec-

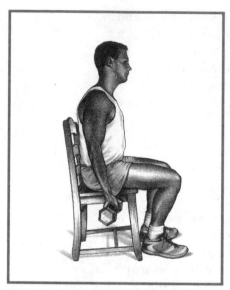

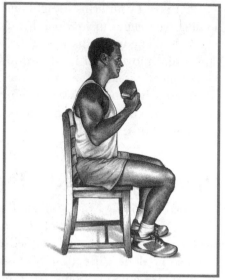

At the start of an arm curl, your arm should be relaxed at your side.

You should feel the tension in your bicep as you bring the weight up to your shoulder.

onds. Repeated five to ten times, this isometric arm curl will aid muscle tone, according to Dr. Stamford.

Repetitions: 6 to 25.

Back-of-the-Upper-Arm Extensions

This basic exercise will help tone the triceps muscles at the backs of your upper arms. You'll need a chair or bench to support your free hand when you lean forward.

1. Stand to the left of the support with your right foot slightly forward and your left foot back. Grasp a weight in your left hand and bend forward at the hips, placing your right hand on the support. Your torso should be almost parallel to the floor, with your back as straight as possible, as shown.

2. Raise your left arm—the one holding the weight—until your upper arm is in line with your torso, with your elbow bent and your forearm hanging straight down. Your arm should be bent at nearly a 90-degree angle at the elbow and pressed lightly against your torso when it's in the correct lift position.

3. Slowly straighten your arm, lifting the weight backward until it's slightly above the level of your buttocks.

4. Slowly return to the starting position.

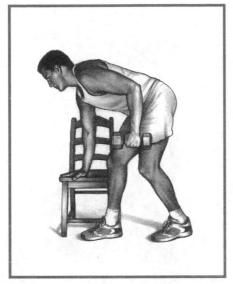

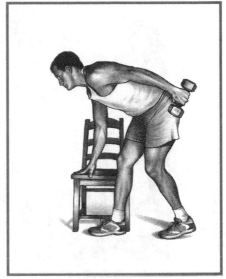

At the start of the extension, your upper arm should be close to your torso and your lower arm hanging straight down.

When you straighten your arm and raise it toward the horizontal, you'll feel the pull in your triceps muscle.

5. Turn around, put the weight in your right hand, place your left hand on the support and repeat the exercise with your right arm.

Repetitions: Alternate left and right, doing six to ten reps with each arm.

Thigh and Buttock Muscle-Toning

You can select any two or three of the following exercises, depending on how much time you have. Just be sure that whichever ones you choose, you go through each exercise correctly, without rushing. As you do these exercises, you'll feel the tension in the area that's getting the workout. You can select the exercises that best target your personal muscle-toning needs.

Modified Knee Bends

This is a great do-it-anywhere leg-strengthening exercise. Although your thighs and buttocks get the biggest benefit, other leg muscles get a workout, too. For best results, you'll

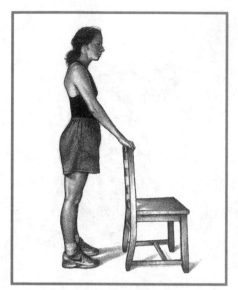

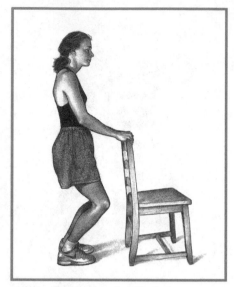

Make sure you're standing erect—not leaning against the chair for support—when you begin to do modified knee bends.

As you bend your knees, keep your body aligned with your heels and your back as vertical as possible.

need to grasp the back of a stable chair, desk or counter for support, as shown.

1. Begin in a standing position, with your feet flat on the floor and shoulder-width apart.

2. Holding on to the support, slowly bend your knees and lower your body until your thighs are almost parallel to the floor. You should feel as if you were sitting in a chair.

3. Return to the starting position.

4. End the movement by raising your heels off the floor so that you're balanced on the balls of your feet.

Repetitions: 6 to 25.

Seated Leg Extensions

For this exercise, you'll need a set of ankle weights, which are available in most sporting goods stores. Select a pair that is comfortably padded and easy to adjust to fit the diameter of your lower leg just above the ankle. Adjustable weights use small rectangular sacks of sand that slide into side compartments to increase the weight in ½- or 1-pound increments. If you have strong legs, you may want to use two ankle weights on each leg.

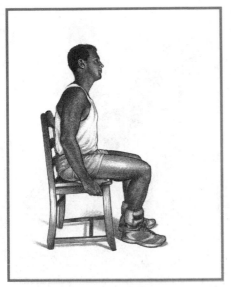

Leg extensions can be done from a seated position on a chair or a bench.

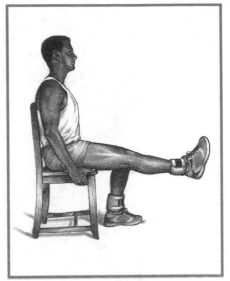

You'll feel the tension all along the top of your thigh as you move your leg forward to a horizontal position.

1. Put on the weights and sit on a chair or bench with your back straight and your feet firmly on the floor. Grasp the sides of the seat with your hands.

2. Raise one knee slightly to lift your foot off the floor. Raise and extend the lower part of your leg, straightening it until the entire leg is parallel to the floor. Hold for a count of 4 or 5.

3. Hold the tension in your leg muscles as you slowly return the leg to the starting position.

4. Do one set of repetitions with one leg, then an equal number with the other.

Repetitions: 6 to 25.

Standing Side Leg Raises

You'll need some support when you do these leg raises. You can use a door frame or put your hand on a desk or tabletop for support. As your legs get stronger, you may use adjustable ankle weights. You can gradually increase the poundage on your ankle weights as your thighs get stronger.

1. Holding on to the support with one hand, raise the opposite foot off the floor and out to the side until you feel tension along the outer muscles of your thigh.

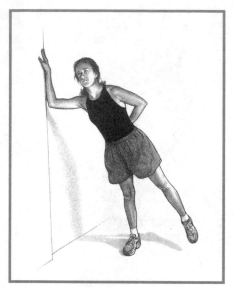

When you're in position for the standing side leg raises, your upraised leg is straight and lifted off the floor.

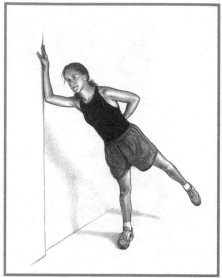

Lean forward against the support as you bring your leg farther up and out to the side, putting tension on the thigh.

2. Hold this position for several seconds.

3. Slowly lower your leg a foot or so, but don't touch the floor.

4. Repeat the lifting movement.

5. After you complete a set of repetitions with one leg, switch positions and do an equal number of repetitions with the other leg.

Repetitions: 6 to 25.

Hip Raises

This simple, effective exercise uses body weight and voluntary contractions to help tone the buttocks area. No weights are needed.

1. Lie on your back with your arms extended directly out from your shoulders and your palms flat on the floor. Bend your knees and place both feet flat on the floor. Your knees and feet should be slightly apart.

2. Slowly raise your hips and upper back while keeping your head, shoulders, hands, arms and feet on the floor.

A Sample Weekly Fast-Firm-Up Schedule

As you look over the muscle-toning exercises in this chapter, you may be wondering how you can fit them all in. The schedule is likely to be different for each individual, but here's a sample schedule that you can follow to maximize your muscle-toning exercises.

Every Day
One Do-It-Anywhere Abdominal-Toning Set
- Transpyramid breathing exercise: 10 repetitions

Monday, Wednesday, Friday
Back-Strengthening Set
- Modified push-ups: 6 to 25 repetitions
- Chest and shoulder raises: 6 to 10 repetitions
- Chest crosses: 6 to 10 repetitions

Upper Arm-Strengthening Set
- Arm curls: 6 to 25 repetitions
- Back-of-the-upper-arm extensions: 6 to 10 repetitions
with each arm

Tuesday, Thursday, Saturday
Complete Abdominal-Toning Set
- Abdominal roll-ups: 25 repetitions
- Exhalation roll-ups: 5 or 6 repetitions
- Twisting exhalation roll-ups: 5 repetitions to each side
- Reverse trunk rotations: 6 to 10 repetitions

Lower Back-Toning Set
- Single knee-to-chest lifts: 6 to 10 repetitions
- Seated lower back stretches: 6 to 10 repetitions
- Pelvic tilt movements: 6 to 10 repetitions

Thigh-Buttocks-Strengthening Set
- Modified knee bends: 6 to 25 repetitions
- Seated leg extensions: 6 to 25 repetitions with each leg
- Standing side leg raises: 6 to 25 repetitions
- Hip raises: 6 to 10 repetitions

Lower Leg Muscle-Toning
- Standing calf raises: 10 to 50 repetitions

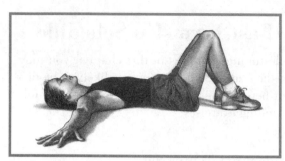

At the start of the hip raise, your torso should be relaxed and flat on the floor.

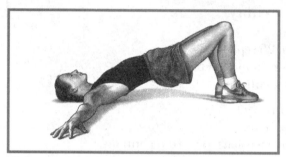

Tighten your buttocks to lift your hips all the way off the floor.

3. Arch your lower back slightly and tense your buttocks. Hold for a few seconds.

4. Slowly return to the starting position.

Repetitions: Six to ten.

Lower Leg Muscle-Toning

You can easily tone the muscles in your lower legs with a single exercise—standing calf raises. These are done without weights, but you will need a piece of wood such as a 2 × 6 board (or a 2 × 8) to support the balls of your feet, plus a pair of straight-backed chairs for support.

Standing Calf Raises

To position yourself for this exercise, place the chairs so that you can hold the backs comfortably with your arms outstretched. Stand between the chairs and hold on to the backs. Step up on the board so that your toes and the balls of your feet are positioned as shown, with your toes pointed straight ahead. Your heels should be parallel to the top of the board, so your entire foot is poised above the floor. Keep your back perfectly straight, but bend your knees very slightly.

1. Lower your heels as far below the level of your toes as is comfortable. Your heels don't have to touch the floor, but you should feel the stretch all along the backs of your calf muscles. Make sure your heels don't roll outward.

2. Slowly rise as high as you can on the balls of your feet until your heels are elevated well above the level of the board.

3. Ease down to the starting position, with your heels lowered as close to the floor as possible.

Variations: For a more advanced version of this exercise, try doing the calf raises with one leg at a time instead of together.

To tone additional lower leg muscles, you might proceed as noted above, but keep your knees straight rather than slightly bent. That will stretch a different group of muscles. (Keep up the repetitions until your calf area feels too tired to continue.)

You can also alter the exercise by bending your knees during the downward motion, when you lower your heels below the level of the board. Then straighten your legs during the upward motion.

Repetitions: 10 to 50.

Max Out the Toning in Your Chores

Even on days when you have no special time to de-

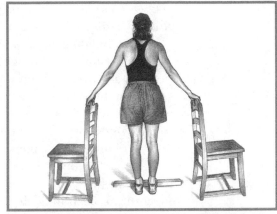

To begin calf raises, lower your heels below toe-level. Your back should be straight, your knees slightly bent and your toes pointing straight ahead.

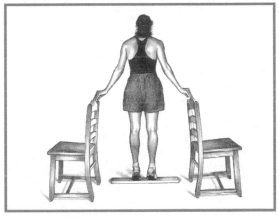

As you raise yourself on the balls of your feet, you'll feel the tension in your calf muscles.

vote to muscle-toning, you can keep in better shape by balancing out the chores you do. You can safely, gradually build more strength while pushing, pulling, turning, lifting and bending during everyday activities. During these chores, try to switch sides to balance your actions. If you're carrying a briefcase or groceries, for example, switch the load from side to side. Or if you're carrying a young child, alternate holding her in your left and right arms. Change your weight-bearing leg from time to time as you work at a counter.

Other activities that can help tone your muscles are weeding the lawn, digging in the garden and shoveling snow.

In short, building and maintaining muscle tone is an integral part of a total fitness program. The benefits go far beyond having a more attractive physique. With healthy, strong muscles, your body is more vigorous, better balanced and better coordinated. And research shows you'll help slow or even reverse the aging process by maintaining muscle tone.

If you're among the thousands of Americans who are already eating a healthy, low-fat diet and doing daily aerobic exercise but are still having a difficult time losing weight, getting stronger means healthfully increasing your metabolism to burn off more excess body fat 24 hours a day, even while sleeping!

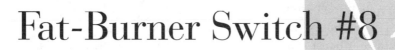

Chapter Eleven

Fat-Burner Switch #8

Catch a Late-Day Second Wind

It's late afternoon. Your mental and physical energy levels have been holding relatively steady—thanks, at least in part, to an afternoon mini-walk and some well-toned muscles. You've had at least one fat-fighting snack since lunchtime.

But as the afternoon wanes, you find that your energy is beginning to flag. Maybe you start to think about an energy recharge. Another snack—one that isn't part of the Low-Fat Living Program? A sweet carbonated drink, perhaps? A cup of coffee for a jolt of caffeine?

Well, hold on. There's actually a name for this mid- to late-afternoon period of tension and tiredness. Chronobiologists call it the breaking point. And there are many almost-effortless ways to fight it and win.

Slump Evasion

The curious thing about this classic afternoon slump is that it can hit you no matter what you're doing. If you're in the office, nearing the end of the day, you might feel the slump just as you're about to leave for home. If you've been running errands or taxiing kids all afternoon, your energy may go "poof" just as you're pulling into the driveway for the last time—facing meal preparations or yet more phone calls before the sun sets. Or if you've worked all day at home, that late-afternoon fogginess may feel like it's moving in.

As you switch on the answering machine, turn off the computer or put away the tools of your trade or the housekeeping items, you may wonder—with a feeling of exhaustion—how you'll ever make it through the next few hours.

Your body's inherent and ancient metabolic patterns go into a wavelike downturn sometime between 3:30 and 5:30 P.M. This common drop-off in alertness and fat-burning power sets up a high-stress fat-forming and fat-storing period that may last all night.

So here's the challenge: to give your energy and metabolism a boost that will help reduce or even reverse this downturn. What you need is a second wind.

Putting Second Wind in Your Sails

Part of the challenge is to make a transition from work time to family time. And the pace of work, for most people, is much different from the pace at home. In addition, your day job may be much more intense than your evening activities.

Many of us have trouble with that transition. Arriving home fatigued and distracted, we may spend much of our evenings on "autopilot." In that mode we go through the motions to care for family members while we're magnetically drawn to eating large, high-fat dinners. Many of us skip exercise at the very time of day that the body needs an energizing, fat-burning boost to keep from packing on the pounds.

Fortunately, your evening doesn't have to be a time of big-meal consumption and end-of-day lethargy. By making some small adjustments in your job routine before you leave for home, followed by some simple tactics when you get there, you can completely avoid the slump and make a smoother transition that will turn on Fat-Burner Switch #8.

Here are several of the simplest, most practical ways I've found to turn things around and catch a late-day second wind.

Smooth Your Transition to Home Life

If you have an office job, it makes sense to arrange your final work minutes so that you reduce the pressure before heading out the door. You need a brief decompression period, so the end of your working day is devoted to your least-taxing tasks. Here are some ideas.

Call only the upbeats. Though you might have quite a few phone messages to return, be selective. Pick through your messages and find someone who's generally supportive, positive and upbeat. You get the chance to end the day with a laugh and a dose of camaraderie—to give and receive a pat on the back.

Clean up tomorrow's welcome mat. Before you go, have a look at your desk. Is this what you want to face bright and early tomorrow morning? Take a minute to rinse out your coffee cup. Throw away the banana peel. Sweep the rye-cracker crumbs off your desk. And while you organize messages and papers, jot down your priority list for tomorrow morning, so all those things are lined up and not swirling around in the "things-to-do" lobe of your brain all evening.

Shake a limb. Why do so many people finish the workday slumped over, then creak to their feet, sigh and head for home? There's no law that says you have to end the day that way. Instead, stretch your muscles a few moments to stretch your mind. Gentle physical movements bring increased blood flow throughout your body and help disentangle you from the thorniest work.

Pause to ask yourself where you are feeling tightness or tension. Then loosen these areas by doing the following exercises smoothly, slowly and with relaxed motions.

Neck rotations. Sitting in a relaxed position, gently and slowly bring your chin forward toward your chest, then gradually rotate your head to the right, back and left, returning to the starting position in a smooth, nonstraining, continuous movement.

Shoulder shrugs. Lift both shoulders simultaneously,

shrugging them as high as possible, then let them relax completely. You'll automatically breathe in on the upward motion and release a nice comfortable breath when you relax.

Torso turns. Stand, raise both elbows as if you were resting them on a chest-high wall, then pivot your upper body slowly to one side. Then pivot in the opposite direction, turning with a smooth, continuous motion. Don't bounce or strain.

Wrist circles. Raise your forearms and keep them steady as you circle your hands around and around from the wrists, as if you were feeling the insides of hollow globes with your fingers.

Knee bends. With your hands on your hips or holding the edge of your desk for balance, slowly lower yourself to a squatting position, then rise. Try to keep your back erect as you move up and down—and don't speed up or strain.

Start fresh. When you head for home, guide your mind first, followed by your body. As you move for the door or step outside your work area, draw in a very deep, smooth breath and let it out slowly, imagining yourself at home. See the sights, hear the sounds, feel the hugs and smiles that bring up your fondest thoughts and feelings about your home life. As you feel your family's caring and comfort, begin winding down, thinking about love, laughter, great food and great sex. Leave your work worries behind. This mental release can be so powerful that in a matter of moments it helps put the day to rest and draws your mind and mood toward the slower rhythms of home. The journey will feel less rushed, the arrival less hurried.

Give up and let go. Whether you are headed directly home or have kids to pick up and errands to run, use the transition period to unwind and slow your pace. We all leave behind a lot of loose ends at the end of the workday. Be confident you'll have the morning energy to wrap things up. And by making that to-do list before leaving, you won't need to worry about forgetting anything. Right now, think ahead to home, and give your mind and heart a boost.

Get a zoom with a view. Somewhere between ending your workday and arriving home, take a few extra moments to look at something beautiful—a flower, a plant, a row of trees or cloud formations in the sky. This break can be an excellent antidote to mental fatigue and promote a more positive mood, according to a study at the University of Michigan in Ann Arbor headed by Rachel Kaplan, Ph.D. Among the benefits described by Dr. Kaplan are increased energy and better health.

And don't neglect this step just because you work at home. We can all use a transition period, and if you have a home office, you need to change your mind-set at the end of the day even though you're not moving from a separate job site to your home. Take a complete break. Step outside or walk a short distance to enjoy a natural scene before you "come home from work."

Use a Time-Out to Energize Your Home Life

Today, more and more of us rush home, hurry to prepare dinner, flip through the newspaper, eat quickly and then either collapse in front of the TV or plunge into another round of scheduled activities—nightly errands, parental duties, catching up on paperwork, preparing reports or paying bills.

What's missing is a brief time-out period to shake off stress and tension and start the evening with extra energy and excitement. And the time-out is more than a luxury; it's a necessity if you want to turn on Fat-Burner #8. Here are some strategies to make it happen.

Buddy up. You and your partner deserve a few minutes of personal wind-down time. If you have children to look after, give each other a break after you greet them, so each of you can change into comfortable clothes and take a brief, relatively quiet interlude. Help put the day to rest. For you, it might be a

Switchbreak
SKILLPOWER NOT WILLPOWER

Ah, it's spring at last—which means, to millions of 9-to-5 Americans, that it's still light outdoors when they leave the office.

But what if you're working late and it's already dark outside? Or you're in the depths of a Minnesota winter and the promise of after-work daylight is still months away?

You can still get more light at the end of the day, even if it isn't 100 percent daylight.

And there's no question that you need it, researchers at Harvard Medical School have discovered. Their studies show that one of the quickest ways to give a quick boost to the brain's alertness and your overall vigor is to turn up the light.

Tomorrow, as you wrap things up at work, click on a few extra lights. If the sun's still out when you step outdoors, plan to walk around for a minute to soak up some rays.

Whether it comes from electricity or solar power, light offers an ancient and powerful way to lift your late-day energy and mood just when they are primed to fall.

hot shower or bath; for your spouse, a relaxing set of exercises. It doesn't need to be long—but make sure there's a coming-home break both of you can count on.

If you're a family with young children, this is a great time to have a high-schooler come over to babysit for an hour or so. The bit of extra help might make all the difference. It will give you some breakaway time to stroll with your partner, sit for a few minutes out on the balcony or deck, putter in the garden or give each other a back rub.

Get a few yuks in. Humor is one of the simplest and most effective ways for the human brain to switch gears and free up your attention for the evening ahead. Bring home at least one offbeat story or look for a chance to play a practical joke.

Does that seem forced? Well, force it—at first. If you can get a laugh, you're making a big difference in the tension level at home and upping your chances of a successful marriage. When psychologists looked at the role of humor in the relation-ships of 50 married couples, they found that it accounted for greater happiness among 70 percent of them. The researchers found that many of the couples who were happiest had learned skills to create and sustain light-heartedness.

In other words, you may have to dust off your ability to clown around and sharpen the way you look at everyday events, searching for the absurdity and humor that always lie just under the surface. (You don't think so? Just look at a Lau-rel and Hardy or Marx Brothers film to see how absurdity ex-plodes from high-stress situations.) Try to make yourself and others laugh—and keep moving ahead toward your goals and dreams.

Move and Munch before Dinner

It seems obvious that to increase fat-burning, you'd want to move around. But you should also have an appetizer.

But won't an appetizer make fat instead of burning it?

Actually, you're doing yourself and your metabolism a favor if you can reinvent and enjoy low-fat appetizers. Accord-ing to scientists, when you stay active in late afternoon and early evening and munch on a few bites of high-taste, low-fat food before the evening meal, chances are your energy and mood will stay higher. In the end, you'll eat less for dinner and consequently store less food as fat.

But who would have thought that you'd also feel less argumentative at the end of the day if you follow this pattern?

It's true. Evidence shows that low blood sugar levels and simple hunger-related tensions may contribute to negative emotions and late-day arguments, according to psychiatrist William Nagler, M.D., of the University of California, Los Angeles, UCLA School of Medicine and co-author of *The Dirty Half Dozen: Six Radical Rules to Make Relationships Last.* Here are some satisfying ways to still the hunger while giving you a quick surge of fat-burning energy.

Dip in to low-fat. Whole-grain rye crackers and pumpernickel bread are the staples of low-fat, low-calorie fare—but what's a cracker or bread without a spread? And here's where you can go right instead of wrong. If you have your crisps or bread with nonfat cream cheese or low-fat bean dip, you'll get great texture and good flavor all in one bite, without turning on any fat-makers. Add some high fiber vegetables such as broccoli, carrots and celery to the platter, and you get still more crunch and snap. You can even have one or two whole-grain fat-free cookies with a half-cup of skim milk or nonfat yogurt—as long as their sweetness doesn't tempt you to eat more.

Soup it up. Probably the best of all appetizers is a cup of tomato soup with several whole-grain rye crackers. According to scientists at Johns Hopkins University in Baltimore, an appetizers of soup can reduce fat cravings and total calorie intake. Not only that, but people who eat soup appetizers take in 25 percent less fat in the meal that follows than those who eat high-fat appetizers. (If you're making canned tomato soup, use the recommended low-fat formula: Make it with 1 percent low-fat or nonfat milk.)

Chuck the cheese. The quintessential appetizer, of course, is the cheese-and-crackers combo that pops up on coffee tables all across America just before dinnertime. With thin slices of low-fat cheese and whole-rye crackers instead of high-fat cocktail crackers, you might be okay. But in the Johns Hopkins study that showed the power of tomato soup to quench appetite and please taste buds, researchers found that regular cheese and crackers did little to dampen the appetite for dinner. And if you go the traditional route of regular high-fat cheese and high-fat crackers, you're getting too much fat before your meal—and doing very little to reduce your appetite.

Catch a Late-Day Second Wind

Chapter Twelve

Fat-Burner Switch #9

Reverse Your Dinner Habits: Make It Early—And Get a Fresh Start on Your Evening

Imagine that you set a goal to get as fat as possible, as efficiently as possible, just to give yourself the greatest chance of having heart disease and other big-time problems. Well, you'd want to eat the biggest, highest-fat meal of the day late in the evening. And after that, you'd want to sit around and snack on high-fat treats until you go to bed.

Sound ridiculous? Of course. Yet that's close to what many Americans do every evening. Without question, this pattern makes us fat. But beyond that, there's evidence that this pattern dulls the mind and drives a wedge into relationships.

The evening meal occurs just as your metabolism is crashing down like a breaking wave. With the approach of night, your biology slows fat-burning and speeds up fat-forming and fat-storing processes. Fortunately, this natural downturn is not inevitable—and it can be delayed until nearer your bedtime.

When you take action to delay that downturn by turning

on Fat-Burner Switch #9, you'll benefit in a number of ways. You'll feel more mental vitality and attentiveness to your personal and family matters, and you'll have a greater tendency to stay active and be in a better mood throughout the evening. As you get the new surge of fat-burning metabolism, there's less chance you'll collapse in front of the television after dinner. For anyone who has been doing that regularly, this Fat-Burner Switch is a rescue vehicle that might literally save your life.

A New Deal on Meals

There are seven simple and practical ways you can reinvent your evening habits. First of all, it's essential to pay attention to when you eat your evening meal, since timing is an important factor. You should also pay attention to the amounts and proportions of fat, carbohydrate, protein and total calories in that meal.

The third factor you might want to consider is how you begin your meal. Some research into the chemistry of the nervous system suggests that you may help turn on Fat-Burner Switch #9 by having protein early in your meal. Fourth, you can change the mood and pace of your eating with some small environmental adjustments that conspire to make you eat less—and therefore, eat less fat. Fifth, I recommend that you delay dessert. That will give you time for the sixth step, which is to get up and get moving for a fresh start on your evening. And the seventh and final strategy is to finish up with a low-fat snack or dessert.

Let's see how these changes fit together to help you turn on Fat-Burner Switch #9.

Make Your Evening Meal Early

For some time, researchers believed that the French have a much lower incidence of heart attack than Americans because they drink far more wine with their meals. But as scientists looked more closely at the evidence, they realized there are other factors as well. For one thing, they found that the French eat their main meal earlier in the day than we do, and they follow that meal with more physical activity.

The typical French person has the largest meal at midday,

consuming 57 percent of total daily calories before 2:00 P.M., according to Boston University School of Medicine scientist R. Curtis Ellison, M.D. Dr. Ellison also found that after the main meal, the French do a variety of physical activities until evening.

In contrast, Americans take in a total of only 38 percent of daily calories before 2:00 P.M. Most of us eat our dinners in the evening—and for most of us, it's the largest, highest-fat meal of the day. The late, heavy meal not only makes us sluggish, it also leads to a related problem. "Eating late in the evening inclines one toward skipping breakfast," according to Dallas Clouatre, Ph.D., author of *The Complete Guide to Anti-Fat Nutrients*.

If you eat a large evening meal that's high in fat, you produce an immediate shift toward fat-forming, fat-storing processes in your body, research has shown. In a study at the University of Minnesota in Minneapolis, researchers demonstrated that people on a 2,000-calorie diet put on weight in very different ways, depending on when they ate. Those who ate most of their calories earlier in the day lost weight, whereas people who ate the same meals later in the day gained—a lot! The average difference between those who lost and those who gained was 2.3 pounds per week.

Even if you don't eat your largest meal at midday, you should eat your evening meal as early in the evening as you can. The ideal time is between 5:30 and 6:00 P.M. Eating between 6:30 and 7:00 is probably fine, at least on occasion. But if you end up eating later than 7:00, you should make it a point to eat small servings. Also be sure to eat more slowly.

Your evening meals should have plenty of vegetables and grains, as do all of Leslie's recipes in part 4. But if you eat late, you should take special care to eat more vegetables and grains and fewer protein-rich and fat-rich foods.

What about weekends? Eat your main meal at midday if you can—or at the latest, by 6:00 P.M. If you're going out to a show or a movie, plan on eating beforehand, with a very light snack afterward. Don't wait until after the show to have a hearty dinner.

Make Your Evening Meal Light and Great-Tasting

To turn on Fat-Burner Switch #9, you need to limit the evening meal to the range of 500 to 600 satisfying and low-fat calories, research suggests. But most of us are amazingly un-

Switchbreak
SKILLPOWER
--►NOT
WILLPOWER

Right now, get a fresh tablet or notebook and write "Evening Food Record" across the top. Then during the next two weeks, write down everything you eat from 5:00 P.M. until bedtime.

At the end of the first week—without looking at your food record—try to remember everything you had each day after 5:00 P.M. Then compare this list of "remembereds" with your record of "actuals."

After the second week, do the same. By keeping these records, you'll not only become more aware of what you're eating but also be able to remember each meal more accurately. This skill will help you decide which high-fat foods to cut from your diet and make you more aware of your actual intake.

aware of much we consume from 5:00 P.M. on into the evening, according to research by Albert F. Smith, Ph.D., a cognitive psychologist who studies memory at the State University of New York at Binghamton. Most of the time, we simply don't remember how much and what we've eaten, according to Dr. Smith.

"The first and perhaps most important change in lifestyle behavior is to keep records," says Kelly D. Brownell, Ph.D., co-director of the Eating and Weight Disorders Clinic at Yale University. A study reported in the *Journal of the American Dietetic Association* revealed that impressive body fat losses are associated with record-keeping. On average, those who kept the most accurate food records lost the most weight.

If you're going to look forward to all your evening meals, they need to be great-tasting as well as light. But obviously, we don't have a lot of time to create delicious gourmet specials every evening. What can you do?

Here some tips to help you put great taste in every meal without tripling your time in the kitchen.

Master the shortcuts. It pays to know time-slashing ways to make quick sauces and super-easy soups. For instance, you can substitute delicious couscous (5 minutes cooking time) for brown rice (45 minutes cooking time). You can trim 50 minutes off the preparation time of nutrient-rich sweet potatoes or yams. And it takes just 10 minutes to make side dishes that taste like a chef's creation—not to mention ready-in-minutes homemade pizza and other fast, low-fat meals. Look at these and some of the other timesaving ideas in chapter 14. With these methods your dinner-in-a-hurry is more fun, more tasty and and far lower in fat.

Fat-Slashing at a Glance

One of the simplest ways to cut grams of fat is to steadily reduce the portion sizes of higher-fat foods you eat while simultaneously increasing your servings of lower-fat or nonfat alternatives. Here are some strategies to make sure you stay on the lean side at every meal.

■ Use plenty of delicious nonfat salad fixings topped with fat-free dressings.

■ Poach, bake or steam vegetables and other foods instead of frying.

■ Increase your intake of fresh and lightly steamed vegetables.

■ On the side, have whole-grain dishes or eat whole-grain bread.

■ Cook or lightly sauté with vegetable broth and a very small amount of oil. Use no-stick sprays and no-stick pans.

■ Accentuate recipe tastes by seasoning foods with pepper, parsley, basil, oregano, jalapeños, garlic, onions, shallots, curry, ginger, horseradish, tarragon and other fresh spices and herbs. (With more flavors, you have less need for the taste and "mouthfeel" of fat in your food.)

■ When you drink milk, make it skim or 1 percent low-fat milk.

■ Choose nonfat yogurt, cream cheese, cottage cheese and sour cream and reduced-fat or nonfat cheeses.

■ Eat less red meat and pork. Substitute beans, peas, lentils, pastas, rice, potatoes and vegetables.

■ Instead of meat, have small servings of poached or baked finfish, canned salmon, water-packed tuna or steamed shellfish.

■ Go for skinless poultry. With turkey, choose breast, drumstick, thigh or ground turkey all without the skin. Or have chicken breast without the skin.

■ Enjoy tasty international recipes—Italian, Japanese, Mexican, Chinese, Greek and Middle Eastern, for example—that combine vegetables or fruits with whole grains and beans and little or no meat.

■ Eat more 100 percent whole-grain foods—breads, crackers, rolls, bagels, tortillas and pastas.

■ On occasion, eat low-fat whole-grain muffins, waffles, pancakes or granola cereals.

Cater to your preferences. The mere sight, smell and taste of great-tasting food may help increase your metabolism and stimulate your body to burn more calories than bland, boring food. Medical researchers in Quebec, for instance, performed repeated animal and human studies to compare nutritionally identical meals that were either tasty or bland. The researchers found that the smell and taste of flavorful food seemed to stimulate the thermic effect of food—the amount of calories burned digesting, absorbing and utilizing it.

What are your favorite main courses, side dishes, fresh vegetables, fruits, soups, breads and pastas? Pinpoint the tastes you love and start searching out—or creating—recipes that accentuate those tastes while gradually reducing fat, refined sugar and cholesterol.

Remember your family matters. Turn the taste challenge into a family affair. Get everyone involved. If the focus is first on savory flavors and second on lowering the fat, it's easier to shift into healthier low-fat living habits.

Spice things up. You'll get a calorie-burning benefit from sprinkling every meal with fat-free seasonings and spices—especially hot stuff. For instance, eating meals laced with hot chili pepper and mustard has been shown to help boost the body's metabolic rate and actually burn more calories. In one study, researchers compared people who ate meals containing three grams of chili and three grams of mustard sauce with those who ate spiceless meals. Though the meals were identical in fat and calories, those who ate the high-spice meals raised their metabolism an average of 25 percent more than the other group.

This benefit doesn't apply to all spices—ginger, for example, does not seem to raise metabolism—but many spicy foods besides chili and hot mustard may have a fat-burning, metabolism-raising effect.

Start Your Meal with Protein-Rich Food

Think about it: One of the main reasons for eating supper is to give you the energy to enjoy your evening. Yet typical high-fat fare does the reverse: If you start the evening with oil-drenched salad, cheese-smothered nachos or a hunk of garlic bread, you're getting a veritable blob of dietary fat that can plunge you into an extended period of mental and physical fatigue.

Though this period is sometimes erroneously perceived as relaxation, it really isn't. But it is a period during which storage of body fat is accelerated. And to make matters worse, too many fat calories at this meal can leave you feeling too tired for evening physical activity or even sex.

Some research suggests that if you start off your evening

meal with high-carbohydrate food such as a chunk of French bread, you may stimulate the production of a brain chemical known as serotonin. This chemical triggers a natural relaxation that sometimes borders on sleepiness. Some evenings, sleep may be just what you want. But if it turns into a daily pattern, the serotonin soothing may pull you away from after-dinner physical activity and, in a related biological effect, block you from deepest sleep.

So you might find that dinner is a more energizing experience if you eat a few bites of low-fat, protein-rich food before you consume the rest of the meal. A number of neuropsychologists and nutritional researchers have suggested that by starting with protein you can stimulate the natural production of neurotransmitters (messenger chemicals) known as catecholamines. These messengers activate the brain to provide feelings of alertness and energy for up to three hours following the meal.

If you want low-fat, protein-rich foods to start your meal, there are many to choose from. I've already mentioned favorites such as tomato soup (made with skim or 1 percent low-fat milk). A small cup of bean or lentil soup is another good starter, or begin with a small serving of a bean or lentil salad or casserole.

Other options include some low-fat or nonfat yogurt, cottage cheese with several slices of fresh fruit or a small glass of skim milk. If you like decaf coffee or a cup of tea with your dinner, lace it with skim milk for the protein boost. Or start your meal with a few bites of a low-fat entrée that features beans or other legumes, skinless chicken breast, turkey or fish.

Adjust Your Pace Setting

Once the meal is under way, everything from the background music to the pace of eating can make a difference in how much you eat. Here are some ways to set the tempo as well as the mood of your dining, so you won't overeat your low-fat fare.

Enjoy some mellow tones. Studies suggest that people eat less and eat more slowly when they listen to soft, slow music. In contrast, "rock 'n' rollers practically inhale food," according to Maria Simonson, Sc.D., Ph.D, director of the Health, Weight and Stress Clinic at the Johns Hopkins Medical Institutions in Baltimore. With slow, soothing music during meals, you're less likely to wolf down your food or grab for second helpings.

Avoid major din. Volume also matters, say scientists at Northern Ireland's University of Ulster. The higher the volume, the more food you're likely to consume. Loud noise, whether loud music or the roar of voices, can increase the rate of eating and the amount eaten, other studies report. So if you're dining out, choose the restaurant with the low-key mood over the high-decibel hangout.

Slow your fork lift. Eat light the easy way—by slowing down your fork. Many people eat more when they eat quickly, and the extra food is more likely to be stored as body fat. Researchers have found that many overweight people are more likely to eat fast, to eat secretly, to nibble at food without being aware of it and to continue eating when full.

A study by Theresa Spiegel, Ph.D., and her colleagues at the University of Pennsylvania in Philadelphia showed that you get fat-burning benefits from eating more slowly and lengthening the meal. Researchers found that those who increased the length of their meals by an average of about four minutes burned more body fat than those who ate more quickly.

Relax and enjoy. As opposed to a hurry-up-and-gulp-it-down pace, you're better off with a less stressed eating style. Your digestion also improves, researchers say. Saliva produces an enzyme called alpha-amylase that initiates the process of digestion. Studies show that stress tends to decrease alpha-amylase activity, whereas relaxation methods significantly enhance the enzyme activity. So if you eat in a highly stressed state, you're less likely to get the full benefit of thoroughly digesting complex carbohydrates and other foods.

Do time between helpings. In the University of Pennsylvania study, Dr. Spiegel and her colleagues found that people who waited 15 minutes before having second helpings felt fuller and more satisfied than those who immediately went back for more. If you still feel hungry after the first course, give yourself some time. You're likely to have a lighter, more satisfying supper because after the wait, you'll probably find that you have no hunger for a second serving.

Delay Dessert

Clearly, when you redesign your evening meal, it may be tough to prevent the calorie count from hurtling over the 500 to 600 mark. Trouble is, if the calories do go too much higher, you're soon into the overeating, fat-forming zone.

One way to prevent this is by getting up from the table without dessert. With a bit of practice, delaying dessert can become fairly easy. By postponing the sweet conclusion to a satisfying meal, you're leaving room for your taste buds to have a treat later on.

Just wait 1½ to 2 hours, until after you've had some brief postdinner physical activity. By then you'll be well into some enjoyable family or personal pursuits, and your dinnertime nutrients will be well on their way through the digestive process.

Don't Just Sit There—Step Out

What you do in the 15 to 30 minutes after eating your evening meal sends a powerful signal to your body, which in turn adjusts your metabolism and sets the stage for deep sleep. What you don't want to do is stay seated—or make your way to the lounge chair and switch on the TV. This promotes only fat-forming, fatigue and grumpiness rather than fat-burning and a pleasant rush of positive evening energy.

According to a study at the Cooper Institute for Aerobics Research in Dallas, the most effective fat-burning exercise after a meal may be slow, sustained walking. And you'll get other benefits as well: A low-intensity exercise like walking can help dissipate harmful stress chemicals and make your mind more resilient under pressure, so stressful events take less of a toll. Plus, a walk after the evening meal may measurably deepen your sleep, according to Peter Hauri, Ph.D., director of the Insomnia Program at the Mayo Clinic Sleep Disorders Center in Rochester, Minnesota.

Other studies support the conclusion that walking is an exercise that helps turn on your Fat-Burner Switches. While carbohydrates are the body's fuel of choice for high-intensity exercise, fat is the best fuel for sustained low-intensity exercise, according to John Duncan, Ph.D., exercise physiologist at the Cooper Institute. So you're more likely to be burning stored fat than carbohydrates when you take an evening stroll after a low-fat meal.

Waiting until after your dinner for that walk is actually a big plus. If you walk after a meal, you may burn 15 percent more calories than if you walk the same time, distance and in-

Walk a Meal Away

Taking a stroll soon after a meal is a high-efficiency way to burn energy, according to studies conducted by researchers in the Department of Exercise Science at the University of South Carolina in Columbia. Evaluating four different groups of women over a three-hour period, researchers found that the women who had a meal and then exercised spent more energy than women in three other groups—those who only exercised, those who only ate a meal and didn't exercise and those who exercised before their meal.

The meal-then-exercise routine increased energy expenditure for the subjects by an average of 30 percent compared with the other routines. Researchers concluded that going for a walk after you eat can bring on "exercise-induced postprandial thermogenesis," which means the production of body heat created by exercising after a meal. And with the increased thermogenesis comes a corresponding increase in fat-burning.

Other researchers report that the combined effect of a walk after a meal can speed up fat-burning heat production by as much as 50 percent. As physiologist Melanie Roffers, Ph.D., former contributing editor to *Medical Selfcare* magazine, puts it: "Exercising at this time of the day elevates the metabolic rate just as it's winding down."

tensity on an empty stomach, according to *Prevention* magazine. "Eating stimulates your sympathetic nervous system," says Bryant A. Stamford, Ph.D., exercise scientist and director of the Health Promotion and Wellness Program at the University of Louisville in Kentucky. "Exercise after eating seems to give a double boost, so it burns more calories."

Light evening exercise may also help ease late-night cravings for high-fat foods, studies have shown. And if a craving does hit, you're better able to choose a nonfattening alternative and bypass the tendency to binge if you've had some low-intensity exercise.

Want to make the most of that after-dinner walk? These suggestions will help you turn on Fat-Burner Switch #9.

Plan on ten—or go for more. A 10-minute walk, started 15 to 20 minutes after the meal is over, is all it takes to stretch your muscles and adjust your metabolism. If time permits, extend your walk to 20 to 30 minutes. But keep the pace comfortable, and above all, enjoy it. That physical activity is giving you a fat-burning bonus that can last all night.

Wear shoes made for walking. You won't get far or enjoy your walk very much if you wear foot-squeezing fashion shoes instead of comfortable walking shoes. Putting on your walking shoes before dinner will save you the trouble of changing and make it just that much easier to head out the door after dinner.

Invite your honey. If you share this after-dinner walk with your partner, you'll have a chance to talk and—yes—even hold hands. Make a practice of it. You'll have a chance to get back in touch with each other, which may help resynchronize your biological romantic rhythms. (These are the wavelike inner brain/body cycles that must be in sync for you and your partner to relax together and experience feelings of strong affection and sustained sexual attraction.)

Gather a gabfest. Some evenings you'll want to include other family members or friends. That after-dinner walk is an ideal chance for some good old-fashioned talk and light-hearted fun—the kind that pulls you closer together.

Time your perambulations. It pays to exercise at approximately the same time each evening. Studies show that people who always go walking at about the same time are more likely to keep doing it night after night and find it enjoyable.

"Your body responds very nicely to habit," explains Frederick C. Hagerman, Ph.D., professor of biological sciences at Ohio University in Athens and physiological consultant to the U.S. Olympic teams. "Do your best to keep your evening exercise scheduled at consistent times."

Enjoy a Midevening Fat-Fighting Dessert or Snack

Almost everyone loves to eat at night. And as bad luck would have it, it's also the peak danger zone for high-fat binges and unconscious nonstop nibbling in front of the television. Fortunately, with some good choices, you can outfox these patterns.

Once you've eaten a light and early dinner and given your metabolism a boost with an after-dinner walk, settle in for some great conversation, music, games, reading or television—then go ahead and have a guilt-free serving of a great-tasting dessert or one of your favorite nighttime snacks.

You'll find a variety of recipes for my family's favorite homemade desserts in chapter 20, with per-serving nutritional analyses. Or for a tantalizing quick-reference list, see the "Low-Fat-Living Desserts" on page 202.

Low-Fat-Living Desserts

Here are some low-fat desserts that are easy to find in your supermarket. If you're buying baked goods, yogurt, ice cream, pudding and other desserts, be sure to check nutrition labels to make sure these foods are low in fat and calories—then limit your servings accordingly. Chew each bite slowly, savoring the taste.

Baked Goods
- Angel food cake
- Fruit pie that is mostly fruit, with a very low fat crust and very little sweetener
- Nonfat, wheat-free multigrain brownies
- Very low fat or fat-free whole-grain cookies (Health Valley is one brand)
- Nonfat granola, very lightly sweetened (such as Walnut Acres)
- Fat-free sponge cake

Yogurt, Light Ice Cream and Pudding
- Very low fat sugar-sweetened or sugar-free ice cream
- Low-fat or nonfat plain yogurt (add your own fat-free granola or fruit)
- Nonfat sugar-sweetened or sugar-free frozen yogurt
- Tapioca pudding, made with skim milk

Fruit
- Any variety of fresh fruit
- Natural, unsweetened applesauce
- Unsweetened orange juice

As you'll see, you have a wonderful variety of low-fat desserts to choose from. But whatever evening treat you select, plan a within-limits serving—one that does not exceed approximately three grams of fat or 300 calories. You need to be especially alert if you select store-bought snacks and desserts: Be sure to read the labels and pay attention to portion size to make sure your late-evening snack meets these requirements.

When you've selected one of your favorites, chew each bite slowly, savoring the taste. After you've finished, brush your teeth right away. Whether you're consciously aware of it or not, brushing helps signal your body that eating time is over—and it can help short-circuit late-night cravings for high-fat foods.

Chapter Thirteen

Fat-Burner Switch #10

Get Deeper, High-Metabolism Sleep and Awaken Invigorated

Even if you get enough sleep to turn off the Fat-*Maker* Switches, are there things you can do to turn on some fat-*burners* during your nightly rest?

The quick answer is yes. Better-quality sleep can speed the building of new muscles and thereby help increase your fat-burning power.

Not only that, there are several simple, specific ways to deepen the quality of your sleep and at the same time increase the chances that your rest is not just more health-promoting but also fat-burning.

The Rest That Builds Muscle Tone

In truth, efficient fat loss and energy-building require that your body get a chance to recover during sleep.

"Recovery ability is defined as the chemical reactions that

are necessary for your body to produce efficient fat loss and muscle-building," explains exercise scientist Ellington Darden, Ph.D., director of research for Nautilus Sports/Medical Industries. "An optimum recovery ability is dependent on adequate deep rest."

When you firm up your muscles you burn more fat calories even while you sleep. But the way you burn those calories is different when you're resting than when you're awake.

During exercise, your muscle tissue itself doesn't actually grow stronger; in fact, it breaks down. But once you lie down to rest, your muscle fibers actually gain tone and thereby increase their metabolic capacity. And the deeper your rest, the better.

So even if you're exercising and toning during the day, you're not giving your muscles a chance to build themselves unless you give them some genuine, no-demands downtime.

Here are several simple action steps to get deeper rest tonight—and to make strides to turn sleep into a greater fat-fighting, energy-restoring ally. (For more help in achieving deep, healthy sleep, you might try *Easing into Sleep*, an audiocassette program by Emmett E. Miller, M.D., or *No More Sleepless Nights*, a book by Peter Hauri, Ph.D., and Shirley Linde, Ph.D. For medical information on sleep treatments and information on accredited sleep disorders centers, contact the American Sleep Disorders Association, 604 Second Street SW, Rochester, MN 55902.)

Shed Your Covers

"Your body will burn significantly more calories each night if you sleep cool," suggests Dr. Darden. "I'm convinced that most people bury themselves under too many covers when they sleep. This prevents their normal thermostats from kicking in and supplying natural body heat."

The more heat your body has to provide, the more fat you'll burn to provide that heat. So Dr. Darden simply recommends that "if you tend to sleep with too many covers, try to eliminate one or two. Try to wean yourself from cranking up the temperature on an electric blanket or using flannel sheets during the winter months." And when summer comes along, Dr. Darden suggests, get rid of the blankets completely and cover up with a single sheet.

Warm Up before Bedtime

Before you go to bed, you need the kind of after-dinner exercise I recommended for Fat-Burner Switch #9. Sleep researchers have come up with some fascinating new information about how this period of exercise helps to induce deeper sleep.

Here's what they've found: Physical inactivity ranks among the prime causes of insomnia. And studies show that the more physically fit you are, the more your sleep improves. But it's not just the exercise itself that's beneficial—it's the increased body temperature.

"If you can increase your body temperature about three to six hours before going to bed, the temperature will then drop most as you are ready to go to sleep," explain Dr. Hauri, director of the Insomnia Program at the Mayo Clinic Sleep Disorders Center in Rochester, Minnesota, and co-researcher Dr. Linde. "The biological 'trough' deepens, and sleep becomes deeper, with fewer awakenings," they note.

Since body temperature is so important, it would seem logical that anything you do to heat up your body several hours before you hit the hay would have a beneficial effect. This conclusion is supported by the research of James A. Horne, Ph.D., a sleep scientist at Loughborough University in Great Britain. According to Dr. Horne, people sleep better when they take a hot bath or shower within three hours of bedtime. So if you happen to skip the warm-up of a good exercise session, try a shower or bath to raise your body temperature a couple of hours before you go to bed.

Don't Go to Bed Hungry

There is evidence that crash diets and low-calorie diets disrupt body temperature. When that happens, it's likely to take much longer for you to fall asleep. According to a study published in the *American Journal of Clinical Nutrition*, hunger disrupts your restorative "slow wave sleep"—the deep kind of sleep that produces long wave patterns in your brain.

When people are dieting, they may attempt a kind of artificial starvation, saying to themselves "If I skip all eating after 5:00 P.M., I'll probably lose more weight." But this attempt at overnight fasting may actually switch off your fat-burner. As far as your metabolism is concerned, going for long stretches without eating is disruptive, even though not as bad as stuffing yourself with high-fat foods in front of the TV.

If you've learned to turn on Fat-Burner Switch #9, you already have a good repertoire of low-fat snacks and desserts that you can eat between 8:00 and 9:00 P.M. Of course, you'll also want to avoid caffeinated drinks such as tea, coffee and sodas, which can keep you fully awake or make you sleep restlessly.

In addition, you may want to test the link between what you eat and the quality of your nightly rest. According to researchers at the Massachusetts Institute of Technology in Cambridge and other institutions, the best advice here is to consistently choose high-carbohydrate, low-fat, low-protein snacks. Since protein in particular may promote alertness, you might start to sleep more deeply almost immediately if you pass on dairy products, which are relatively high in protein.

What if you're staying up late tonight and you're wondering what to do if you get hungry again before bed? Can you eat a second small snack several hours after your midevening snack or dessert?

Of course. But stick to a few bites of low-fat, low-protein, high-carb fare. Reach for two rye crackers and a piece of just-ripe fruit, for example. Or have a couple of low-fat, high-fiber cookies with a small glass of orange juice. Nighttime foods such as these may actually help deepen your sleep by increasing the brain messenger chemicals that promote a relaxed state of mind and calm emotions.

Sleep Deeper—With No Clock in Sight

To truly sleep well, it's not enough to touch a level of deep, metabolism-enhancing rest if it's sustained for only a short time. What you really need is deep rest during your entire sleep period.

You can do at least one thing to your environment to better ensure that you get such rest, according to research at the Mayo Clinic Sleep Disorders Center. "For most people the bedroom should be a time-free environment," says Dr. Hauri. "Set the alarm if you must, but put the clock where it can be heard but not seen."

This is especially important for people who have insomnia, according to Dr. Hauri. With the clock out of sight, you won't wake up again and again during the night to find yourself staring at the figures on the dial. "People sleep better without time pressure," says Dr. Hauri.

Put Aside Your Problems at the End of the Day

Stress and sleep don't mix. Neither do work and sleep—or family problems and sleep.

If you want the best possible rest, and especially if you suffer from insomnia, make it a family rule that your bedroom is reserved as a comfortable, relaxing haven. It's for either restful sleep or a warm, positive sexual relationship. Nothing else. Keep heated discussions, intense brainstorming, computer work and monthly finances out of your bedroom, since they accustom your body to a learned association with sleeplessness.

The associations with work and stress can be stronger than you're aware of, once those wake-up forces invade the peace and privacy of your bedroom. If you find that you often lie awake and that your problems and tensions rush in as soon as you put your head on the pillow, your environment could be the reason. Even in the dark, a place that has gathered stressful associations can rob you of pleasant relaxation.

Set Your Weekend Wake-Ups to Your Weekday Role

One widely celebrated American habit is "sleeping in" on weekends. Unfortunately, the habit of slamming off the alarm on Saturday morning and turning over to catch 80 more winks is a saboteur of deep sleep. That's because sleeping in actually confuses your body's biological clock. It creates a jet lag–like disruption pattern known as free running.

According to sleep researchers, free running tends to lower your energy rather than raise it. In addition to feeling worn out

---

Switchbreak
SKILLPOWER
NOT ◀--
WILLPOWER

Right now, have a look around your bedroom for subtle, invasive reminders of business or personal pressures.

Are the glowing digits of your alarm clock shining toward your pillow? Turn the clock the other way.

Is your checkbook on the dresser with a pile of bills right next to it? Retire your financial worries—along with all that paperwork—to the next room.

Do you have an open briefcase on the chair? A laptop computer humming away? A work-related magazine open to a half-finished article you promised to read by morning?

Right now, exile all of these items to other rooms. Then, when you go to bed tonight, you'll fall asleep in the lowest-stress zone of your house.

and less alert after too much sleep, you may also have more difficulty falling asleep the next night.

Even if your night's sleep has been poor or has been cut short for some reason, it makes sense to get up at about the same time every day to help synchronize your body's biological rhythms.

Yes, at times you may want to sleep in. But when you do, it's a good idea to limit your extra time in bed to no more than an hour or so. Open the curtains to expose yourself to daylight as soon as you wake up and immediately start turning on Fat-Burner Switch #1—getting light, some exercise and a superb low-fat breakfast. All these actions help stabilize your sleep/wake rhythm.

Feeling particularly groggy some mornings?

If possible, wake up at least a minute or two earlier to lie in bed, blink your eyes and move your arms and legs. Allow your body to gradually adjust to being wide awake. The way you spend these first wakeful minutes can have a significant influence on your energy and performance all day long.

Reminder List: Turn On the Fat-Burners

Fat-Burner Switch #1: Quick-Start Your Morning Metabolism

Fat-Burner Switch #2: Eat Low-Fat, High-Fiber Snacks

Fat-Burner Switch #3: Drink Water and Other Fat-Fighting Beverages

Fat-Burner Switch #4: Enjoy Do-It-Anywhere Active Minutes and Low-Intensity Aerobics

Fat-Burner Switch #5: Have a Fat-Fighting Lunch

Fat-Burner Switch #6: Use On-the-Spot Distress Blockers

Fat-Burner Switch #7: Count on Fast Firm-Ups: Quick and Easy Muscle-Toning

Fat-Burner Switch #8: Catch a Late-Day Second Wind

Fat-Burner Switch #9: Reverse Your Dinner Habits: Make It Early—And Get a Fresh Start on Your Evening

Fat-Burner Switch #10: Get Deeper, High-Metabolism Sleep and Awaken Invigorated

---

Reprogram Your Kitchen and Fight Fat When You Dine Out

rue or false: Delicious, healthful, low-fat food takes way too long to cook.

False! And the tips in these chapters prove it.

Yes, it's true that some foods like homemade bread, traditional brown rice and slow-cooked dried beans do take their own sweet time. But there are countless quick and healthy versions of many dishes that you can easily make without spending most of your evening in the kitchen.

Just what you've been looking for?

You're not alone. It's a fact of life today that busy schedules limit time for meal preparation. But as Leslie and I have discovered in our home, fixing fast meals doesn't mean you're stuck with the fat. In the time it takes to heat a TV dinner in the oven or to make a run to the nearest take-out restaurant, you can prepare a variety of healthful, fast meals.

As we've added to our repertoire of low-fat recipes, Leslie and I have also kept a list of tricks we've developed to get in and out of the kitchen as fast as possible, with a minimum amount of preparation and cleanup time.

Part

3

Chapter Fourteen

Meals in Minutes: Low-Fat Fast Food at Home

The key to quick low-fat cooking is to plan ahead. For instance, having a well-stocked pantry, with all the items you need right at your fingertips, gives you the feeling of being in control of your kitchen and your family's nutrition. (And we'll give you some tips for doing that in chapter 17.) Also, you need to think ahead to what you'll be having for the week, so you can consolidate your shopping and avoid making time-consuming multiple trips to the store. And you can plan: If you decide on fresh fish for one meal, for instance, you'll know which day you need to swing by the fish store on your way home from work.

Of course, for people who love to cook—and my wife, Leslie, is among them—lingering over preparation is just as enjoyable as lingering over the tastefully prepared low-fat meal that emerges from the oven. But that's not true every day. Often we just want to get in and out of the kitchen as quickly as possible. And yet we want the food to be very tasty, so we'll constantly be motivated to follow our Low-Fat Living Program. It's essential that we have a collection of recipes that we can draw upon for our daily standby menus.

When speed is desired and easier is better, here are some of the timesaving tactics you can use in your household.

Each weekend, invest ten minutes planning the meals ahead. You'll receive an amazing timesaving payoff when you devote a few minutes each weekend to choosing the coming week's main meals.

By planning ahead you streamline your shopping lists and help minimize the stressful "What should we eat tonight?" question that keeps cropping up when there's no advance plan.

You might even invest a few weekend minutes precooking beans and other legumes. Or make some bread dough that can be frozen and then thawed, raised and baked later in the week when you want a quick loaf of delicious homemade bread.

Delegate kitchen responsibilities. If you have children, dividing kitchen tasks saves time and brings the family members closer together. As soon as the children are old enough, they can set and clear the table, wash dishes and even help prepare food. In many homes, these shared minutes are a simple, valuable daily ritual of connection.

At our house, one of Leslie's satisfactions is that she can prepare a fast, special low-fat meal, knowing that she's all finished in the kitchen when the meal arrives at the table. The other tasks are taken care of: Our children help set and clear the table, and I do the cleanup and the dishes.

Keep a step-saver list on hand. Whenever you start to run out of an ingredient, write it down immediately on an easy-access grocery list. Don't wait until you run out; that's how you end up making one-item raids on the grocery store. It makes life easier—and saves trips to the supermarket— when you write down everything that's on "low" before it's on "empty."

Add personal notes to recipes. Whenever you change a recipe, pencil the change in the margin. If you substitute an ingredient, adjust cooking time or change the seasonings to meet your family's preferences, jot down the change right away. Then, when you next prepare that meal, you won't have to wonder what you did last time.

Reprogram Your Kitchen

Cut down on cooking time. Use your microwave to speed up defrosting and reheating foods. The microwave can be your best ally when you want to reduce preparation and cooking times. It's especially useful when there are items that cook slowly, such as casseroles, sauces, squash and some beans and other legumes.

A pressure cooker is another valuable kitchen tool to consider. There is no faster way to cook legumes. Two hours of simmering can be shortened to 30 minutes of pressure-steaming if you use a pressure cooker instead of a regular pot. And the time it takes to cook other dishes—brown rice, sauces, soups and chili, for example—can be reduced to one-third of the usual time if you use a pressure cooker. Despite the speed of cooking, there's no loss of flavor.

Get two meals from one recipe: Double it. In our home we often prepare a double recipe when cooking soups, chili, casseroles and other dishes that freeze well. After we've served the meal and the food has cooled down, we put the leftovers— enough for another whole meal—in containers with tight-fitting lids and place them in the freezer. Voilá—an entire "frozen dinner" ready to go.

On days when we are running late and don't have time to cook, we thaw and bake (or microwave) the frozen food, then add a quick salad and some bread, and dinner is ready. We've found that these low-fat meals taste far better—and are far less expensive—than any frozen meal-in-a-box from the supermarket.

Freeze your favorite loaves. Keep one or two loaves of your favorite whole-grain bread and a package or two of rolls in the freezer for quick defrosting. This can round out a meal in minutes.

Soak ahead for legume recipes. Many of the most healthful and delicious recipes for beans and other legumes require some quick and simple advance preparation, such as soaking overnight. This is where planning ahead will help. If the beans have already been soaked, they don't take long to cook.

In a pinch, canned beans are a good last-minute substitute. Their one drawback is that they're high in salt, because they're packed in a high-sodium brine. But there's a simple way to reduce the sodium in canned beans: Simply drain them and rinse in a colander.

Low-Fat Homework Made Easy: Scanning Labels to Find the Fat

Food labels give you the facts—and with a little practice, one glance will tell you whether the label you're looking at describes a low-fat food.

Serving Size

Ask yourself whether you'll actually eat the amount shown on the label. If you will, then you don't need a calculator to figure out how much fat and how many calories you're getting. But if you're going to eat twice that much, remember to double everything.

Calories and Total Fat

This is where it's better to look at the absolute numbers rather than the percentages. If you know how many calories and how much fat you're allowing yourself every day, these numbers tell you instantly whether you're within your range for the meal or snack you're about to have.

Saturated Fat and Cholesterol

No more than 10 percent of your calories should come from saturated fat. As for cholesterol, the American Heart Association recommends no more than 300 milligrams daily.

Sodium

Although it's not a factor that directly affects your low-fat diet, high sodium can pose another health risk for some people by leading to high blood pressure.

Dietary Fiber

The more, the better. Foods that are high in fiber help keep your digestive system working smoothly. And since they make you feel full longer, high-fiber foods ultimately help you eat less food in general and therefore less fat and fewer calories.

Nutritional Facts

Serving Size 1 Container (227g)

Amount Per Serving

Calories 240   Calories from fat 25

	% Daily Value*
Total Fat 3g	5%
Saturated Fat 1.5g	8%
Cholesterol 15mg	5%
Sodium 135mg	6%
Potassium 500mg	14%
Total Carbohydrate 46g	15%
Dietary Fiber 1g	4%
Sugars 44g	
Protein 9g	

Vitamin A 4%	Vitamin C 10%
Calcium 35%	Iron 0%

*Percent Daily Values are based on 2,000 calorie diet

Enjoy more salad greens—with less work washing them. Do you love salads but find yourself skipping them because of the time it takes to clean the fixings?

When you bring home fresh greens from the market, wash enough for several meals. Then, because dry greens stay fresh longer than wet ones, remove all the water with a salad spinner. Gently wrap the greens in a clean cotton kitchen towel, place them in a plastic produce bag and refrigerate until needed. This way, you have only one cleanup, and the washed-and-dried salad fixings stay fresh for about three to four days.

Hoard the makings of quick sauces and soups. When you're stocking up on canned nonfat chicken or vegetable broth, always buy more than you need, so you have an ever-ready supply on the shelf. The cans take only an instant to open, and either kind of broth adds instant flavor to many dishes.

Standbys to Swear By

Back in the days of high-fat living, many moms had their standbys for each day of the week. Meat loaf on Monday. Chicken on Tuesday. Spaghetti and meatballs on Wednesday, and so on. Not much variation—but these reliable, familiar recipes were easy to prepare.

Well, the fat focus has changed, and with it the nature of the meals. But there's still a lot to be said for reliable standbys that you can count on. What follows are some of our substitutes for the old high-fat main courses, side dishes and even desserts. And because we love new flavors in our household, these standbys never get old, as often as we've served them, because we're always adding new spices to keep the tastes interesting. They're fast, easy and delicious—and very low in fat.

Pizza and Pita-za Specials

Many grocery stores now carry whole-wheat pita breads and traditional and whole-grain Italian focaccia flatbreads. They're especially easy to store in your freezer, since they lie flat and take up little space. With these you can whip up a homemade pizza anytime, with less fat than a to-go meal from your neighborhood pizzeria.

In fact, making lean pizza takes less time than a pizza delivery. To make a pita-bread pizza, for example, heat the oven to 350° and bake the pita until it's slightly crisp. Add tomato sauce, chopped vegetables and seasonings and then bake briefly until the add-ons are heated through. You'll add tasty variations such as low-fat cheese, but basically, that's all there is to it. It's cheaper than delivered pizza, more tasty and a lot lower in fat.

Premier Pasta—With Variations

Pasta is one of our family's most popular fast dinners. But to keep the tastes bright and new, we have several different pasta varieties on hand: traditional and whole-grain spaghetti, linguine, rotini and wagon wheels (the favorite of our five-year-old). We also vary the sauces.

A simple tomato sauce, whether store-bought or made from one of the recipes in this book, is easy to modify and spark up with new flavors. We sometimes add leftovers—cooked chicken or seafood, tofu, cooked beans, vegetables, fresh herbs, onions and garlic. And with a bit of skim milk or evaporated skim milk you can transform a traditional tomato sauce into a creamy red sauce.

Memorable Almost-Instant Pilaf

A pilaf has the most simple ingredients, but they're all low-fat and nutritious, so you can make up an Eastern-style, exotically flavored meal in record time.

We like to sauté some onions and garlic, then add a quick-cooking grain like brown rice or barley, defatted chicken or vegetable stock and a few pinches of herbs. It takes about ten minutes to simmer, and then we sprinkle it with a little finely grated orange or lemon rind.

Oriental Expressions

For another great fast-meal option, cook or reheat some brown rice, add Chinese or soba (buckwheat) noodles and top with quickly sautéed vegetables with or without chicken, seafood, tofu or legumes. Add some low-sodium soy sauce or teriyaki sauce as a nonfat seasoning or quick marinade.

Appealing Rapid-Bake Poultry

You can broil skinless chicken or turkey breasts in just a few minutes, and almost instantly, you have the foundation of a fast low-fat meal.

And the side dishes for this meal don't take much longer. It takes five minutes to make couscous (a delicious grain dish) and about the same amount of time to steam vegetables. Serve with a tossed salad made with low-fat or nonfat dressing and some whole-grain bread, and you have a very complete meal in under a half-hour.

Believe-It-or-Not Beanwiches

Heat up homemade or canned refried (but fat-free) beans and spread a layer inside a whole-wheat pita bread. This is one of the fastest of the low-fat standbys in our home. We top our beanwiches with nonfat sour cream, salsa, tomatoes, lettuce or sprouts, a little low-fat Cheddar cheese, green chili peppers and diced onions. It's a great-tasting low-fat sandwich that takes about ten minutes to make.

Quick-Mex in Minutes

For a variation on beanwiches, use whole-wheat tortillas or low-fat soft or hard taco shells. Make them with the same fillings as the beanwiches, or check out the taco meal in chapter 19, which doesn't take much longer to prepare.

Low-Fat Burgers on Buns

If you have ground turkey breast on hand or a quick low-fat "veggie burger" mix, you're ready to cook a quick meal anytime. Keep some whole-grain buns in the freezer and thaw them in the toaster oven or microwave while you're getting the condiments ready. We love to add tomatoes, lettuce or sprouts, onions and pickles; you can choose other favorite ingredients to go on top. To create a homemade low-fat burger meal like this takes about 15 minutes.

Mama's High-Speed, Low-Fat Antipasto

Keep your refrigerator and pantry stocked with cans of white beans, black beans, water-packed tuna, pimentos, baby corn, artichoke hearts (packed in water, not oil), pick-

The Alpha of Omega-3's

Many people realize that there's a type of beneficial oil called omega-3 fatty acids in certain fish. But how do you pick a fish that supplies omega-3's? And what does that "fish oil" actually do for you?

First of all, fish carry widely varying amounts of the beneficial omega-3's. In some, only about 5 percent of the fat is omega-3 fatty acids; in others, the content can range as high as 40 percent.

While omega-3's are technically a collection of different fatty acids, there's one in particular that may help reduce heart disease and heart attack risk. This acid helps the clotting action of your blood, reduces levels of LDL ("bad" cholesterol) and raises levels of HDL ("good" cholesterol). All these potential benefits come from an organic chemical with an almost impossible name: eicosapentaenoic acid, or EPA for short.

The fish that contain significant EPA are generally deep-water fish, notably salmon, albacore tuna, mackerel, herring and sardines. EPA is also present in lesser concentrations in cod, whitefish, bonito, shad, pompano, halibut, bluefish, bass, trout and some other varieties.

Since omega-3's with their EPA make up only part of the fat in fish, you can't consume seafood willy-nilly just to get the heart-protective benefits. In fact, as with any source of fats, it's important to choose very small portions.

You can get omega-3's from some nonfish sources, though in smaller doses. Among the excellent alternatives are dried beans, tofu (which is made from soybeans), butternuts and walnuts.

Several studies suggest that you can get some minor protection against cardiovascular disease by eating EPA-rich foods just once or twice a week. And people who have diabetes or arthritis may also benefit.

led red beets and other quick side dishes and garnishes. All of these fast-to-the-table items are low in fat. If you drain and rinse the canned items that come in brine, they'll be light on the sodium.

Arrange a decorative selection of your favorites on a large plate lined with fresh green-leaf lettuce. Sprinkle with lemon juice or balsamic vinegar and fresh herbs.

Prime-Time Fruit Purees

Keep peeled and sliced fruit in plastic bags in your freezer. Any time you're ready for dessert, put a fruit mixture in the food processor, puree until smooth, then serve immediately. Our favorite candidates for this instant puree are peaches, kiwifruit, raspberries, blackberries, blueberries and strawberries, but just about any fruit works well.

Fast Fish

Fresh fish fillets cook so quickly that they're done before you know it. Just be sure to choose uniformly thin fillets, which cook the fastest.

Preheat the oven to broil (450° to 500°). Put the fish in to broil, then check after three minutes and baste evenly with your favorite juice (orange or lemon juice or spicy vegetable-tomato cocktail) or nonfat marinade.

Flavor-Packed Instant Couscous

This side dish packs great taste, goes with everything and is simple to prepare. Sauté some chopped onions and minced garlic in a little olive or canola oil.

Stir in some couscous (or bulgur), chicken or vegetable broth and a little seasoning such as parsley, basil or curry powder. Cover, remove from the heat and let stand for ten minutes. Fluff with a fork and serve.

For variety, add some diced tomatoes, water chestnuts or sliced roasted red peppers.

Short-Order Shortcuts for Time-Pressed Cooks

Every cook develops quick tricks that make recipes simpler and faster to prepare. These shortcuts are important, because once you start using them, you'll find it's just as easy to prepare fresh fruits, vegetables and garnishes as it is to use prepared foods or prepackaged items. Here are some of the shortcuts we use that shave minutes off preparation time.

Peel Garlic in Seconds

Place individual cloves on a cutting board. Smash them with the flat side of a broad knife such as a chef's knife. The peels should slip right off. Then press them through a good-quality garlic press.

Low-Fat Dishes for Fast-Paced People

All the following recipes take 10 to 60 minutes to prepare and cook, though some (marked with asterisks) require additional time to marinate or chill.

Pastas and Pasta Sauces

Angel Hair Pasta with Fresh Tomato Sauce (page 320)—Preparation: 35 minutes

Couscous Pilaf (page 333)—Preparation and cooking: 10 minutes

Fettuccine with Roasted Red Pepper Sauce (page 336)—Preparation and cooking: 15 minutes

Lemon Linguine Parmesan (page 313)—Preparation and cooking: 10 to 20 minutes

Linguine Frittata with Broccoli (page 271)—Preparation and cooking: 20 to 30 minutes

Oriental Noodles (page 299)—Preparation and cooking: 30 minutes

Pasta Rustica (page 342)—Preparation and cooking: 30 minutes

Salads and Salad Dressings

Balsamic Splash (page 348)—Preparation: 5 minutes

Caesar-Style Salad (page 344)—Preparation: 5 minutes

Chicken Salad with Peaches and Pecans (page 277)—Preparation and cooking: 20 minutes

Citrus-Season Salad with Ginger-Horseradish Dressing (page 307)—Preparation: 15 minutes

Creamy Garlic Dressing (page 314)—Preparation: 5 minutes

Cucumber and Red Grape Salad (page 282)—Preparation: 10 minutes

Dilled Cucumber Salad (page 285)—Preparation: 10 minutes

European Mixed Vegetable Salad (page 347)—Preparation: 10 minutes

Four-Bean Salad with Balsamic Vinaigrette* (page 290)—Preparation: 10 minutes

Fresh Green Bean Salad* (page 330)—Preparation: 20 to 25 minutes

Greek Pasta Salad (page 286)—Preparation: 15 minutes

Greens with Baby Beets, Toasted Walnuts and Maple-Raspberry Vinaigrette (page 354)—Preparation: 10 minutes

Israeli Salad* (page 276)—Preparation: 10 minutes

Mesclun Greens with Italian Parmesan Vinaigrette (page 327)—Preparation: 5 minutes

Mixed Green Salad with Creamy Fresh Basil Dressing*(page 321)—Preparation: 10 minutes

Mixed Greens with Peach and Pecan Dressing (page 274)—Preparation: 10 minutes

Red- and Green-Leaf Lettuce with Maple-Walnut Dressing (page 351)—Preparation: 10 minutes

Red-Leaf Lettuce with Pine Nuts, Cherries and Dried-Tomato Vinaigrette (page 338)—Preparation: 10 minutes

Salad Nouveau (page 314)—Preparation: 10 minutes

Spinach Salad with Pears, Walnuts and Warm Mustard Vinaigrette (page 334)—Preparation and cooking: 10 minutes

Tex-Mex Pasta Salad (page 294)—Preparation: 20 minutes

Vegetables, Beans and Rice

Baked Yams with Nutmeg Cream (page 318)—Preparation: 5 minutes; baking: 35 to 45 minutes

Broccoli Lemon Amandine (page 347)—Preparation and cooking: 15 minutes

Brown Basmati Rice with Lemon (page 318)—Preparation and cooking: 45 to 50 minutes

Colorful Corn Relish* (page 297)—Preparation: 10 minutes

Honey-Glazed Baby Carrots (page 334)—Preparation and cooking: 25 minutes

Mashed Potatoes with a Difference (page 346)—Preparation and cooking: 20 to 25 minutes

Middle Eastern Baked Falafel (page 283)—Preparation: 15 minutes; baking: 20 minutes

Quesadillas (page 288) with Sweet Pea Guacamole (page 289)—Preparation and cooking: 40 minutes

Southwestern Black Beans (page 323)—Preparation: 10 minutes

Specialty Green Beans (page 337)—Preparation and cooking: 20 minutes

Spicy French Potatoes (page 330)—Preparation: 10 minutes; baking: 20 minutes

Tacos (page 315)—Preparation and cooking: 15 minutes

Soups and Stews

Autumn's Acorn Cheddar Soup (page 296)—Preparation: 10 minutes; baking: 45 minutes

Hot-and-Sour Soup (page 341)—Preparation and cooking: 25 minutes

Old-Fashioned Chicken and Vegetable Stew (page 352)—Preparation and cooking: 45 minutes

(continued)

Low-Fat Dishes for Fast-Paced People—Continued

Roasted Chestnut and Wild Rice Soup (page 292)—Preparation and cooking: 1 hour

Southwestern Chicken Chili (page 303)—Preparation: 10 minutes; cooking time: 1 hour

Thick and Zesty Gazpacho* (page 268)—Preparation: 15 to 20 minutes

Poultry

Chicken Cutlets with Raspberry Vinaigrette (page 312)—Preparation and cooking: 35 minutes

Santa Fe Chicken Fajitas (page 322)—Preparation and cooking: 25 minutes

Turkey Burgers (page 329)—Preparation and cooking: 20 to 30 minutes

Seafood

Picante Seafood Veracruz (page 317)—Preparation and cooking: 40 minutes

Pepper-Seared Sea Scallops (page 336)—Preparation and cooking: 15 minutes

Thai Stir-Fry (page 339)—Preparation and cooking: 45 minutes

Breads, Chips and Sandwiches

Cracked-Wheat Quick Bread (page 280)—Preparation: 5 minutes; baking: 45 minutes

Gingerbread Muffins (page 298)—Preparation: 10 minutes; baking: 20 minutes

Green Chili and Cheddar Buttermilk Biscuits (page 270)—Preparation: 10 minutes; baking: 12 to 15 minutes

Hummus-in-Pita Sandwiches (page 275)—Preparation: 15 minutes

Lentil Spread in Pita Pockets (page 305)—Preparation: 10 minutes; cooking: 45 minutes

Oatmeal Soda Bread (page 273)—Preparation: 15 minutes; baking: 30 to 40 minutes

Old-Fashioned Cornbread (page 304)—Preparation: 10 minutes; baking: 20 minutes

Peasants' Salad Pita Pockets (page 291)—Preparation: 15 minutes

Ratatouille and Grilled Mozzarella Sandwiches (page 281)—Preparation and cooking: 45 minutes

Cook Yams in Minutes

To slice 50 minutes off the cooking time of nutrient-packed yams or sweet potatoes, first cut the unpeeled tubers into big cubes. Boil the cubes about ten minutes, or until tender. Drain and serve.

Or for variety, cut yams or sweet potatoes into ½-inch-thick slabs and coat them with low-sodium soy sauce mixed with a few drops of olive or canola oil. Grill until crisp and golden brown.

There's a microwave option, too: Pierce the sweet potatoes several times with a fork and microwave until tender. One potato takes about 4 to 5 minutes. With four in the microwave, the cooking time is more likely to be 10 to 12 minutes.

Have Your Squash in Ten

Your microwave stands ready to make tender, tasty squash in under ten minutes. Cut the squash in half and pierce the skin with a fork. Spaghetti squash takes eight minutes to cook in the microwave. Butternut or acorn squash, cut in half this way, cooks to perfection in ten minutes.

Find a Rice Substitute

Brown rice needs to be boiled a full 45 minutes before it's ready. If you haven't got time for that—and you don't have any precooked brown rice stored in the refrigerator—try one of these other quick-cooking grains, which are ready to eat in 5 to 12 minutes.

- Bulgur wheat: 7 minutes
- Quick-cooking barley: 12 minutes
- Couscous: 5 minutes
- Quick-cooking brown rice: 10 minutes

Chapter Fifteen

Phase Out Fat
in Every Meal

Many of us have vivid memories of enticing aromas wafting from our mothers' or grandmothers' kitchens. There is something so special, so loving and supportive, about enjoying and passing down recipes and traditions from one generation to another. Throughout history, food has served as a symbol of caring, sharing and providing.

Unfortunately, many recipe favorites may be loaded with fat. Does that mean you have to give them up?

No—especially not if you learn simple ways to keep all the great taste while phasing out the excess fat.

As we've discovered in our kitchen, you can create new, more healthful versions of your old favorites. This chapter offers a collection of quick, practical tips that you can begin using in your kitchen today.

In this chapter you'll also find guidelines for preparing whole-grain breads and cereals as well as legumes—beans, peas and lentils. It's no secret that these foods are your best friends when you take up the Low-Fat Living Program. Nutritious, delicious, filled with fiber and carrying all the essential nutrients, grains and legumes are filling and satisfying. Most are easy to cook, and they contain little or no fat. Yet many

Slick Moves: Should You Change Your Oil?

Okay, the frying pan's in front of you. The salad stands ungarnished. Some oil seems to be called for. But which are the healthiest?

From a health standpoint, it looks as if two of the better choices in oils for cooking and salads are olive and canola oils, but only if they're used in limited quantities.

Why these two?

Both are high in monounsaturated fatty acids, which have been found to help control cholesterol. Additionally, olive oil may help protect against cardiac disease, according to studies at Stanford University. Researchers have found that olive oil can help reduce formation of unwanted blood clots that lead to stroke and heart attack. Plus, several studies on breast and colon cancer report that olive oil apparently doesn't promote tumors the way other oils can.

Many people use canola oil when they don't like the flavor that olive oil gives certain foods, particularly sweet baked goods. But a small amount of olive oil is delicious in a salad dressing. And you can use a small amount in frying, too, particularly for fish, or add just a few drops to the water when you're cooking pasta.

Quick bread and muffin recipes work well with the substitution of applesauce for three-quarters of the fat called for in the recipe. If a muffin recipe calls for ½ cup of butter, for instance, you can substitute two tablespoons of butter and six tablespoons of applesauce to make up for the loss of fat.

Then do a taste test. If the muffins have a good flavor and texture, try cutting back on the fat even more the next time. If they seem to lack some flavor, next time add more sweetener, vanilla, lemon or spices like cinnamon and nutmeg. Just look at the original recipe and figure out which spices and flavors you can enhance by adding more.

When making recipe substitutions, always watch the cooking times— especially when baking. Cooking times may vary according to the type of ingredient being substituted. If you substitute honey or maple syrup for sugar, for example, lower the oven temperature by 25°. These sweeteners brown faster than sugar.

people seem to think they're too much trouble to prepare.

But if you want to eat your fill of a healthful diet, you'll want to get used to preparing meals that include lots of whole grains and legumes. Peer into the low-fat pantry, and you'll find short-grain and long-grain brown rice; hot-cereal grains like rolled oats, millet, cream of rye and cream of brown rice; whole-grain flours like barley, oats, cornmeal, rye and buckwheat; and legumes like lentils, black-eyed peas, chick-peas and black, kidney, pinto and white beans.

We've provided many hints for success with these ingredients. You'll find cooking methods, cooking times and quality guidelines for the various legumes. There's also advice for baking quick breads that will be helpful when you get to the recipes in part 4. Of course, all these methods for phasing out fat in favorite recipes and using more whole grains and legumes are based on firsthand testing in our kitchen.

Tips on Trade-Offs

The truth is, successfully preserving taste while reducing fat takes experimentation. You'll find that some recipes are better-suited than others to little or no fat.

Since fat and salt are common flavor enhancers, when both of these ingredients are reduced or eliminated you may find the recipe a bit bland. Simply compensate by increasing the types and amounts of herbs and spices, which will bring out more flavor. (And in sweet-tasting recipes, you can add more sweetener.) When substituted for refined grains—white flour or white rice, for example—healthful whole grains not only bring unique flavors to recipes, they're also more filling and satisfying.

Eliminating the oil in some sauces will not alter the flavor very much, but cutting back the fat in baked goods can render them dry and tasteless if you're not careful. In other recipes, you'll find that you can easily cut the butter, margarine or oil in half with good results. And it's easy to make changes like substituting two egg whites for one whole egg or nonfat milk for whole milk.

Health from the Ground Up

One important part of the process for reducing fat in your family's favorite recipes is to reduce the quantity of
(continued on page 230)

Send in the Subs

This table will give you some good basic ideas on how even the simplest trade-offs in recipe ingredients can reduce the fat. Some of the suggested ingredient changes are direct substitutions—exchanging skim milk for whole milk, for example, which saves you eight grams of fat per cup. Others are rather cre-

Instead of...	Substitute...	Fat Reduction (grams)
Condiments, Sauces, Flavorings and Sweeteners		
⅔ cup mayonnaise	⅔ cup reduced-calorie mayonnaise	63
White sauce made with 1 cup whole milk and 2 Tbsp. flour and 2 Tbsp. margarine	White sauce made with 1 cup 1% low-fat milk and 2 Tbsp. flour	28
1 oz. unsweetened chocolate	1 oz. cocoa powder	15
1 oz. baking chocolate	3 Tbsp. unsweetened cocoa	13
1 Tbsp. mayonnaise	1 Tbsp. nonfat mayonnaise	11
4 Tbsp. fudge topping	4 Tbsp. fat-free fudge topping	8
Dairy Products and Eggs		
1 cup sour cream	1 cup nonfat sour cream	48
½ cup heavy cream	½ cup evaporated skim milk	44
4 oz. cream cheese	4 oz. nonfat cream cheese	40
4 oz. cream cheese	4 oz. Neufchâtel cheese	33
1 cup sour cream	1 cup reduced-fat sour cream (1 g. fat/Tbsp.)	32
8 oz. whole-milk ricotta cheese	8 oz. 1% fat cottage cheese	29
4 oz. Cheddar cheese	4 oz. reduced-fat Cheddar cheese (4 g. fat/oz.)	22
4 oz. Swiss cheese	3 oz. reduced-fat Swiss cheese slices, plus 1 oz. Swiss cheese	18
½ cup whole-milk ricotta cheese	½ cup nonfat ricotta cheese	16
1 cup whole milk	1 cup skim milk	8

ative—and are certainly worth a bit of experimentation.

What matters most is finding ingenious ways to keep the taste. Fortunately, taste often depends more on naturally low-fat or fat-free ingredients than on high-fat ones.

Instead of...	Substitute...	Fat Reduction (grams)
1 large egg	2 egg whites	5
10 oz. Cheddar cheese	10 oz. part-skim Cheddar cheese	4

Fats and Oils

1 cup oil	1 cup applesauce	218
½ cup butter, margarine or oil	¼ cup butter, margarine or oil	46
1 Tbsp. butter or margarine	1¼-second spray of vegetable spray	10

Meats and Fish

4 oz. regular ground beef, broiled	4 oz. ground turkey breast, broiled	22
1 lb. lean pork shoulder (before cooking)	1 lb. swordfish (before cooking)	20
4 oz. oil-packed light tuna	4 oz. water-packed light tuna	8
4 oz. chicken breast with skin, roasted	4 oz. skinless chicken breast, roasted	4

Snacks, Side Dishes and Desserts

1 cup buttered oil-popped popcorn	1 cup unbuttered air-popped popcorn	15
1 oz. dry-roasted peanuts	1 oz. roasted chestnuts	13
1 baked potato with 1 Tbsp. butter	1 baked potato with 1 Tbsp. nonfat sour cream and chives	11
1 croissant	1 bagel	10
1 oz. potato chips	1 oz. nonfat potato chips	10
½ cup vanilla premium ice cream	½ cup vanilla premium frozen yogurt	8
1 slice pizza with cheese and pepperoni	1 slice pizza with cheese and mushrooms	4
2 small chocolate chip cookies	2 fig bars	4

Phase Out Fat in Every Meal

The Youth Truth: Veggies Pare Off Years

Naturally, the snacks and recipes we recommend for low-fat living include lots of fresh fruits and vegetables. That makes sense, since they have little or no fat and are high in many nutrients that you need for energy.

But there's another bonus as well. They also contain substances that may slow aging processes in your cells, according to researchers.

Many fruits and vegetables contain vitamins and other natural substances that can help neutralize free radicals, molecular fragments that can harm body cells. And blocking free radicals is crucial to protecting your body from degenerative diseases and premature aging.

In other words, all those fruits and vegetables that help you maintain your good health while you're fighting fat can also help you look and feel younger.

But what exactly are free radicals, and how do certain nutrients stand in the way of their insidious attacks?

According to the widely accepted "free radical theory," unstable, highly reactive pieces of molecules darting among our cells react easily with oxygen, creating oxidation. And oxidation is what erodes things, causing metal to rust and fruit to rot. The free radicals in cells set off chain reactions, creating a destructive effect that biochemists call a cascade. The predominant damage is to DNA, the genetic material inside the nucleus of the cell. When DNA gets damaged, the aftereffects can lead to cancer, heart disease and premature aging.

When you get fresh fruits and vegetables in your diet, you're absorbing some substances called antioxidants. These are free radical quenchers that can short-circuit the oxidation process. These substances interfere with the madcap destruction caused by free radicals. The antioxidants in fresh produce are beta-carotene—which is found in brightly colored and dark green fresh vegetables—and vitamin C.

Other substances that help restrain free radicals are important B vitamins (B_1, B_6 and pantothenic acid), cysteine (an amino acid), zinc, selenium, catechols and indoles—protective substances found in potatoes and bananas. Add the radical-control benefits you get from chlorophyll, which is found in most green vegetables, and it's clear that fresh fruits and vegetables turn into all-around cell protectors.

beef, pork and other meats that you consume each week.

If you're not yet on a low-meat diet, we'll give you some guidelines for getting there gradually. It's often easier than most of us first imagine, and eating little or no meat is an important and health-enhancing dietary change.

A growing number of researchers and health organizations now advise moving toward a vegetarian diet that includes whole grains, beans and legumes, fruits, vegetables and low-fat or nonfat dairy products. Others recommend a semivegetarian diet, which allows room for limited amounts of skinless poultry or fish but includes little or no beef or pork.

The arguments in favor of a vegetarian or semivegetarian diet are supported by research. In a study at the University of Kuopio, Finland, medical researchers followed new vegetarians for seven months and found that their total blood cholesterol levels dropped by an average of 9 percent. The levels of HDL ("good" cholesterol) went up, which improved total cholesterol ratios by 2.5 percent. After seven months, 38 percent of the people who had recently gone on vegetarian diets reported that they felt more alert and vigorous and less fatigued.

A vegetarian cuisine can also affect mood. Researchers in a five-year Family Heart Study in Portland, Oregon, have reported that many people who adopt a diet low in fat and fried foods and rich in low-fat whole grains, fruits, vegetables and legumes experience fewer day-to-day feelings of "the blues." They also exhibit fewer feelings of anger. The study suggests that healthful low-fat eating—tending toward more vegetarian meals—may help people cope more effectively with everyday stresses.

In the past, some people have shied away from a vegetarian or semivegetarian diet on the assumption that meat provides nutrients that can't be found in fruits and vegetables. But medical researchers, after carefully studying tens of thousands of vegetarians over decades, have concluded that they are generally well-nourished. Better yet, this group has significantly fewer chronic degenerative diseases than the rest of the U.S. population.

As a group, vegetarians have been found to have lower blood pressure and more ideal blood cholesterol levels. Among vegetarians there is lower incidence of heart disease, osteoporosis, obesity, arthritis, diabetes and kidney disease. If you switch from a high-fat meat diet to low-fat vegetarian cuisine, you're likely to lower your risk of certain cancers, and you'll have a generally stronger immune system, studies show.

One reason vegetarian diets lower cancer risk is that fruits and vegetables contain fewer mutagens, substances that can lead to cancer. "Our working hypothesis is that mutagens in fried and broiled meats initiate, and high-fat diets promote, cancers of the breast, prostate and colon," say scientists at the American Health Foundation in Valhalla, New York. "Fried potatoes and similar foods contain some mutagens, but meats contain a thousand times more."

Painless Steps toward Lower-Meat Living

Day by day, you can take deliberate steps to trim the fat in your diet by shifting away from meat. Whether or not you cut it out entirely, you'll discover that what starts out as a bit of a challenge can become an enjoyable new habit. Here's how you can start to make it happen.

Eat fresh-baked bread and rolls. Consider making it a pleasurable weekly habit to bake some homemade bread. The aroma of bread baking is one of life's pleasures.

If you're short on time you might want to invest in one of the many kitchen bread-baking machines that are now available. Or check the Yellow Pages for your nearest whole-grain bakery (Great Harvest Bakery is one nationwide chain). Look for new flavors: Try some of the delicious fresh-baked 100 percent whole-grain, rye and pumpernickel breads, rolls and breadsticks.

Every meal can be accompanied by 100 percent whole-grain baked goods. The natural flavor of whole-grain bread is often so delicious that you'll be able to go light on the margarine or butter—and then, before long, skip it entirely.

Cut back on portions of red meat. Begin mathematically. Eat one-fifth less red meat this week. Take off another fifth next week. Perhaps, at the same time, you can substitute low-fat chicken or turkey breast or fresh fish for beef or pork. As you continue to reduce your portions, you can gradually turn meat into a mealtime "garnish."

A realistic step? Yes it is, at least for most of us. You might set an initial goal of having no more than one serving of lean meat, fish or poultry a day, limiting your portion to three or four ounces (the size of a deck of cards).

Go for more flavor enhancers. No one wants to change his diet unless the new meals and snacks have fresh, knockout tastes. Keep a condiment tray in the refrigerator, stocked with your favorite hot and spicy fixings—garlic, spices, salsas, chutneys and chow-chows—and flavor each meal the way you want it to taste.

Add variety—and zip—to your salads. Look for vegetables with color and great new flavors. When you stop by your local produce stand or explore the farmers market, be on the lookout for hundreds of possible additions to mealtime salads. Deep green spinach, purple kale and arugula are some increasingly popular options. You can always count on carrots, tomatoes, onions, broccoli and cauliflower. But what about a light sprinkling of diced apples, chopped nuts or very low fat shredded cheese for added taste?

Be willing to try new fat-free salad dressings as they show up in the supermarket, and watch for them in gourmet shops. Once you've identified the flavors you like, you can always make your own. In addition to the low-fat dressings in part 4, you have the option of making a quick dressing with a very small amount of olive oil followed by a good splash of balsamic vinegar or lemon juice, plus your favorite seasonings.

Fill in with fruits and veggies. By adding fresh produce to foods you already enjoy, you make a shift to low-fat eating while hanging on to some flavors you love. If tuna or chicken salad is your favorite, try making it with fat-free mayonnaise and chopped green or red peppers. Then add slices of tomatoes, onions or cucumbers—or all three. Serve on a bed of fresh green-leaf or romaine lettuce. In less than a minute, you can have an extra serving of vegetables while preserving the main part of your favorite-tasting salad or sandwich.

In stews and casseroles, add less meat and put in some extra vegetables, grains or pasta. If you're used to high-fat slices of ham or salami served on thin bread or crackers, replace the meat with crispy fresh slices of cucumbers, carrots, celery or zucchini. If you're serving an appetizer, try some broccoli or cauliflower florets, along with some guiltless spicy salsas and low-fat or fat-free creamy dips.

Shop the specialty foods section. Plan more low-meat or meatless meals with your favorite ethnic foods—flavorful Mexican, Tex-Mex, Asian, Italian and others.

Keep your kitchen well-stocked with vegetable soups, fat-free canned beans, low-fat whole-grain crackers, pastas, frozen fruit juices, just-ripe fruits and fresh spices. Broaden your menus with small sample servings of side dishes, soups or casseroles containing "exotic" new foods such as basmati rice, kasha, bulgur wheat, couscous, quinoa and soy tempeh.

Also consider trying some quick meals by stir-frying in a wok without meat and with little oil. As so many Americans have already discovered, your taste preferences may change faster than you think.

Create new low-fat meatless recipe favorites. Flip through your favorite cookbooks to find new recipes that call for little or no meat. Experiment with other low-fat substitutes—and pencil in your changes for future reference.

Update the heirlooms. Every family has favorite recipes, and some have been passed down through the generations. Transforming those culinary heirlooms to meet today's low-fat nutritional guidelines is a way to combine the best of both worlds. Keep the old recipes for sentimental value (Leslie attaches them to the back of the newly transformed version), but apply the principles in this chapter to cut the fat.

Each time you prepare an updated recipe, make sure you have a pencil handy to add any further revision ideas. When you hand these recipes down to the next generation in your family, you're not only passing on a tradition but also sharing a lower-fat version that promotes good health and good memories.

Cooking with Whole Grains

In addition to tailoring your recipes to make them lower in fat, you'll also want to use as many low-fat, high-nutrition, high-fiber ingredients as possible when you cook. For this purpose, you can't do better than whole grains.

Whole grains are a vital part of an optimal diet. Along with legumes, whole grains are the main constituent in the diets of long-lived, healthy people throughout the world. And the flour that's made from those grains is equally rich in nutrients.

Unfortunately, many people have a short supply of whole grains on their kitchen shelves. The grain products most commonly used in America are white rice, white all-purpose flour and small amounts of rolled oats for an occasional bowl of hot oatmeal or an oatmeal cookie.

As modern technology has spread to the food industry, refined grains have become more available and unrefined grains less so. And we definitely lose something when whole grains go through processing. When nutritious whole wheat is milled into white flour, we lose essential nutrients like the outer fiber-rich bran and highly nutritious germ that are ground off in the processing. White flour is often chemically bleached, which may entail problems of its own. Yet even though the end product is a pale imitation of the original whole-grain food, refined white flour is the only kind that many Americans use.

Rice, another important whole grain, also loses a lot when it's refined. Though the original brown rice is rich in fiber and nutrients, it reaches most kitchens as white rice. During processing, the outside of the rice is polished, removing the fiber-rich bran coating. Relatively few nutrients remain by the time it's cooked and served.

Your local supermarket may not have some of the whole grains that are such an important part of low-fat living, so to stock up, you may need to visit a natural foods, gourmet or ethnic gocery store. Or you can order some grains by mail. (See chapter 17 for a list of sources.) Once you have sources, you can buy grains in quantity, since they store well. Just be sure they're stored in tightly covered containers in a cool, dark, dry place. To store for more than a few months, keep whole grains and flour in the refrigerator or even the freezer, so they don't go rancid.

Cooking Grains for Entrées and Side Dishes

Cooking grains is simplicity itself. All you need are boiling water and the grain you're going to cook.

Different grains require different cooking times. At first it's a challenge to figure out how much dry grain you need in order to end up with the right amount to serve.

As a general guideline, you can plan on using about ½ cup of cooked grain per person. You'll find that you may want to use more or less, depending on the meal, the grain and personal preferences. For specific yields and cooking times, see the "Whole-Grain Cooking Chart" on page 236.

(continued on page 238)

Phase Out Fat in Every Meal

Whole-Grain Cooking Chart

Grain (1 cup raw)	Main Course/Side Dish Grains			Hot Cereal		
	Water (cups)	Cooking Time (min.)	Yield (cups)	Water (cups)	Cooking Time (min.)	Yield (cups)
Amaranth	2	15–25	2–2½	3	15–25	2½
Barley, hulled	2–2½	45–50	2–3	3	20–25	3
Brown rice	2	35–45	2–3	4	5–10	4
Buckwheat, hulled	2	15–20	2½–4	5	10–12	4
Cornmeal	3–4	25	3–4	4	5–10	4
Millet	2	20–25	2–3	3–4	20–30	4
Oats	2	45	2–2½	2	10–15	1¾
Quinoa	2	10–15	3	—	—	—
Rye	3–4	90	2⅔	3	10	3
Wheat	4	120–180	2½	4	15	4
Wild rice	2–3	35–45	3	4	45–60	4

Flour	Additional Comments
May be used as a thickener similiar to cornstarch or arrowroot. Good for sauces.	May be popped like popcorn. Use a frying pan without oil.
Similiar texture and flavor to wheat. Little gluten. A good substitute for wheat if eliminating gluten is desired.	Use barley flakes for hot cereal. The outer bran coating is polished off pearl barley; use only if hulled isn't available.
Granular, crumbly texture. Short-grain rice is best. Good combined with oat, millet, and barley flour.	Use rice ground into grits for hot cereal. Rice flakes also work well for hot cereal.
Dark, heavy, distinctive flavor. Good in buckwheat pancakes. Use unhulled buckwheat for flour.	White buckwheat is hulled and un-roasted—the best choice. Use flakes for hot cereal. Whole grain also works well.
Best used in cornbread or mixed whole-grain breads. High-lysine cornmeal is a good choice.	Use cornmeal for hot grain cereal. Use cornmeal or flour as a main-course grain—polenta.
Cakey texture. Good in sauces. Best mixed with rice, oat and barley flours.	Whole grain is used as a main-course grain and for hot cereal.
Moist texture. Unhulled oats are ground into flour. Rolled oats may be ground in blender to make flour.	Use rolled oats for hot cereal. Grits, groats and quick oats may also be used for hot cereal.
Whole grain may be ground into flour and used mixed with other whole-grain flours.	Just recently available in the U.S. Used mostly as a main-course grain.
Dark rye flour is best. Light rye has the outer bran coating removed.	Use quick-cooking flakes for hot cereal. Groats and regular flakes may also be used.
Significant gluten content. Best flour for yeast breads.	Use quick-cooking flakes for hot cereal. Use whole-wheat pastry flour for quick breads.
Moist texture. Best used with other whole-grain flours.	Use whole grain for cooking hot cereal.

Here's the basic procedure for cooking any grain.

1. Bring the required amount of water to a boil in a saucepan.

2. Slowly add the grain and bring to a boil again.

3. Reduce the heat to low, cover and simmer for the recommended amount of time, or until all the water is absorbed. The grains should be chewy, not pasty, tough, crunchy or hard.

4. Remove the pan from the heat and let stand, covered, for five to ten minutes. This produces a lighter, less sticky texture.

5. Gently fluff the grain with a fork and serve.

In addition, here are some tips that will help ensure your grain dishes are well-cooked, along with some ideas for adding more flavor.

■ Rinse grains only if they look dirty or have pieces of debris or if rinsing is called for in a recipe. Otherwise, it's not necessary. (One exception: Wild rice does have to be rinsed and drained before cooking.)

■ Don't stir grains during cooking. This makes them sticky and gummy instead of fluffy.

■ For additional flavor, add vegetable or chicken broth along with—or instead of—the cooking water. Or you can add some dry white wine to the cooking water.

■ Experiment with all sorts of herbs, spices and chopped vegetables, adding them to taste. Herbs and spices can be added to the water at any time during the cooking process. To make sure fresh vegetables stay crisp and don't get overcooked, add them near the end of the cooking time. If you're using frozen vegetables, they'll need only a couple of minutes in the pan at the end of the cycle, giving them just enough time to heat through.

Cooking Hot Whole-Grain Cereals

Eating a whole-grain cereal for breakfast is one of the best ways to start your day, and it takes only a few quick steps to mix up a bowlful. Use the "Whole-Grain Cooking Chart" on page 236 for the proportions and cooking times. Then follow these steps for cooking cereal.

1. Place the required amount of water in a saucepan.
2. Bring the water to a boil and stir in the cereal.
3. Bring to a boil again while stirring.
4. Reduce the heat to low and cook for the recommended time, stirring occasionally until the cereal attains a smooth, creamy consistency.
5. During the last few minutes of cooking, add your choice of sweetener, skim milk, nonfat yogurt, fresh or dried fruit, spices or ground nuts.
6. Remove from the heat and serve.

You can create infinite combinations of ingredients. Add fresh fruits that are in season. Try your whole-grain cereal with different flavors of yogurt and a wide variety of seasonings. Some people come up with a favorite—like the Bircher-Benner Muesli described in "The 'Master Breakfast' from Switzerland" on page 77—and stick with it. Others never get tired of trying new ingredients. It gives a fresh start to every day.

Making Quick Breads with Whole-Grain Flours

In part 4 you'll find two dozen recipes for delicious yeast breads that are made with whole-grain flours. In addition to being used to make yeast-risen breads, whole-wheat and other whole-grain flours may be used very successfully for quick breads that don't contain yeast and don't require kneading. Some of the most popular quick breads are in the form of muffins and biscuits, while others look like small loaves of regular bread when they're done.

Quick breads are made from batter that is poured into pans and baked immediately. The rising action comes from baking powder, baking soda or both. But since they don't contain yeast, quick breads tend to have a cakey texture. They usually are relatively sweet and somewhat higher in fat than yeast breads. And as the name implies, they take less preparation time because you don't have to allow time for the dough to rise, nor do you have to knead it before baking.

Whole-wheat pastry flour gives quick breads an excellent overall texture, but you can use any whole-grain flour, and a combination of flours works very well.

You'll find specific recipes for quick breads throughout the lunch and dinner menus in part 4. Once you have the knack of making quick breads, you'll find it's easy to come up with your own recipes, using any combination of grains, herbs, fruits and nuts that appeals to you. To help you out, here are several general tips for making any quick bread successfully.

■ Work quickly and do not overmix the batter.

■ Mix the dry ingredients and the wet ingredients in separate bowls. Use a large bowl for the dry ingredients, including flour, baking powder, baking soda, spices and dry sweetener. Use a smaller bowl for the wet ingredients, such as butter, margarine or oil, liquid sweeteners, milk, extracts and eggs. While the wet ingredients are still separate from the dry, oil the pans and preheat the oven.

■ Combine the wet and dry ingredients just before you're ready to pour the batter into the pan and pop it in the oven. Quickly pour the wet ingredients into the dry. With a rubber spatula, mix only until a smooth batter is formed and all the ingredients are incorporated.

■ When you think the bread is ready or when the timer rings, test the center of the loaf, muffin or cake with a toothpick. If the toothpick comes out dry or with a small bit of crumb on it, the bread is finished. But it needs to bake longer if the toothpick comes out wet.

Note: When you're testing a quick bread that's very low in fat, you can expect the toothpick to come out moist. But if there's uncooked batter on it, let the bread bake longer.

■ Once the quick bread is finished, remove it from the oven and let it cool for a few minutes. Then take it out of the pan and cool it on a rack. The bread should be cool to the touch before you cut it.

■ When you're making quick breads at high altitudes, you may need to slightly decrease the amounts of baking powder and sweetener and slightly increase the liquid called for in recipes.

Many quick bread recipes make two loaves. Whenever possible, I like to double the recipe to make four loaves. Quick breads freeze well, and you can thaw a frozen loaf quickly in the microwave. If you're more likely to be using one or two slices at a time, just slice the bread before freezing.

Over the years I've developed my own favorite whole-grain flour mix—the one I use for many of my quick breads, cookies, muffins and cakes. I've found that you can use this mix whenever a recipe calls for whole-grain flour or whole-wheat pastry flour. Simply mix equal amounts of barley flour, brown rice flour, oat flour and millet flour.

The flours can be mixed ahead, then stored in a tightly sealed container in a cool, dark, dry place. How much you mix, of course, depends on how often you bake bread. But as long as the flour is kept in a tightly sealed container, it's good for up to several months.

Selecting and Cooking Dried Legumes

Like whole grains and whole-grain foods, legumes are a staple for many of the world's healthiest and longest-lived people. Because they're highly nutritious and high in fiber, with very little saturated fat, legumes are an important part of a low-fat diet.

Legumes are the edible mature seeds that grow inside the pods of leguminous plants. This important food group, known for centuries as poor man's meat, includes beans, peas and lentils. Nearly all are inexpensive and easy to prepare. Dried legumes like navy beans, kidney beans and dried peas must be cooked a fairly long time to make them digestible. But some fresh legumes, including peas, green (string) beans and lima beans, cook very quickly, and some can even be eaten raw or lightly blanched.

Like grains, dried legumes are easy to store. Just make sure they're in tightly covered containers in a cool, dark, dry place. As long as moisture doesn't get to them, they should keep for months.

Legumes are usually sold in clear plastic bags, making it easy to check the quality before you buy. But you need to know what to look for. Here are some hints.

■ Choose bright, uniformly colored legumes. The ones that have a dull or faded color have been stored a longer time. It doesn't mean they've gone bad, but they may take a long time to cook.

■ Look for consistent size. The larger the size, the longer they take to cook. If different sizes are mixed together, some of the legumes will be undercooked while others will be overcooked.

■ If some of the legumes are cracked or shriveled or have pinholes, they may have insect damage.

The Presoak Method

It's no secret that the largest group of legumes—beans—is notorious for causing flatulence. But there's one cooking method that minimizes this problem. If you soak the beans in water, then discard the soaking water and add fresh water before cooking, you'll remove most of the indigestible carbohydrates called alpha-galactosides or trisaccharides, the villains that produce intestinal gas. Although some water-soluble vitamins may be lost by discarding the soaking water, the more easily digested legumes are still nutrient-rich.

These are the simple steps to preparing dried beans.

1. Measure out the quantity you need, using the amount given in your recipe or 1 cup.

2. Sort through the beans, removing any pebbles, dirt or grit. Also toss any that look cracked, shriveled or discolored.

3. Place the beans in a strainer or colander and rinse them under running water. Pour them into a large pot and fill the pot to the top with warm water.

4. Cover the pot and let the beans soak overnight. It's best to put the pot in the refrigerator if there's room.

5. In the morning, pour off the soaking water and refill with fresh water. Then let the beans soak in this water until you're ready to cook them.

When you're ready to start, pour off the soaking water and refill the pot with fresh water, using the minimum amount suggested in "Cooking Dried Legumes" as a guideline. Place the pot on the stove, bring the water to a boil, then reduce the heat to low. Partially cover the pot with the lid, but be sure to leave it slightly ajar. Some beans (especially chick-peas and soybeans) produce foam that will spill over the side if you cover the pot completely. During cooking, you can remove the foam easily with a large spoon.

6. Check the beans regularly to make certain they don't

Cooking Dried Legumes

This table gives cooking times for a variety of legumes, including beans, lentils, lima beans and split peas. It also shows the approximate yield of cooked legumes when you begin with one cup of dry measure.

Dry Legumes (1 cup)	Minimum Water (cups)	Cooking Time (hr.)*	Yield (cups)
Adzuki beans†	4	¾–1½	2½
Black (turtle) beans	4	1½–2	2–2½
Black-eyed peas	3–4	1	2
Chick-peas (garbanzos)	4	2½–3	3¼–4
Fava beans	3–4	1–1½	2½
Great Northern beans	3–4	1	2
Kidney beans	3	1½	2–2½
Lentils	3	¾–1	2–2¼
Lima beans, baby	2	1½	1¾
Lima beans, large	2	1½	1¼
Mung beans	3–4	3	2½
Navy or pea beans	2–3	1	2
Peas, whole	2–3	1–1½	2–2½
Pinto beans	3	2–2½	2
Red or pink beans, small	3	2½	2
Soybeans	3–4	3	2
Split peas	3	¾–1	2

*Cooking times may vary.
†Also called aduki or azuki beans.

overcook. (The "Cooking Dried Legumes" table also lists approximate cooking times.) To test whether they're done, lift one out with a spoon. Let it cool slightly and pinch it between your fingers or teeth. If the inside is soft and easy to press, with a texture similar to that of a well-cooked baked potato, remove the pot from the heat. Drain the beans, and they're ready to serve.

When cooking beans for use in salads, make sure they are firm but tender by keeping a careful watch on the pot and removing them at the appropriate time.

Quick-Cook Method

If you forget to soak the beans or if you've planned a meal too late for overnight soaking, here's a quick alternative.

1. Sort and rinse the beans as directed in Steps 2 and 3 above.

2. Put them into boiling water in a large pot. Or you can begin with cool water, put the beans in the pot and bring them to a rapid boil.

3. Boil for two to five minutes. Turn the heat off, cover the pot and let stand for at least one hour.

Pour off the soaking water, replace with fresh water and cook, using the quantities and times listed in "Cooking Dried Legumes" as general guidelines. Beans that have been prepared using this quick method may require a little more cooking time than ones that have been presoaked.

Unless a recipe indicates otherwise, you should always make sure the beans have almost finished cooking before you add most other ingredients. That's because fat, salt, broth, wine and acidic ingredients like tomatoes, vinegar, lemon and molasses will toughen the skins of the beans and create longer cooking times. But you can add garlic, onions, herbs and spices at any point without affecting the preparation time.

Cooked beans are easy to store. They keep in the refrigerator for up to a week and can be frozen for up to six months. So make a large batch each time you cook them and store the extra quantity. It's just an extra three steps to freeze your cooked legumes.

1. After cooking, drain the legumes well in a colander or strainer.

2. Let the legumes dry slightly and then put them into a tightly covered container.

3. Label and date the container and place it in the freezer.

Buying Precooked Legumes

Since soaking and relatively long cooking times are needed to prepare many legumes, one alternative is to buy precooked legumes that come in cans or jars. Since they're already prepared, all you need to do is heat them up.

Companies now sell legumes packed in plain water, without sodium. But often you'll find that salt has been added, so check the labels. If you would like to reduce the sodium content, rinse them under running water before heating them.

For salads and other cold dishes, just pour the cooked legumes into a colander. Rinse, then drain and serve without any further preparation. This is a convenient way to include these nutritious foods in your diet more often.

It's a good idea to check the labels for added ingredients besides sodium. Be on the lookout for preservatives, sugar, fats and artificial colors. Even if the can or jar says "all natural" on the front, you need to read the ingredient list, since the beans could have sugar, fats and other additions that may be natural but are definitely unnecessary and undesirable. My advice is that you simply choose other products.

Chapter Sixteen

Fight Fat When You Eat Out

Today, American families spend an average of 40 percent of their household food budgets at restaurants. Therefore, low-fat living is not only in our own hands but in the pots, pans and buffets controlled by chefs in America's 620,000 restaurants.

Chances are that your busy lifestyle often makes it necessary for you to eat meals and snacks away from home. But there's no reason why dining out has to be a dietary disaster. While many menu items are still loaded with fat and cholesterol, making healthy choices is becoming easier. Restaurants are adding more fresh salads, seafood, baked potatoes, grain/legume casseroles and side dishes, whole-grain breads and lower-fat pasta recipes to their menus. Nonetheless, you still need to watch out for hidden fats, especially in prepared cookies, muffins, piecrusts, cream sauces, soups and cheeses.

Here are some dining-out strategies that will help you meet your low-fat standards.

■ Skip all-you-can-eat buffets and smorgasbords.

■ Order à la carte, since full-course "bargain dinners" encourage overeating and tend to be too high in fat and protein.

■ If possible, look over the menu in advance or call ahead to ask about featured recipes and daily specials.

■ Don't be shy about making requests over the phone or in person. Many restaurants will eliminate salt, cook with half the fat (or no added fat) and cut back on cheese, eggs and whole-milk dairy products.

■ Look for restaurants that are listed by the American Heart Association as serving low-fat meals. You can write to 7300 Greenville Avenue, Dallas, TX 75231, for a printed list of restaurants in your area that serve low-fat meals.

■ Look for menus displaying small American Heart Association heart symbols on items that are "heart-healthy"—certified to be low in fat, cholesterol and sodium.

Giving Orders

Okay, you're seated inside your chosen restaurant, or you've approached the counter for takeout. You're scanning the menu, considering what looks good—and low-fat. Unfortunately, nothing on the menu tells you how many grams of fat you'll get from each serving. So what are the criteria for your choices? Here's a beginning.

Avoid all fried foods. Even if the restaurant claims that the food is fried in "healthy" vegetable oils, the frying process may produce trans-fatty acids that have been linked to a variety of health problems.

Curb your appetite for appetizers. Keep a watchful eye on high-fat items disguised as appetizers and positioned at the beginning of the menu. They're a common downfall when you're famished and you want "just a little something" to tide you over until the rest of the meal arrives.

Potato skins, tempura, deep-fried zucchini, mushrooms and mozzarella tempt us all with their crispy jackets of solid fat. If you want something while you're waiting, opt instead for ice water or iced tea and a slice or two of fresh-baked whole-grain bread. Or if the restaurant has a vegetable broth or non-creamy tomato soup, order that. Sip the beverage first and then savor each bite of the fresh bread or spoonful of soup.

Keep a salad watch. In many restaurants it pays to be a bit of a culinary detective when ordering salads. Salad bars are always a good choice if you choose the fresh vegetables, but stay away from the premixed salads (including coleslaw) that have a cream or heavy oil base, since they are usually high in fat. There are a couple of fixings you need to avoid, too: Olives have ⅓ to 1 gram of fat, and half an avocado contains over 30 grams of fat.

Dress for less excess. Unless you know a dressing is non-fat, order it on the side. One tablespoon of oil (of any kind) has 14 grams of fat.

Any dressing made with regular mayonnaise is a threat to your fat-watch, since everyday mayo weighs in at about 12 grams of fat per tablespoon. To keep control of the fat content of your salad dressing, you might request lemon or oil and vinegar, separately and on the side. That way you can gauge how much fat you're consuming by going very light on the oil (or drizzling lemon juice over the salad instead) and selecting a rich-tasting gourmet vinegar such as balsamic, champagne, raspberry or white or red wine.

French dressings in a heavy tomato base can be relatively low in fat. If you just sprinkle some on with a spoon, you can control the quantity. You might also want to take a small container of one of your own favorite dressings from home.

Do some fat subtraction from the main attraction. On to the entrée. When you're dining out, one of the major sources of fat can be a thick slab of beef or pork, fried fish or chicken or a dish swimming in cream, butter, margarine, cheese or oily sauce. Ask for foods prepared the low-fat way, such as sauce on the side, fish or skinless poultry cooked without any added fat and little or no cheese.

In general, choose entrées that are steamed, poached, broiled, roasted, baked or cooked in their own juices. Good restaurants will broil seafood or poultry dry (without fat) and unsalted. And if you want a low-fat sauce, just ask; the chef may be able to prepare one that's to your liking.

Savor suitable soup. The best restaurant soups are vegetable-based. Stay away from cream- and meat-based soups, since they're usually high in fat.

Don't cream the pasta. Any pasta is a good choice if it's served with tomato, wine or another low-fat sauce. But avoid thick, creamy, high-fat sauces.

Be grateful for grain. Whole-grain breads, rolls, bagels and low-fat muffins are delicious sources of fiber and complex carbohydrates. But skip the nut spreads, mayonnaise, butter and margarine.

If you're having breakfast in a restaurant, choose hot cereals such as oatmeal and multigrain varieties and whole-grain dry cereals. Have your cereal with skim milk, and count on fruit for added flavor.

Defat the dessert. When you choose to have dessert, make the portion small—or better yet, take a low-fat dessert home with you for an evening treat after you've had your walk. A slice of home-baked pie or cake is all right as a once-a-month option, but not more. If you really don't want fresh fruit, look for fruit-based desserts on the menu and order frozen sorbet, nonfat frozen yogurt or low-fat or nonfat pudding.

Watch quantities. Many eateries serve extra-large portions of food, which is a particular problem if you eat out often. If you're dining with other people, consider having a fresh salad with a bean, vegetable or grain side dish and a piece of whole-grain bread. When you know main servings are going to be large, split your entrée with another person.

Eat the World's Treats

Many ethnic and specialty restaurants offer exquisite-tasting cuisines that feature whole grains, legumes, vegetables and fruits and recipes supplemented with fish or poultry. Any cuisine that's new to you can tempt or challenge your taste buds— and if you go for meatless fare, you'll get low fat along with high flavor. Here are several insights about a number of our favorite cuisines.

Italian

Delicious low-fat foods with a pleasing array of tastes make Italian restaurants a good choice for dining away from home. Pasta with marinara (tomato-based), vegetable, red clam or wine sauce is first-rate. *Shrimp al vino blanco* (sautéed in white wine) gets high marks, too, for its low fat content.

If you see *pollo cacciatore* on the menu, it's another good option—boneless chicken breast served in a tomato and mushroom sauce. The list also includes nonmeat (vegetable) lasagna, but you need to ask for low-fat cheeses or less cheese. Or try cioppino—fisherman's stew with a variety of seafood and vegetables in a tomato-based stock—if you first make certain the stock is low in fat.

Enjoy pizza? Hold the olives, and ask for extra vegetables but one-half or one-third the normal amount of cheese. Onions, green peppers and mushrooms are good low-fat toppings, but you'll also want to try fresh spinach, garlic, tomatoes, artichoke hearts, beans, seafood, skinless turkey or chicken breast and other ingredients for an inviting change of pace.

Mexican

When chosen with care, Mexican food is inexpensive, delicious, high in complex carbohydrates and low in fat. Beans, rice, unfried corn tortillas, salsa, fish and salads are common staples. Vegetable-bean burritos, fresh fish marinated in lime sauce and beans with rice are low-fat specialties.

Some authentic Mexican recipes include distinctive vegetables with unique flavors. Jícama is a tropical fruit that looks similar to a rutabaga and tastes delicious. Occasionally, squash blossoms are served as a garnish. Whenever you have the opportunity, try tomatillos (similar to small, naturally green tomatoes), chayote (a pear-shaped squash) and nopal cactus. And of course, Mexico is famous for its delightful array of fresh peppers.

A good practice when selecting a new Mexican-style restaurant is to call ahead and ask if the chef uses lard, coconut oil or another oil in the refried beans. Many eateries have switched to small amounts of soybean oil or, ideally, add no fat at all.

Skip the sour cream, guacamole, red meat, pork and egg dishes as well as fried foods, and request no more than half the usual amount of cheese.

French

Each region of France can be recognized by its distinctive culinary riches. In recent years, food from the warm and sunny south of France—grilled seafood, vegetables, garlic and spices, cooked or served with splashes of olive oil—has become popular in America.

More French chefs than ever before are preparing nouvelle cuisine, including a special variety called *cuisine minceur* ("cuisine of slimness"). To create these low-fat specialties that preserve the French touch, chefs use culinary techniques such as steaming or poaching seafood or poultry in vegetable juices and wine and serving side dishes of fresh vegetables, potatoes and grains.

When you're offered dessert in a French restaurant, skip the tempting pastries and request fresh fruit. While it may seem hard to ignore the pastry tray, your meal will end on a wonderful high note if you choose poached fruit (usually peaches or pears). It's cooked in a light wine sauce, which adds a delightful flavor with few calories.

Spanish

A variety of culinary specialties from Spain emphasize beans, rice, fresh seafood or poultry, potatoes, peppers, garlic and fresh vegetables, with the flavor of olive oil that characterizes so much Mediterranean cooking. Spanish appetizers called *tapas* have gained popularity in America. Traditionally, these snacks include a wide range of hot and cold morsels—such as seafood, vegetables, olives and salads—served as midday and early-evening appetizers on large platters. Just be sure to bypass the egg dishes, fried foods and dishes that are loaded with sausage and other meats.

Indian

Recipes used in many Indian restaurants often include vegetables, legumes, yogurt and lots of spices. Avoid dishes soaked in coconut oil or ghee, which is clarified butter.

One popular recipe is *murg jalfraize*—chicken or legumes flavored with fresh spices and sautéed with onions, tomatoes and bell peppers. For the lowest-fat version of this dish, ask that it be sautéed without butter or oil.

Chinese

Some menu items at Chinese restaurants are good choices because of the emphasis on rice and vegetables, with only small amounts of seafood or poultry. Bypass the appetizer dishes such as egg rolls and spring rolls, they're usually deep-fried and just brimming with fat. And whatever you do, avoid duck: Just 3½ ounces of Peking duck has 30 grams of fat.

Stir-fried dishes generally get good low-fat ratings. They tend to be cooked quickly in a lightly oiled, very hot wok, and the vegetables retain more vitamins than those cooked the traditional American way. Also, the oil is usually peanut, which is high in monounsaturates—but always ask that the chef use as little oil as possible. One favorite low-fat stir-fry is *moo goo gai pan*, a combination of mushrooms, bamboo shoots, water chestnuts and chicken, seafood or tofu served over rice.

Japanese

Generally low in fat, Japanese cuisine is based on protein-rich soybean products such as tofu and tempeh as well as on seafood, vegetables, noodles and rice. The seaweed used in Japanese soups and stews is high in minerals. One top entrée choice is *yosenabe*, a vegetable dish with seafood.

American

Once you get away from American fast-food places and into some regional and specialty restaurants, you find healthful dishes and an array of dining options. Many restaurants in New England and on the West Coast have unbeatable selections of their own fresh seafood specials, served with salads that feature fresh vegetables and greens from nearby farms. Cajun restaurants are sprouting up all over—but beware the deep-fried food. Instead, order Cajun gumbos and other red-hot dishes; you'll get new flavors that quell your appetite while challenging your taste buds.

Restaurants that feature California cuisine—low-fat dishes with lots of fresh vegetables and beans—are also cropping up nationwide. Serving sizes are reasonable, and many cooks are exploring wonderful new ways to bring out the best flavors in fresh foods and legumes.

Delicatessen

Neighborhood delis are now everywhere. These make-it-to-order eating establishments range from bagel shops to full-service restaurants.

Delis usually have a wide variety of sandwich fixings. Good low-fat choices include fresh-roasted turkey breast and chicken breast and low-fat Swiss cheese. In many delis you'll also find vegetable fixings, gourmet spices, fresh-baked breads, salads and beverages, plus snacks and the best-tasting pickles in the United States. But stay away from the creamy prepared salads like potato salad, coleslaw and pasta salad, unless you find out for certain that they're made with low-fat or nonfat mayo.

Vegetarian

Although vegetarian restaurants serve nonmeat and even nondairy meals, many dishes tend to be high in fat. Watch for hidden cheeses and avoid items heavy with oil, butter or cream.

To discover new taste treats, choose fresh, whole-grain breads and grain/legume casseroles and side dishes. Many vegetarian cooks are doing great things with rice and pasta dishes, preparing them with low-fat sauces and a variety of fresh seasonal vegetables.

Taking Your Low-Fat Show on the Road

When you travel—for business or pleasure—you may find, as we have, that it really pays to preplan meals and snacks to reduce stress and keep your energy high.

Making a fast-food stop every time you want a drink or snack is a costly tactic not only in dollars but also in fat. Be prepared to stay hydrated and satisfy your appetite by taking along mineral water, iced tea, fruit juice and some of our low-fat snacks.

For full meals, if time is tight or your restaurant options are limited, prepare some low-fat picnic food in advance. Have a light meal in the car or stop at a scenic spot. If there's a slow-down due to weather or a traffic delay, you can pause for your on-the-road meal while you wait it out.

We often pack a small cooler with sandwiches and marinated salads in plastic containers, along with a few servings of a low-fat dessert. When Leslie and I are traveling by air on business, we slip a few sandwiches and snacks into briefcase, purse and boarding bag. And when the whole family goes along, we take a separate "food bag."

Packing low-fat food for a trip is fun, and it has made traveling the low-fat way feel more like a picnic. We never feel that we have to put up with bland, high-fat airport fare and roadside fast food.

Chapter Seventeen

Restock Your Pantry

It's no secret that one of the best and simplest ways to set yourself up for success is to re-engineer your environment, making it easy and convenient to choose low-fat foods at home. If your shelves are filled with high-fat goods, now is the time to clean them out and to stock up on ingredients that you'll find in the following lists.

Keeping ingredients on hand for low-fat meals and snacks means fewer trips to the store, saving both time and money. If you live in a small apartment, your pantry and freezer space may be very limited. But that's no reason to live with constant shortages of supplies you need.

Consider rearranging things, putting up some additional shelves and cleaning out part of a closet for some extra storage space for canned goods, grains and pastas. As you make the shift to low-fat living, keep making new lists of ingredients you need to have on hand. As you try the recipes in this book and create your own favorite low-fat meals by altering traditional recipes, you'll find that you'll need nearly all the ingredients listed here.

The Best Goods

As I've mentioned, you should keep a shopping list posted in plain sight, so it's handy to make notes whenever you notice you're running low on something. This consolidates supermarket trips and makes cooking much more enjoyable (few things are as irritating as deciding on a great recipe for a meal or snack and then discovering—in midrecipe—that someone has to run to the store or to a neighbor's house for a key ingredient).

Here's a very basic list of the essential ingredients we keep on hand for meals in minutes and for the recipes in part 4.

Breads and Pasta Products

Storage tip: Breads can be stored in the freezer and thawed as needed.

- Low-fat and nonfat whole-grain crackers
- Pastas (such as linguine, fettucine, spaghetti, angel hair, ziti, corkscrew, mostaccioli, shells, macaroni and spirals)
- Rye crackers (such as Wasa Crispbread, Ry-Krisp, Finn Crisps, Kavali and others without added fat)
- Whole-grain breads (if you don't have time to bake your own, consider a bread-baking machine or look in the Yellow Pages for bakeries that use 100 percent whole grains)
- Whole-wheat or corn tortillas or chapatis (Indian whole-wheat flatbreads)
- Whole-wheat pita bread

Canned Goods

- Artichoke hearts (packed in water)
- Chopped green chili peppers
- Cooking spray (olive oil and canola oil)
- Crushed or pureed tomatoes
- Evaporated skim milk
- Fruit (packed in fruit juice, without added sweeteners)
- Fruit juice

- Italian-style or regular whole tomatoes
- Legumes (such as chick-peas, black-eyed peas and navy, pinto, black and kidney beans)
- Pimentos
- Nonfat, low-sodium chicken broth
- Nonfat vegetable broth
- Pink or red salmon
- Refried beans (without lard or other fat)
- Salsa or picante sauce
- Tomato and/or vegetable juice
- Tomato paste
- Tomato sauce (with little or no added oil, fat or sodium)
- Tuna (packed in water)
- Water chestnuts

Dairy Products

- Low-fat Swiss cheese (such as Jarlsberg light)
- Nonfat cream cheese
- Nonfat or low-fat cultured buttermilk
- Nonfat or low-fat ricotta cheese
- Nonfat or 1 or 2 percent cottage cheese
- Nonfat plain yogurt
- Nonfat sour cream
- Parmesan cheese
- Part-skim Cheddar cheese
- Part-skim mozzarella cheese
- Skim milk
- Unsalted butter

Dry Goods

- Active dry yeast
- Arrowroot (which can be used instead of cornstarch)
- Baking powder
- Baking soda
- Carob powder or cocoa powder (regular and Dutch process)
- Dried fruits (such as raisins, currants and dates)
- Dried legumes (such as lentils, black-eyed peas, chick-peas and black, kidney, pinto and white beans)
- Low-fat or nonfat whole-grain cookies

- Nonfat dry milk
- Nonfat granola and a variety of low-fat whole-grain breakfast cereals
- Nuts and seeds (such as almonds, walnuts, pine nuts, pecans, pumpkin seeds, sunflower seeds, poppy seeds and hulled sesame seeds; stock and use them in small quantities, when they're as fresh as possible)
- Peanut butter (without added oil or sweetener)
- Taco shells
- Tahini (sesame-seed butter)
- Very low fat or nonfat snacks (such as pretzels and baked tortilla chips)

Grains and Flours

Storage tip: It's generally a good idea to keep flour in the freezer in an airtight bag.

- Brown rice (try short-grain for risotto and long-grain, such as brown basmati rice, for most other dishes)
- Couscous
- Hot-cereal grains (such as old-fashioned rolled oats, millet, cream of rye and cream of brown rice)
- Hulled barley
- Popcorn
- Unbleached flour
- Whole-grain flours (such as whole-wheat flour, whole-wheat pastry flour, barley, oat, cornmeal, rye, buckwheat, millet and brown rice flours)

Herbs, Spices and Dry Seasonings

- Allspice
- Basil
- Bay leaves
- Caraway
- Cayenne pepper
- Celery seeds
- Chili powder (there are many varieties, from mild to extra-hot)
- Cinnamon
- Cloves
- Coriander
- Cream of tartar

- Cumin
- Curry
- Dill
- Garlic (granulated or powdered)
- Ginger
- Marjoram
- Mustard powder
- Nutmeg
- Oregano
- Paprika
- Peppercorns (either black peppercorns or a mixture of different types)
- Red-pepper flakes
- Rosemary
- Saffron (very expensive, but a little goes a long way; be sure to get real saffron, which is made from crocus-flower stigmas, not safflower)
- Sage
- Salt
- Tarragon
- Thyme
- Turmeric

Miscellaneous Perishables

- Eggs (grade A large) or egg substitute
- Fresh fruit
- Fresh herbs (such as parsley, basil and cilantro)
- Fresh or frozen poultry
- Fresh or frozen seafood
- Fresh or frozen vegetables
- Frozen fruit (such as unsweetened berries and peaches)
- Garlic
- Lemons and limes
- Mushrooms
- Onions (yellow, white and red)
- Potatoes and yams
- Tomatoes

Oils, Condiments and Wet Seasonings

- Applesauce, unsweetened (a great substitute for fat in some baked-good recipes)

- Canola oil
- Chili puree with garlic (for added seasoning in Asian dishes)
- Flavored natural extracts (especially vanilla, lemon, orange and almond)
- Hot-pepper sauce
- Jam (all-fruit), jelly, conserves, preserves and spreads
- Ketchup
- Liquid smoke (to add the flavor of ham or bacon without added fat)
- Mustard (such as Dijon-style and country or stone-ground)
- Nonfat and low-fat mayonnaise
- Nonfat marinades
- Nonfat salad dressings
- Olive oil
- Soy sauce (reduced-sodium is best)
- Steak sauce (such as A-1)
- Very low fat and nonfat soups
- Vinegars (such as balsamic, white wine, red wine, champagne, raspberry and rice wine; good-quality, well-flavored vinegars make it easier to reduce the amount of oil needed in salads and dressings)
- Wine for cooking (dry red and white and cooking sherry)
- Worcestershire sauce

Sweeteners

- Brown sugar
- Honey
- Maple syrup
- Molasses
- Sugar

Wielding the Right Utensils

The right kitchen tools are essential—and in the long run they make preparation time shorter and easier. There are some custom-designed utensils you'll want for low-fat cooking. Here's a short list of those that are indispensable in our kitchen because they make cooking tasks easier and faster.

Food processor. Shop around to choose the kitchen marvel that best suits your needs and budget. A food processor saves you time when chopping, slicing, mixing and pureeing.

Garlic press. This is one of the tools used most often in our kitchen. For fresh garlic in any recipe, remove a clove of garlic from its head and lightly crush it under a cutting board or by using your palm to crack the skin. Peel the clove, place it inside the press and squeeze. The traditional method of chopping the garlic into fine pieces takes minutes longer.

Handheld electric mixer. This low-cost item comes in handy. We use ours to beat the yeast and a little flour, for example, when making whole-grain bread or rolls; this technique helps develop the gluten and creates a better texture. The mixer is also handy for beating egg whites.

Kitchen knives. There are many advantages to having a set of good-quality kitchen knives. Once you've chosen a set, keep them sharp. A wooden block that holds the knives is a good investment; the knives stay in much better condition if they aren't clanging against each other in a drawer. Use a chef's sharpening steel to keep your knives razor-sharp.

Lemon juicer. For several dollars you can get a little contraption that squeezes juice from lemons while screening out the seeds. It's a good time-saver.

No-stick pans. We love our no-stick frying pans, and other no-stick pans help to eliminate or dramatically lower the amount of fat necessary to prevent foods from sticking to the cooking surface.

Salad spinner. Available in most kitchen and hardware stores, this gadget is a big help whenever fresh lettuce and other salad greens are called for. After washing the lettuce, you spin it dry in the easy-turn container. No more wet towels and wasted time hand-drying each leaf before making a salad.

Shopping Cart Blanche: Meals and Wares by Mail

Every low-fat cook needs access to supplies, and there's no guarantee that your neighborhood has the fresh-stocked foods or utensils you need. If you have any trouble finding the freshest, best-tasting ingredients for some of our recipes, here are some of our favorite mail-order companies, which offer everything from organic whole grains and spices to canned products, fresh produce and balsamic vinegar. Some of these companies are also excellent sources of quality cooking utensils.

■ American Spoon Foods (P.O. Box 566, Petoskey, MI 49770). Tucked away in rural northern Michigan, this company offers a memorable array of the state's wild and domestic fruits, honeys, nut-meats, wild mushrooms, fruit preserves, jellies, conserves, fruit butters and dried fruits.

■ The Chef's Catalog (3215 Commercial Avenue, Northbrook, IL 60062). Offers professional-style kitchen equipment and useful home-kitchen utensils, from knives and wine racks to pasta machines, food processors, garlic presses and all sorts of obscure but immensely useful kitchen gadgets.

■ Dean and Deluca (560 Broadway, New York, NY 10012). A great mail-order source for high-taste foods and ingredients from around the world, including everything from pastas, grains, beans, teas, oils and specialty vinegars to cookware and kitchen tools.

■ Diamond Organics (P.O. Box 2159, Freedom, CA 95019). Shopping for the freshest organic produce has never been easier. Order with a credit card, and Diamond Organics will ship freshly picked fruits, vegetables and herbs (backed by an unconditional guarantee) by overnight delivery. Other than those from our own garden, the best salad fixings we've ever eaten have come from Diamond Organics. Consider splitting an order with friends or neighbors to divide the shipping costs.

■ Southwest Gourmet Gallery (Sinagua Plaza, Suite D, 320 North Highway 89A, Sedona, AZ 86336). Far and away our favorite mail-order source for fresh, flavor-packed salsas, sauces, marinades, mustards and seasoning spices.

■ Walnut Acres (Penns Creek, PA 17862). Walnut Acres has been farming organically since 1946. The catalog includes over 40 pages filled with foods grown on this farm or carefully selected from reputable outside suppliers.

Fresh-Start Recipes for Low-Fat Living

The truth is, all the nutritional guidelines in the world won't result in better health and energy if you can't bring the low-fat dietary principles to life in your kitchen. "What we need," wrote the late Jean Mayer, Ph.D., an internationally known nutritionist and former president of Tufts University in Medford, Massachusetts, "are practical examples . . . in the preparation of delicious light cuisine. And well-written recipes can give consumers all the information they need to do this, right down to the portion sizes."

I believe that the following pages are a shining example of what Dr. Mayer called for. These recipes and sample menus for low-fat living were prepared, tested and written by my wife, Leslie (author of *America's New Low-Fat Cuisine*). Leslie and I and our children have been following the Low-Fat Living Program for years, getting renewed energy and enjoying wonderful flavors every time we make these recipes.

No matter how busy or hectic our lives have been, the meals and snacks that you'll discover on the pages ahead have contributed much enjoyment to our days. My enthusiasm for these

Part

4

recipes is confirmed by the many people who have attended Leslie's courses and who have tested the menus with their own families and friends.

Feasting on Fruits of the Earth

Consistent with the low-fat recommendations of various health organizations, many of the recipes in this section of the book are vegetarian. But Leslie has also included delicious options for meals with seafood and poultry. Every daily menu offers a great-tasting variety of nutrient-packed vegetables, whole grains, legumes and other healthy foods.

You can mix and match meals and menus for added variety, using our suggestions as a starting point for creating more of your own new favorite recipes. Each recipe has a full analysis, including fat, saturated fat, cholesterol, total calories and fiber, as well as other nutritional information.

In each of the complete meals, no more than 25 percent of calories come from fat. For some of the individual recipes, however, the amount of calories from fat is somewhat higher. To be sure that the total meal is low-fat, be sure you don't exceed the recommended serving size for each part of the meal.

What's it like to taste the results of Leslie's cooking skills? Let's just say I'm lucky. She's an exceptional chef who has passionately and insightfully studied culinary traditions from around the world. In our kitchen, she has designed and created the most pleasurable and memorable low-fat meals and snacks I've ever tasted.

These recipes and meal plans have made everyday low-fat living more achievable and enjoyable than I ever imagined it could be.

To my mind and heart this is not just a special section of recipes. It's a bright and timely nutritional invitation to you and your loved ones to begin a lifetime of highly enjoyable low-fat living. And that's one of the best investments you can make.

Chapter Eighteen

Fresh-Start Recipes for Low-Fat Lunches

S oups, salads and sandwiches are standard lunchtime fare for many families. And that's fine for low-fat living. But I like to remind people of the wonderful variety of combinations and flavors that you can pack in a lunchtime menu. From Thick and Zesty Gazpacho to Citrus-Season Salad with Ginger-Horseradish Dressing, here are two weeks of favorite lunch menus. Some of these recipes are best if made with fresh ingredients, so you'll want to check your local supermarket for the fruits and vegetables that are in season. Others can be prepared any time of year. In addition to a variety of soups, salads and sandwiches, you'll also find some easy-to-prepare "imports," such as baked falafel, quesadillas and oriental noodles.

For easy reference, here are the 14 fresh-start lunch menus in this chapter.

Day 1

Thick and Zesty Gazpacho (page 268)
Green Chili and Cheddar Buttermilk Biscuits (page 270)

Day 2

Linguine Frittata with Broccoli (page 271)
Oatmeal Soda Bread (page 273)
Mixed Greens with Peach and Pecan Dressing (page 274)

Day 3

Hummus in Pita Sandwiches (page 275)
Israeli Salad (page 276)

Day 4

Chicken Salad with Peaches and Pecans (page 277)
or Chicken and Wheat Berry Salad (page 278)
Cracked-Wheat Quick Bread (page 280)

Day 5

Ratatouille and Grilled Mozzarella
Sandwiches (page 281)
Cucumber and Red Grape Salad (page 282)

Day 6

Middle Eastern Baked Falafel (page 283)
Dilled Cucumber Salad (page 285)

Day 7

Greek Pasta Salad (page 286)
Whole-Wheat French Bread (page 399)

Day 8

Quesadillas (page 288)
Sweet Pea Guacamole (page 289)
Four-Bean Salad with Balsamic Vinaigrette (page 290)

Day 9

Peasants' Salad Pita Pockets (page 291)
Roasted Chestnut and Wild Rice Soup (page 292)

Day 10

Tex-Mex Pasta Salad (page 294)

Day 11

Autumn's Acorn Cheddar Soup (page 296)
Colorful Corn Relish (page 297)
Gingerbread Muffins (page 298)

Day 12

Oriental Noodles (page 299)
Wonton Chips (page 300)

Day 13

Thick and Hearty Vegetable Chili (page 302)
or Southwestern Chicken Chili (page 303)
Old-Fashioned Cornbread (page 304)

Day 14

Lentil Spread in Pita Pockets (page 305)
Citrus-Season Salad with Ginger-Horseradish Dressing
(page 307)

Day 1

Thick and Zesty Gazpacho
Green Chili and Cheddar Buttermilk Biscuits

This meal has lots of flavor.

You can make the soup ahead of time and keep it refrigerated, and the biscuits are quick and easy to make.

Serve two biscuits with a bowl of soup.

NUTRITIONAL ANALYSIS FOR LUNCH

Per serving: 414 calories, 10.7 g. total fat (23% of calories), 2.9 g. monounsaturated fat, 0.8 g. polyunsaturated fat, 4.2 g. saturated fat, 17.8 g. protein, 67.2 g. carbohydrate, 8.3 g. dietary fiber, 16 mg. cholesterol, 1,267 mg. sodium

Thick and Zesty Gazpacho

FRESH-START COOKING TIP
If you substitute dried herbs for fresh, remember that they are much stronger; use only one-quarter to one-third as much.

Gazpacho is a delicious chilled, tomato-based vegetable soup. It makes a perfect summer's meal. You can take it along on picnics if you chill it well beforehand and pour it into a widemouthed Thermos.

Like other uncooked, cold soups, gazpacho relies on the vegetables for thickness and flavor. In the recipe below, you'll find that I've suggested a number of variations to produce different flavors—vegetable juice cocktail instead of tomato juice, chopped red peppers or pimentos and either fresh or dried herbs.

As the name suggests, my interpretation is slightly spicy (you can increase or decrease the seasoning) and filled with chunks of vegetables.

Even though the recipe has quite a few ingredients, it's very fast and easy to make.

To shorten the chilling time, refrigerate the juice and vegetables ahead of time.

Garnish the soup with whole-wheat croutons and chopped chives, if desired.

4 cups tomato juice or vegetable juice cocktail

1 large onion, finely chopped

1 green pepper, chopped

1 cucumber, chopped

2 tomatoes, finely chopped

1½ cups cooked chick-peas or 1½ cups canned chick-peas, rinsed and drained

¼ cup chopped roasted red peppers or pimentos

2 large cloves garlic, minced

2 tablespoons red-wine vinegar

2 tablespoons minced fresh parsley

⅓ teaspoons minced fresh cilantro

1 tablespoon olive oil

1 tablespoon honey or sugar

1 tablespoon minced fresh basil or 1 teaspoon dried

1 tablespoon minced fresh dill or 1 teaspoon dried

½ teaspoon dried tarragon

½ teaspoon dried thyme

¼ teaspoon ground cumin

Freshly ground black pepper

Hot-pepper sauce

6 tablespoons nonfat sour cream or yogurt

PREPARATION TIME: 15–20 MINUTES

CHILLING TIME: 1–2 HOURS OR MORE

In a large bowl, mix the tomato juice or vegetable juice cocktail, onions, green peppers, cucumbers, tomatoes, chick-peas and red peppers or pimentos.

Add the garlic, vinegar, parsley, cilantro, oil, honey or sugar, basil, dill, tarragon, thyme, cumin and black pepper and hot-pepper sauce to taste.

Mix well.

Chill for 1 to 2 hours or more.

Serve in 6 individual bowls. Top each serving with 1 tablespoon of the sour cream or yogurt.

Per serving: 198 calories, 3.9 g. total fat (17% of calories), 1.7 g. monounsaturated fat, 0.3 g. polyunsaturated fat, 0.4 g. saturated fat, 8.6 g. protein, 35.2 g. carbohydrate, 3.7 g. dietary fiber, 0 mg. cholesterol, 621 mg. sodium

Serves 6

Low-Fat Lunches

Green Chili and Cheddar
Buttermilk Biscuits

Biscuits are traditionally made with white flour and lots of butter, creating a very tasty yet high-fat addition to a meal. I've worked years on developing a low-fat whole-grain biscuit that has light crumbs, a semitraditional flavor and airy texture.

Here I've added green chili peppers and Cheddar cheese to the basic recipe, giving the biscuits a southwestern flair. If you can find low-fat sharp Cheddar, it works exceptionally well.

1¾	cups whole-wheat pastry flour
1	tablespoon baking powder
1	teaspoon sugar
¼	teaspoon baking soda
¼	teaspoon salt
2	tablespoons unsalted butter or margarine
1	cup nonfat buttermilk
3	ounces low-fat Cheddar cheese, shredded
2	ounces canned green chili peppers, chopped

In a medium bowl, mix the flour, baking powder, sugar, baking soda and salt.

Preheat the oven to 450°.

Using a pastry blender or 2 knives, cut the butter or margarine into the flour mixture to make fine crumbs.

Using a fork, very gently stir the buttermilk, Cheddar and peppers into the flour mixture; stir only until mixed.

Using a large spoon, drop the mixture into 12 mounds on a baking sheet. Bake for 12 to 15 minutes, or until the biscuits are lightly browned on top. Serve at once.

Per 2 biscuits: 216 calories, 6.8 g. total fat (27% of calories), 1.2 g. monounsaturated fat, 0.5 g. polyunsaturated fat, 3.8 g. saturated fat, 9.2 g. protein, 32 g. carbohydrate, 4.6 g. dietary fiber, 16 mg. cholesterol, 646 mg. sodium

Makes 12

Day 2

Linguine Frittata with Broccoli
Oatmeal Soda Bread
Mixed Greens with Peach and Pecan Dressing

Eggs can fit nicely into a healthy, low-fat meal plan if you cut back on the number of yolks you eat and combine them with egg substitute. They supply good-quality protein. Eggs are also a good source of iron, especially if you eat them with fruits and vegetables high in vitamin C, which enhances the absorption of iron.

Frittata is an Italian version of a French omelet, although it's a bit drier and easier to make.

The delicious Oatmeal Soda Bread takes less than 1 hour from start to finish.

For a quicker lunch, you can substitute any crusty whole-grain bread and nonfat salad dressing.

NUTRITIONAL ANALYSIS FOR LUNCH

Per serving: 479 calories, 11 g. total fat (21% of calories), 2.4 g. monounsaturated fat, 2.3 g. polyunsaturated fat, 1.5 g. saturated fat, 29.5 g. protein, 71.8 g. carbohydrate, 13 g. dietary fiber, 116 mg. cholesterol, 553 mg. sodium

Linguine Frittata with Broccoli

The filling is what gives a frittata its uniqueness, and the eggs are what bind it together.

Just about anything can go into a frittata—vegetables, dried tomatoes, potatoes, seafood, cheese, fresh herbs and virtually anything else that sounds appealing.

Frittatas are a great way to use up last night's leftover pasta. The filling ingredients are combined with the eggs and then cooked slowly in a frying pan.

The final touch is placing the frying pan under the broiler to finish cooking the eggs until golden.

Frittatas are good served hot or at room temperature.

PREPARATION
AND COOKING
TIME: 20–30
MINUTES

2   eggs
1   cup fat-free egg substitute
2   tablespoons nonfat sour cream
½   cup shredded low-fat Swiss cheese
1   cup cold cooked linguine
2   tablespoons sliced roasted red peppers
    Salt
    Freshly ground black pepper
1   shallot, chopped
1   clove garlic, minced
1   cup broccoli florets, broken into small pieces

In a medium bowl, whisk together the eggs, egg substitute and sour cream until smooth.

Stir in the Swiss, linguine and red peppers. Season with the salt and black pepper. Set aside.

Lightly coat a large no-stick, oven-safe frying pan with no-stick spray. Add the shallots, garlic and broccoli. Cook over medium heat for 5 minutes, or until the shallots are wilted and the broccoli is bright green.

Stir the broccoli mixture into the egg mixture and quickly pour it back into the frying pan. Cook the mixture over medium-low heat. Be sure the heat is low enough to cook the eggs slowly and not burn the bottom. Rotate the pan several times during cooking, so the bottom of the frittata cooks evenly.

Preheat the broiler and place the top rack at least 5″ from the heating unit.

When the bottom of the frittata begins to brown and the sides begin to cook, transfer the frying pan to the broiler. Cook the frittata for a few minutes, until the top begins to brown.

If the center of the frittata is not fully cooked, place it back beneath the broiler on the bottom rack to finish cooking.

Cut the frittata into 4 wedges. Serve slightly cooled or at room temperature.

FRESH-START COOKING TIP
You can eliminate the fat and cholesterol in many recipes by substituting two egg whites for each whole egg—a savings of five grams of fat per egg yolk. In most recipes, nonfat egg substitute also works well.

Per serving: 176 calories, 6.3 g. total fat (32% of calories), 1 g. monounsaturated fat, 0.4 g. polyunsaturated fat, 0.8 g. saturated fat, 15.8 g. protein, 14.8 g. carbohydrate, 1.2 g. dietary fiber, 116 mg. cholesterol, 147 mg. sodium

Serves 4

Oatmeal Soda Bread

This is a quick and easy bread to make. As the name suggests, it's made with baking soda as a leavening agent. This recipe calls for whole-wheat pastry flour, but you can use any whole-grain flour. The loaf has a very decorative crust, covered with rolled oats. If you don't have buttermilk, make your own by adding 2½ tablespoons lemon juice to 1¼ cups warm skim milk.

FRESH-START COOKING TIP
Keep extra loaves of bread in the freezer. You can quickly defrost a loaf of bread to round out a fast meal, adding extra fiber and complex carbohydrates.

3	cups whole-wheat pastry flour
1	teaspoon baking soda
1	teaspoon baking powder
½	teaspoon salt
1	tablespoon honey
¾	cup rolled oats
1½	cups nonfat buttermilk

PREPARATION TIME: 15 MINUTES

BAKING TIME: 30–40 MINUTES

Preheat the oven to 375°. Lightly coat a baking sheet with no-stick spray. In a large bowl, combine the flour, baking soda, baking powder, salt, honey and ½ cup of the oats.

Make a well in the center of the flour mixture. Pour in the buttermilk and stir to combine.

Spread the remaining ¼ cup oats onto a countertop or another clean, flat surface. Turn the dough out onto the oats and knead a few times. The dough should be smooth, round and covered with a thick layer of oats.

Place the dough on the prepared baking sheet. Using a sharp knife, cut an X about ½" deep on the top. Lightly coat the top with no-stick spray.

Bake for 30 to 40 minutes, or until the bread sounds hollow when tapped on the bottom.

Place the bread on a rack to cool slightly before slicing.

Per serving: 234 calories, 1.9 g. total fat (7% of calories), 0.4 g. monounsaturated fat, 0.7 g. polyunsaturated fat, 0.4 g. saturated fat, 10.2 g. protein, 46.8 g. carbohydrate, 7.6 g. dietary fiber, 0 mg. cholesterol, 328 mg. sodium

Serves 4

Low-Fat Lunches

Mixed Greens with Peach and Pecan Dressing

You can use any mild oil in this dressing, but walnut oil creates the nicest flavor.

PREPARATION TIME: 10 MINUTES

8	cups mixed greens torn into bite-size pieces
1	peach, quartered
1½	tablespoons white-wine vinegar
1½	tablespoons nonfat chicken broth or water
1	teaspoon walnut oil
¼	teaspoon sugar or honey
⅛	teaspoon dried thyme
⅛	teaspoon freshly ground black pepper
3	pecan halves

Divide the greens among 4 individual salad plates. Set aside.

In a blender or food processor, combine the peaches, vinegar, broth or water, oil, sugar or honey, thyme, pepper and pecans. Mix until smooth. Spoon over the greens to serve.

Per serving: 69 calories, 2.8 g. total fat (32% of calories), 1 g. monounsaturated fat, 1.2 g. polyunsaturated fat, 0.3 g. saturated fat, 3.5 g. protein, 10.2 g. carbohydrate, 4.2 g. dietary fiber, 0 mg. cholesterol, 78 mg. sodium

Serves 8

Day 3

Hummus in Pita Sandwiches
Israeli Salad

This sandwich-and-salad meal is easy to fix and keeps well in the refrigerator. Though traditional hummus is made with quite a bit of oil, here's a lower-fat version.

NUTRITIONAL ANALYSIS FOR LUNCH

Per serving: 315 calories, 6.9 g. total fat (20% of calories), 1.1 g. monounsaturated fat, 0.5 g. polyunsaturated fat, 0.3 g. saturated fat, 13.4 g. protein, 53.4 g. carbohydrate, 4.6 g. dietary fiber, 0 mg. cholesterol, 242 mg. sodium

Hummus in Pita Sandwiches

Hummus is a spread made from chick-peas (also known as garbanzo beans) and tahini (sesame-seed paste). It's the perfect filling for pita bread. This Middle Eastern sandwich is delicious any time of year. It is very easy to make and provides a great fast meal if you use canned chick-peas.

2 cups cooked chick-peas or 2 cups canned chick-peas, rinsed and drained
¼ cup lemon juice
2 cloves garlic
2 tablespoons unroasted tahini
2 tablespoons minced fresh parsley
¼ teaspoon ground cumin
¼ teaspoon ground coriander
 Freshly ground black pepper
 Ground red pepper or hot-pepper sauce
 Salt (optional)
6 whole-wheat pita breads
3 tomatoes, sliced
½ small onion, thinly sliced
12 leaves leaf lettuce
 Alfalfa sprouts (optional)

PREPARATION TIME: 15 MINUTES

In a blender or food processor, combine the chick-peas, lemon juice, garlic, tahini, parsley, cumin, coriander and black pepper, red pepper or hot-pepper sauce and salt (if using) to taste. Puree until very smooth and creamy. Add a little water to thin slightly, if necessary.

Cut the pitas in half and spread the hummus inside each pocket. Add the tomatoes and onions and fill with lettuce and sprouts (if using).

Per serving: 266 calories, 5 g. total fat (16% of calories), 0.05 g. monounsaturated fat, 0.2 g. polyunsaturated fat, 0.05 g. saturated fat, 12 g. protein, 45.4 g. carbohydrate, 2.6 g. dietary fiber, 0 mg. cholesterol, 233 mg. sodium

Serves 6

PREPARATION TIME:
10 MINUTES

MARINATING TIME: 1 HOUR OR MORE

Israeli Salad

In season, the outdoor markets in Israel are filled with an abundance of juicy red tomatoes, crunchy cucumbers and very inexpensive red and yellow peppers.

This salad is crisp, light and refreshing, not oily. For an added burst of color, use a mixture of green, red and yellow peppers.

FRESH-START COOKING TIP

Fresh herbs such as basil and cilantro can easily be frozen. They're almost as good as fresh when you take them out of the freezer to use in soups, stews or casseroles. For freezing, remove the large stems from the herbs, rinse and dry well. Pack the herbs, whole, into a pint-size resealable freezer bag. Squeeze out as much air as possible, label the bag and store in the freezer. To use, remove from the freezer and crush the herbs in the sealed bag. Use as much as you need and return the rest to the freezer.

2	large cucumbers, peeled and cubed
2	tomatoes, cubed
1	small red onion, chopped
1	green, red or yellow pepper, diced
1	yellow summer squash, cubed
¼	cup nonfat chicken broth
2	tablespoons olive oil
2	tablespoons lemon juice
1	large clove garlic, minced
1	tablespoon minced fresh basil or 1 teaspoon dried
½	teaspoon dried oregano
	Salt (optional)
	Freshly ground black pepper

In a large bowl, combine the cucumbers, tomatoes, onions, green, red or yellow peppers and squash. Set aside.

In a small cup, mix the broth, oil, lemon juice, garlic, basil, oregano and salt (if using) and black pepper to taste. Pour over the vegetables and toss gently.

Cover and marinate at room temperature for at least 1 hour (the longer the salad marinates, the more flavor it will have); toss occasionally.

Taste to adjust seasonings before serving.

Per serving: 49 calories, 1.9 g. total fat (31% of calories), 1.1 g. monounsaturated fat, 0.3 g. polyunsaturated fat, 0.3 g. saturated fat, 1.4 g. protein, 8 g. carbohydrate, 2 g. dietary fiber, 0 mg. cholesterol, 9 mg. sodium

Serves 6

Day 4

Chicken Salad with Peaches and Pecans
or Chicken and Wheat Berry Salad
Cracked-Wheat Quick Bread

There are so many ways to make chicken salad, I had a hard time choosing just one recipe for this menu—so here are two, with options to add or substitute ingredients as you desire, creating your own new recipes. Serve the chicken salad over a bed of greens with 1½ slices of bread on the side. Or you can serve the chicken salad in pita bread with lettuce, tomato and sprouts or as a regular sandwich on bread or a bagel.

NUTRITIONAL ANALYSIS FOR LUNCH

Per serving (with Chicken Salad with Peaches and Pecans): 445 calories, 9.6 g. total fat (19% of calories), 4.8 g. monounsaturated fat, 2.6 g. polyunsaturated fat, 1.3 g. saturated fat, 27.7 g. protein, 63.8 g. carbohydrate, 6 g. dietary fiber, 47 mg. cholesterol, 688 mg. sodium

Per serving (with Chicken and Wheat Berry Salad): 426 calories, 7.7 g. total fat (16% of calories), 3.7 g. monounsaturated fat, 2.2 g. polyunsaturated fat, 1.1 g. saturated fat, 21.2 g. protein, 71.1 g. carbohydrate, 6.5 g. dietary fiber, 31 mg. cholesterol, 888 mg. sodium

Chicken Salad with Peaches and Pecans

In this recipe, nonfat sour cream and nonfat mayonnaise make a traditional-tasting dressing without the usual amount of fat.

For variety, add some cooked wild rice to the salad. To make the wild rice, bring 1½ cups water to a boil and add ½ cup wild rice. Reduce the heat and simmer for 45 minutes. Drain any excess water and stir the wild rice into the salad.

You may substitute any fresh or canned fruit for the peaches. Some of my family's seasonal favorites are grapes, cherries, strawberries, blueberries and kiwifruit.

PREPARATION
AND COOKING
TIME: 20
MINUTES

1   pound boneless, skinless chicken breasts
2   stalks celery, chopped
½   cup nonfat sour cream
½   cup nonfat mayonnaise
¼   cup coarsely chopped pecans
¼   teaspoon dried tarragon
    Salt (optional)
    Freshly ground black pepper
1   cup cubed peaches

Place the chicken between pieces of wax paper or plastic wrap. Using a meat mallet, pound slightly to an even thickness.

In a no-stick frying pan over medium heat, cook the chicken for 10 minutes, or until it is cooked through. Add a little water to prevent burning. Remove the chicken from the pan. Allow to cool slightly and cut into cubes.

In a large bowl, combine the chicken, celery, sour cream, mayonnaise, pecans, tarragon and salt (if using) and pepper to taste. Mix well.

Gently fold in the peaches. Refrigerate the salad until ready to serve.

Per serving: 210 calories, 6.6 g. total fat (28% of calories), 3.5 g. monounsaturated fat, 1.6 g. polyunsaturated fat, 0.9 g. saturated fat, 19.7 g. protein, 17.7 g. carbohydrate, 1.4 g. dietary fiber, 46 mg. cholesterol, 477 mg. sodium

Serves 4

Chicken and Wheat Berry Salad

This salad is unique in that it uses cooked wheat berries for the base. It has a slightly sweet flavor and a wonderfully crunchy texture. The wheat berries take a while to cook, but you can make them ahead of time and refrigerate them until needed.

You can also soak the uncooked wheat berries overnight to reduce the cooking time to 30 minutes. (You can find

FRESH-START COOKING TIP
Most of the fat in poultry comes from the skin. In removing the skin you save about five grams of fat per three-ounce serving.

wheat berries at a natural foods store or a specialty foods shop.) The remainder of the salad can be put together in 20 minutes.

PREPARATION AND COOKING TIME: 1–2 HOURS

1	cup uncooked wheat berries
1	pound boneless, skinless chicken breasts
1¼	cups nonfat mayonnaise
2	stalks celery, chopped
1	small apple, chopped
1	small red onion, finely chopped
4	tablespoons chopped pecans or walnuts
½	cup chopped fresh parsley
1½	teaspoons maple syrup
1	tablespoon champagne vinegar or white-wine vinegar
½–1	tablespoon apple juice
	Salt (optional)
	Freshly ground black pepper

Bring 3 cups water to a boil. Add the wheat berries and lower the heat.

Simmer, covered, for 1½ to 2 hours (or for 30 minutes if the berries are presoaked), or until the water is absorbed and the berries are tender. Set aside.

Meanwhile, place the chicken between pieces of wax paper or plastic wrap. With a meat mallet, pound slightly to an even thickness.

In a no-stick frying pan over medium heat, cook the chicken for 10 minutes, or until it is cooked through. Add a little water to prevent burning. Remove the chicken from the pan. Allow to cool slightly and cut into cubes.

In a large bowl, combine the wheat berries, chicken, mayonnaise, celery, apples, onions, pecans or walnuts, parsley, maple syrup, vinegar, juice and salt (if using) and pepper to taste. Taste to adjust the seasonings and chill until ready to serve.

Per serving: 191 calories, 4.7 g. total fat (22% of calories), 2.4 g. monounsaturated fat, 1.2 g. polyunsaturated fat, 0.7 g. saturated fat, 13.2 g. protein, 25 g. carbohydrate, 1.9 g. dietary fiber, 30 mg. cholesterol, 677 mg. sodium

Serves 6

Low-Fat Lunches

Cracked-Wheat Quick Bread

This bread has the ingredients typical of a yeast-raised dough yet uses baking powder and baking soda for the leavening. It has a mildly sweet flavor and a texture somewhere between that of a yeast bread and a quick bread.

PREPARATION TIME:
5 MINUTES
BAKING TIME:
45 MINUTES

1½	cups whole-wheat flour
¾	cup unbleached flour
½	cup rolled oats
½	cup sugar
2	tablespoons cracked wheat
1½	teaspoons baking powder
½	teaspoon baking soda
¼	teaspoon salt
1–1¼	cups skim milk
1	tablespoon canola oil
2	egg whites

Preheat the oven to 350°. Lightly coat an 8½" × 4½" loaf pan with no-stick spray.

In a large bowl, combine the whole-wheat flour, unbleached flour, oats, sugar, cracked wheat, baking powder, baking soda and salt.

In a medium bowl, whisk together the milk, oil and egg whites.

Make a well in the center of the flour mixture and pour in the milk mixture. Stir until the dry ingredients are just moistened.

Pour the batter into the prepared pan and bake for 45 minutes, or until a toothpick inserted into the center comes out clean. Remove the bread from the pan and let stand on a rack until cool.

Per 1½ slices: 235 calories, 3 g. total fat (11% of calories), 1.3 g. monounsaturated fat, 1 g. polyunsaturated fat, 0.4 g. saturated fat, 8 g. protein, 46.1 g. carbohydrate, 4.6 g. dietary fiber, 1 mg. cholesterol, 211 mg. sodium

Makes 9 slices

FRESH-START COOKING TIP

Bread crumbs are easy to make and are a great way to use leftover bread. Store bread slices in the freezer until you're ready to make crumbs. Then put the bread in a food processor and process until the bread is in fine crumbs. If the crumbs are too moist, spread them on a baking sheet and bake at 300° for three to five minutes. If frozen, the bread crumbs will last up to a year, and you can use them directly from the freezer.

Day 5

Ratatouille and Grilled Mozzarella Sandwiches
Cucumber and Red Grape Salad

Ratatouille is a French mixed-vegetable dish often made from the summer's abundance of garden-fresh vegetables. It can be served hot, at room temperature or chilled.

NUTRITIONAL ANALYSIS FOR LUNCH

Per serving: 433 calories, 9.9 g. total fat (21% of calories), 3 g. monounsaturated fat, 0.8 g. polyunsaturated fat, 3.4 g. saturated fat, 20.4 g. protein, 72.9 g. carbohydrate, 10.5 g. dietary fiber, 16 mg. cholesterol, 555 mg. sodium

Ratatouille and Grilled Mozzarella Sandwiches

Ratatouille can be served in many ways: on top of cooked grains, pasta, pizza or baked or mashed potatoes; in crêpes, pita bread or lasagna; or with crackers. I like to serve it on a hero-style roll with slices of grilled mozzarella.

1	tablespoon olive oil
1	large onion, chopped
6	large cloves garlic, minced
1	green pepper, cut into strips
1	red pepper, cut into strips
1	medium eggplant, cubed
2	cups mushrooms, thickly sliced
3	small zucchini, thickly sliced
4	tomatoes, cubed
1	cup low-sodium tomato puree
¼	cup dry red wine or sherry
4	tablespoons minced fresh basil or 2 teaspoons dried
1	tablespoon lemon juice
2	teaspoons dried thyme
1	teaspoon dried oregano
1	teaspoon ground cumin
	Freshly ground black pepper
	Salt (optional)

PREPARATION AND COOKING TIME: 45 MINUTES

(continued)

¼ cup chopped fresh parsley
6 small whole-grain hero-style rolls
6 ounces mozzarella cheese, cut into 12 slices

Warm the oil in a very large no-stick frying pan or medium pot over medium heat.

Add the onions and cook for 5 minutes.

Add the garlic, green peppers, red peppers, eggplant, mushrooms, zucchini, tomatoes, tomato puree, wine or sherry, basil, lemon juice, thyme, oregano, cumin and black pepper and salt (if using) to taste. Stir well and cover.

Reduce the heat to medium low and cook for 20 minutes, stirring occasionally. Add the parsley and cook for 10 minutes more.

Cut the rolls in half lengthwise. Spread each piece with a thick layer of ratatouille and top with 1 slice of the mozzarella. Place the rolls under the broiler for a few seconds, until the mozzarella has melted.

Serve the sandwiches open-faced with plenty of napkins.

Per serving: 334 calories, 9.3 g. total fat (23% of calories), 3 g. monounsaturated fat, 0.6 g. polyunsaturated fat, 3.3 g. saturated fat, 16.6 g. protein, 50.8 g. carbohydrate, 7.2 g. dietary fiber, 16 mg. cholesterol, 475 mg. sodium

Serves 6

Cucumber and Red Grape Salad

This simple salad is full of flavors and textures—sweet, crunchy, cool and tangy. It tastes wonderful on a warm summer's day.

PREPARATION TIME: 10 MINUTES

3 cucumbers, peeled and thinly sliced
2 cups seedless red grapes
2 stalks celery, chopped
½ cup nonfat sour cream or yogurt
1 tablespoon apple cider vinegar or white-wine vinegar
1 teaspoon dried dill
1 teaspoon dried chives
1 teaspoon Dijon mustard

1   teaspoon honey or sugar
    Freshly ground black pepper

In a large bowl, combine the cucumbers, grapes and celery. Set aside.

In a small bowl, mix the sour cream or yogurt, vinegar, dill, chives, mustard, honey or sugar and pepper to taste. Pour over the cucumber mixture. Toss gently and chill until ready to serve.

Per serving: 99 calories, 0.6 g. total fat (5% of calories), 0.02 g. monounsaturated fat, 0.2 g. polyunsaturated fat, 0.1 g. saturated fat, 3.8 g. protein, 22.1 g. carbohydrate, 3.3 g. dietary fiber, 0 mg. cholesterol, 80 mg. sodium

Serves 4

> **FRESH-START COOKING TIP**
> In many recipes you can enjoy creamy sauces without a lot of fat. Skim milk, evaporated skim milk, nonfat sour cream, low-fat or nonfat cream cheese or yogurt and part-skim cheeses can be substituted for fattier ingredients.

Day 6

Middle Eastern Baked Falafel
Dilled Cucumber Salad

In Israel, falafel is sold in little shops, much as pizza is sold in America. Traditional falafel balls are deep-fried and then covered with a heavy tahini sauce. I have created a low-fat variation: baked falafel with a light yogurt-tahini dressing. Both the falafel balls and the sauce can be made ahead of time. Leftovers store well in the refrigerator.

NUTRITIONAL ANALYSIS FOR LUNCH

Per serving: 312 calories, 5.5 g. total fat (16% of calories), 0.1 g. monounsaturated fat, 0.2 g. polyunsaturated fat, 0.2 g. saturated fat, 14.9 g. protein, 53.3 g. carbohydrate, 4 g. dietary fiber, 0 mg. cholesterol, 252 mg. sodium

Middle Eastern Baked Falafel

For a fast-meal alternative, prepackaged falafel mix is available in many natural foods stores.

Instead of frying the falafel as directed on the package, try lightly browning the balls over medium heat in a no-stick frying pan (coat the pan with no-stick spray first).

PREPARATION TIME:
15 MINUTES
BAKING TIME:
20 MINUTES

Falafel

2½ cups cooked chick-peas or 2½ cups canned chick-peas, rinsed and drained
2 large cloves garlic, minced
2 tablespoons minced fresh parsley
2 teaspoons ground coriander
2 teaspoons ground cumin
½ teaspoon chili powder
Ground red pepper
Freshly ground black pepper
Salt

Yogurt-Tahini Sauce

2 tablespoons nonfat yogurt
2 tablespoons tahini
1 tablespoon lemon juice
1 small clove garlic, minced
1 teaspoon minced fresh parsley
Ground red pepper or hot-pepper sauce
½ cup water

Topping

2 tomatoes, chopped
½ cup minced onions

Assembly

6 whole-wheat pita breads
3 cups shredded romaine lettuce

To make the falafel: Preheat the oven to 400°.

In a blender or food processor, combine the chick-peas, garlic, parsley, coriander, cumin, chili powder and red pepper, black pepper and salt to taste.

Process until the ingredients form a thick paste.

Lightly coat a baking sheet with no-stick spray. Roll the chick-pea mixture into 1″ balls and place on the sheet. Lightly coat the balls with no-stick spray. Bake for 20 minutes, or until the balls are lightly browned. Set aside.

To make the yogurt-tahini sauce: Meanwhile, in a blender or food processor, combine the yogurt, tahini, lemon juice, garlic and parsley. Add enough red pepper or hot-pepper sauce to make the sauce spicy.

With the motor running, pour in enough of the water to make a thin dressing.

Transfer the mixture to a bowl and refrigerate until ready to use. (The sauce will thicken as it chills. If it becomes too thick, add a little more water before serving.)

To make the topping: In a medium bowl, combine the tomatoes and onions.

To assemble the falafel: Cut the pitas in half and fill each pocket with the lettuce, falafel balls, dressing, tomato-onion mixture and more dressing.

> *Per serving: 283 calories, 5.3 g. total fat (17% of calories), 0.1 g. monounsaturated fat, 0.1 g. polyunsaturated fat, 0.04 g. saturated fat, 13.2 g. protein, 47.4 g. carbohydrate, 2.4 g. dietary fiber, 0 mg. cholesterol, 238 mg. sodium*

Serves 6

Dilled Cucumber Salad

Here's a cool, crisp low-fat salad that takes advantage of the summer's abundance of fresh cucumbers. Peel the cucumbers if the skin is bitter or waxed.

2	large cucumbers, peeled and thinly sliced or cubed
2	scallions, thinly sliced
1	tablespoon white-wine vinegar or lemon juice
¼	cup nonfat yogurt
½	teaspoon dried dill
⅛	teaspoon garlic powder
	Freshly ground black pepper
	Salt

PREPARATION TIME: 10 MINUTES

In a large bowl, combine the cucumbers, scallions, vinegar or lemon juice, yogurt, dill, garlic powder and pepper and salt to taste. Mix well.

Cover and refrigerate until ready to serve.

> *Per serving: 29 calories, 0.2 g. total fat (6% of calories), 0.01 g. monounsaturated fat, 0.07 g. polyunsaturated fat, 0.2 g. saturated fat, 1.7 g. protein, 5.9 g. carbohydrate, 1.6 g. dietary fiber, 0 mg. cholesterol, 14 mg. sodium*

Serves 4

Day 7
Greek Pasta Salad
Whole-Wheat French Bread (page 399)

This pasta dish is a meal in itself. Add two slices of crusty Whole-Wheat French Bread, and you're set.

NUTRITIONAL ANALYSIS FOR LUNCH

Per serving: 596 calories, 11 g. total fat (17% of calories), 4.5 g. monounsaturated fat, 1.4 g. polyunsaturated fat, 3.8 g. saturated fat, 24 g. protein, 101.8 g. carbohydrate, 11.8 g. dietary fiber, 17 mg. cholesterol, 833 mg. sodium

FRESH-START COOKING TIP
When choosing pasta, whether it's fresh or dried, be sure to look for the kinds that are made without eggs and oil.

Greek Pasta Salad

This salad actually improves in flavor over time, so you can make it in advance and keep it refrigerated until you're ready to serve it. It's easy to make. To speed preparation you can buy prewashed fresh spinach.

A good-quality feta cheese is important for flavor in this recipe.

Serve the salad at room temperature or slightly chilled.

PREPARATION TIME: 15 MINUTES

1	pound spinach fettuccine
½	cup nonfat chicken or vegetable broth
2	tablespoons olive oil
2	tablespoons balsamic or white-wine vinegar
3	cloves garlic, minced
1	teaspoon dried basil
1	teaspoon dried oregano
4	ounces feta cheese, crumbled
8	ounces spinach, washed, dried and chopped
1	cucumber, peeled and chopped
½	small red onion, very thinly sliced
	Freshly ground black pepper
	Salt (optional)
10	cherry tomatoes, quartered

Cook the fettuccine in a large pot of boiling water for 8 minutes, or until al dente.

Meanwhile, in a small bowl, mix the broth, oil, vinegar, garlic, basil and oregano.

Drain the fettuccine and place it in a large bowl.

Add the broth mixture, feta, spinach, cucumbers and onions. Toss well.

Season with the pepper and salt (if using).

Taste and add more broth, vinegar, pepper or salt as desired. Add the tomatoes and toss gently.

Per serving: 386 calories, 9.8 g. total fat (23% of calories), 4.3 g. monounsaturated fat, 1 g. polyunsaturated fat, 3.6 g. saturated fat, 15 g. protein, 57.4 g. carbohydrate, 4.2 g. dietary fiber, 17 mg. cholesterol, 297 mg. sodium

Serves 6

Day 8

Quesadillas
Sweet Pea Guacamole
Four-Bean Salad with Balsamic Vinaigrette

This meal is quite eclectic, yet the individual parts go together well. I've taken traditional high-fat guacamole to new heights with the use of sweet peas instead of avocados and other high-fat ingredients; the result is unique and surprisingly delicious.

The quesadillas (*kay-sa-DE-as*), often served as a Mexican appetizer, can be filled with any number of ingredients to suit your taste.

To complete the meal, serve a salad made of four types of legumes that are marinated in a balsamic vinaigrette. The recipes make six servings, but you can cut them in half if you wish.

NUTRITIONAL ANALYSIS FOR LUNCH

Per serving: 624 calories, 13.8 g. total fat (20% of calories), 3.2 g. monounsaturated fat, 1.3 g. polyunsaturated fat, 3.2 g. saturated fat, 30.1 g. protein, 97.8 g. carbohydrate, 10.1 g. dietary fiber, 12 mg. cholesterol, 1,163 mg. sodium

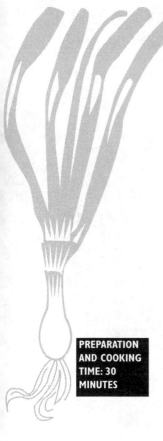

Quesadillas

To make quesadillas, you sandwich a variety of ingredients between flour tortillas and grill the "package" quickly. Try adding cooked chicken or seafood, beans, olives, peppers, pimentos, mild green chili peppers, hot peppers or other chopped vegetables.

12   flour tortillas
1½   cups shredded low-fat Cheddar cheese
 2   tomatoes, chopped
 1   bunch scallions, chopped
     Sweet Pea Guacamole (opposite page)
 6   tablespoons nonfat sour cream
     Salsa

Preheat the oven to 200°. Place a baking sheet in the oven.

Heat a no-stick frying pan over medium-high heat for 1 minute.

Place a tortilla in the pan and top with ⅙ each of the Cheddar, tomatoes and scallions. Place another tortilla on top.

Cook for about 2 minutes, or until the bottom tortilla is lightly browned.

PREPARATION AND COOKING TIME: 30 MINUTES

Using a long spatula, turn the quesadilla over and cook until the other tortilla is lightly browned. (Watch them carefully, as they burn quickly.) Transfer the quesadilla to the baking sheet in the oven to keep warm.

Repeat with the remaining 10 tortillas, Cheddar, tomatoes and scallions to make a total of 6 quesadillas.

Cut each quesadilla into quarters. Place 4 quarters on individual plates and place a heaping scoop of the guacamole in the center of each plate.

Spoon 1 tablespoon of the sour cream on top of the gaucamole; add the salsa on the side.

Per serving: 288 calories, 7.8 g. total fat (24% of calories), 0.02 g. monounsaturated fat, 0.1 g. polyunsaturated fat, 2.4 g. saturated fat, 12.4 g. protein, 42.4 g. carbohydrate, 2.3 g. dietary fiber, 12 mg. cholesterol, 427 mg. sodium

Serves 6

Fresh-Start Recipes

Sweet Pea Guacamole

Traditional guacamole is made from mashed avocados, which are very high in fat. In fact, there is approximately 30 grams of fat in 1 avocado.

Well, here's a great alternative. In this recipe I've used frozen sweet peas and cilantro to create a unique yet somewhat familiar feeling. And there's an added bonus: If you've made regular guacamole, you know it's hard to get avocados when they're just ripe enough but not too ripe. With frozen peas, of course, you never have that problem.

For more spiciness, add extra green chili peppers. You can use this guacamole as an accompaniment for any Mexican dish or as a dip for baked tortilla chips.

½	cup chopped fresh cilantro
2	tablespoons lime juice
2	tablespoons canned chopped green chili peppers
1	tablespoon olive oil
1	pound frozen sweet peas, thawed
½	teaspoon salt
¼	teaspoon ground cumin
¼	cup finely chopped red onions
1	tomato, chopped
	Freshly ground black pepper

PREPARATION TIME: 10 MINUTES

In a blender or food processor, combine the cilantro, lime juice, chili peppers and oil.

Add the peas, salt and cumin. Puree until smooth.

Pour into a serving bowl and stir in the onions and tomatoes.

Season with the black pepper. Refrigerate until ready to serve.

Per serving: 97 calories, 2.6 g. total fat (23% of calories), 1.7 g. monounsaturated fat, 0.3 g. polyunsaturated fat, 0.3 g. saturated fat, 4.6 g. protein, 14.6 g. carbohydrate, 0.4 g. dietary fiber, 0 mg. cholesterol, 218 mg. sodium

Serves 6

Low-Fat Lunches

Four-Bean Salad
with Balsamic Vinaigrette

This is a very fast and easy recipe, although the flavors are anything but simple. The longer the legumes marinate, the more they pick up "snap" from the balsamic dressing. Just about any type of legumes can be used—black-eyed peas, navy beans, pinto beans and so on. It also tastes great served on top of mixed greens.

PREPARATION TIME:
10 MINUTES

MARINATING TIME: 2 HOURS OR MORE

1	can (15 ounces) kidney beans, rinsed and drained
1	can (15 ounces) Great Northern beans, rinsed and drained
1	can (15 ounces) chick-peas, rinsed and drained
1	cup fresh green beans, lightly steamed
½	cup water or nonfat chicken broth
¼	cup red-wine vinegar
3	tablespoons balsamic vinegar
3	tablespoons minced fresh parsley
2	tablespoons chopped shallots
2	tablespoons olive oil
	Freshly ground black pepper
	Salt
	Pinch of sugar

In a wide, shallow bowl, place the kidney beans in an even layer. Add the Great Northern beans in an even layer and cover with even layers of the chick-peas and green beans. Set aside.

In a medium bowl, whisk together the water or broth, red-wine vinegar, balsamic vinegar, parsley, shallots, oil and pepper, salt and sugar to taste. Pour over the beans.

Cover and marinate for at least 2 hours, or until ready to serve. Stir the beans occasionally while marinating. Taste to adjust the seasoning before serving.

Per serving: 239 calories, 3.4 g. total fat (12% of calories), 1.5 g. monounsaturated fat, 0.9 g. polyunsaturated fat, 0.5 g. saturated fat, 13.1 g. protein, 40.8 g. carbohydrate, 7.4 g. dietary fiber, 0 mg. cholesterol, 518 mg. sodium

FRESH-START COOKING TIP
Beans are high in fiber and protein but low in fat. If you're using canned beans, rinse them well to remove the excess sodium.

Serves 6

Day 9

Peasants' Salad Pita Pockets
Roasted Chestnut and Wild Rice Soup

This sandwich and hearty soup have distinctive flavors that complement each other well. This is an easy meal to prepare ahead, and leftovers are delicious.

NUTRITIONAL ANALYSIS FOR LUNCH

Per serving: 617 calories, 13.6 g. total fat (20% of calories), 3.2 g. monounsaturated fat, 1.3 g. polyunsaturated fat, 10 g. saturated fat, 26.6 g. protein, 99.8 g. carbohydrate, 10.1 g. dietary fiber, 37 mg. cholesterol, 1,488 mg. sodium

Peasants' Salad Pita Pockets

The inspiration for this recipe comes from Bacino's restaurant in Naperville, Illinois, which has one of the most creative, varied and delicious salad bars I've ever seen—as well as good pizza. The combination of ingredients in this recipe is unique, and the salad contains no added oil. It's moistened with balsamic vinegar, which soaks into the bread and coats the vegetables.

You can eat the salad by itself, tossed on salad greens, served on crackers or crostini or packed into pita pockets as I've suggested here. For variety, add Creamy Garlic Dressing (page 314) or nonfat ranch-style dressing to the pitas.

4	cups cubed whole-grain French bread
½	small red onion, quartered and very thinly sliced
1½	cups small broccoli florets
1	cup small cauliflower florets
½	red pepper, thinly sliced
½	yellow or green pepper, thinly sliced
1	cucumber, peeled and cubed
5	cherry tomatoes, halved, or 1 large tomato, cubed

PREPARATION TIME: 15 MINUTES

(continued)

4 ounces mushrooms, thinly sliced
4 ounces feta cheese, crumbled
6 tablespoons balsamic vinegar
¼ cup minced fresh basil or 2 tablespoons dried
¼ cup minced fresh oregano or 2 tablespoons dried
½–¾ teaspoon salt
  Freshly ground black pepper
6 whole-wheat pita breads

In a very large bowl, mix the bread cubes, onions, broccoli, cauliflower, red peppers, yellow or green peppers, cucumbers, tomatoes, mushrooms, feta, vinegar, basil, oregano, salt and black pepper to taste. Toss well. Let the salad marinate for more flavor.

Cut the pitas in half and stuff the salad inside each pocket. Serve with garlic or ranch dressing, if desired.

Per serving: 299 calories, 6.7 g. total fat (19% of calories), 1.2 g. monounsaturated fat, 0.8 g. polyunsaturated fat, 3.1 g. saturated fat, 12.5 g. protein, 49.7 g. carbohydrate, 7 g. dietary fiber, 17 mg. cholesterol, 841 mg. sodium

Serves 6

Roasted Chestnut and Wild Rice Soup

Chestnuts are available in a variety of ways: fresh, in jars, in cans and dried. I prefer them fresh, roasted in the oven. They are usually a seasonal item, sold most often around the Christmas holidays.

Chestnuts have barely any fat and are high in fiber, making them a great snack option. If you're using fresh chestnuts in this recipe, be sure to buy extras, since occasionally several are moldy inside and need to be discarded.

To roast chestnuts, preheat the oven to 425°. Use a sharp knife to cut an X on the flat side of each chestnut. Place the chestnuts on a baking sheet and bake for about 15 to 20 minutes. Let them cool slightly and then peel.

For variety, you can omit the chestnuts and use 2 large potatoes to create Wild Rice and Potato Soup.

PREPARATION AND COOKING TIME: I HOUR

1¼	cups water
½	cup wild rice, rinsed and drained
2	tablespoons unsalted butter or margarine
2	small onions, chopped
1	large potato, peeled and cubed
12	chestnuts, roasted
2¼	cups nonfat chicken or vegetable broth
1½	cups evaporated skim milk
½–1	teaspoon salt
	Freshly ground black pepper
1	tablespoon cooking sherry
4	teaspoons minced fresh chives

Bring the water to a boil in a small saucepan.

Stir in the wild rice and reduce the heat to medium low.

Cover and cook for 45 minutes, or until the water is absorbed.

Meanwhile, in a soup pot, melt the butter or margarine over medium heat.

Add the onions and cook for 5 minutes.

Stir in the potatoes and chestnuts. Cook for 2 to 3 minutes longer.

Add the broth and milk.

Bring to a boil, then reduce the heat to low and simmer for 30 minutes.

Working in batches, transfer the mixture to a blender or food processor and blend until smooth.

Pour back into the soup pot.

Stir in the wild rice and season with the salt, pepper and sherry. Warm through.

Serve garnished with the chives.

Per serving: 318 calories, 6.9 g. total fat (19% of calories), 2 g. monounsaturated fat, 0.5 g. polyunsaturated fat, 6.9 g. saturated fat, 14.1 g. protein, 50.1 g. carbohydrate, 3.1 g. dietary fiber, 20 mg. cholesterol, 647 mg. sodium

Serves 4

Day 10

Tex-Mex Pasta Salad

This pasta salad is a meal in itself, but I recommend serving it with store-bought baked tortilla chips. There are several varieties that have no added fat and can be found in most grocery and natural foods stores.

Per serving (including 1 ounce baked tortilla chips): 605 calories, 12.3 g. total fat (18% of calories), 5.1 g. monounsaturated fat, 1.2 g. polyunsaturated fat, 2.7 g. saturated fat, 22.3 g. protein, 104.7 g. carbohydrate, 7 g. dietary fiber, 8 mg. cholesterol, 1,236 mg. sodium

Tex-Mex Pasta Salad

PREPARATION TIME: 20 MINUTES

Although the tricolor pasta in this recipe creates an especially festive-looking dish, you can use any color or shape of pasta. The salad makes a great cool-weather or warm-weather meal.

Be sure to make some extra, so you have leftovers. The leftovers are delicious even after several days in the refrigerator.

Serve the salad with baked tortilla chips.

FRESH-START COOKING TIP
Tossing cooked pasta in a little nonfat chicken broth before adding the sauce lends the same silky texture to the pasta as adding oil, with none of the fat. The broth coats the strands of pasta, keeping them from sticking together. And don't add oil to the cooking water when making pasta. Just stir the pasta a few times while it's cooking.

1	pound tricolor corkscrew pasta
3	tablespoons olive oil
3	tablespoons nonfat chicken or vegetable broth
5	tablespoons white-wine vinegar
3	tablespoons nonfat low-sodium tomato sauce
2	cloves garlic, minced
1	tablespoon chili powder
1	teaspoon salt
¼	teaspoon dried oregano
½	cup finely chopped onions
½	green pepper, finely chopped
1	cup frozen corn, thawed
¼	cup chopped fresh parsley

1 can (4 ounces) green chili peppers, chopped
4 ounces pimentos, sliced
1 can (15 ounces) kidney beans, rinsed and drained
4 ounces low-fat Cheddar cheese, cubed
1 tablespoon finely chopped fresh cilantro
Freshly ground black pepper

Cook the pasta in a large pot of boiling water for 4 to 8 minutes, or until al dente; do not overcook.

In a small cup, whisk together the oil, broth, vinegar, tomato sauce, garlic, chili powder, salt and oregano. Set the cup aside while mixing the other ingredients.

In a large bowl, combine the onions, green peppers, corn, parsley, chili peppers, pimentos, beans, Cheddar, cilantro and black pepper to taste. Stir in the pasta

Pour in the oil mixture and toss gently to combine.

Per serving: 495 calories, 11.3 g. total fat (18% of calories), 5.1 g. monounsaturated fat, 1.2 g. polyunsaturated fat, 2.7 g. saturated fat, 19.3 g. protein, 80.7 g. carbohydrate, 5 g. dietary fiber, 8 mg. cholesterol, 1,096 mg. sodium

Serves 6

Day 11

Autumn's Acorn Cheddar Soup
Colorful Corn Relish
Gingerbread Muffins

This is a perfect meal for the cool days of autumn, when squash is at its best. The entire meal makes wonderful leftovers: The soup is easily reheated, the flavor of the salad improves as it marinates, and the muffins are great snacks.

**NUTRITIONAL
ANALYSIS
FOR LUNCH**

Per serving (including 1 muffin): 507 calories, 13 g. total fat (23% of calories), 4.7 g. monounsaturated fat, 1.3 g. polyunsaturated fat, 4.7 g. saturated fat, 23.5 g. protein, 82 g. carbohydrate, 7.2 g. dietary fiber, 20 mg. cholesterol, 1,237 mg. sodium

Low-Fat Lunches

Autumn's Acorn Cheddar Soup

This soup has a subtle yet hearty flavor and conjures up images of crisp fall days. The creamy orange color is very appealing to the eye, and the texture is smooth, rich and thick. You can prepare the squash in the microwave to shorten the cooking time.

PREPARATION TIME: 10 MINUTES

BAKING TIME: 45 MINUTES

2   medium acorn squash
1   tablespoon unsalted butter or margarine
3   cups nonfat chicken or vegetable broth
¼–½ teaspoon dried sage
1   teaspoon garlic powder
6   ounces low-fat Cheddar cheese, shredded
1½   cups evaporated skim milk
      Salt
1–2   teaspoons freshly ground black pepper
      Ground nutmeg

Preheat the oven to 475°.

Using a sharp knife, cut the squash in half. Scoop out the seeds with a spoon and place the squash cut side down on a baking sheet with edges (to prevent the juice from dripping into your oven). Bake for 45 minutes, or until the squash is soft.

Spoon the pulp into a food processor and puree until smooth. Mix in the butter or margarine, broth, sage and garlic powder.

Transfer the puree to a medium soup pot and cook over low heat for several minutes.

Slowly add the Cheddar and milk, stirring until the cheese has melted. Thin with additional milk if necessary. Add the salt and pepper to taste and sprinkle with the nutmeg. Serve immediately or hold over the lowest heat until ready to serve.

FRESH-START COOKING TIP
Because fat not only provides richness but amplifies flavor, your low-fat dishes need more seasonings. Use the recipe recommendations as a starting point, then increase the seasonings to suit your own taste.

Per serving: 227 calories, 6.5 g. total fat (24% of calories), 0.6 g. monounsaturated fat, 0.3 g. polyunsaturated fat, 3.8 g. saturated fat, 13.9 g. protein, 31.2 g. carbohydrate, 3 g. dietary fiber, 20 mg. cholesterol, 717 mg. sodium

Serves 6

Colorful Corn Relish

As the name suggests, this salad makes an appealing presentation. It is fast and easy to prepare and can be made several days in advance.

The longer the relish marinates, the more the flavor is enhanced. Adjust the seasonings to your personal preference, adding more or less green chili peppers, cilantro, lime, vinegar or salt.

3	cups frozen corn, thawed
½	cup finely chopped red onions
½	green pepper, finely chopped
1	can (15½ ounces) black-eyed peas, rinsed and drained
4	ounces pimentos, diced
1	can (4 ounces) green chili peppers, chopped
¼	cup minced fresh parsley
1	tablespoon minced fresh cilantro
2	tablespoons olive oil
3	tablespoons lime juice
2	tablespoons white-wine vinegar
2	teaspoons garlic powder
1	teaspoon dried basil
¼	teaspoon ground cumin
	Freshly ground black pepper
	Salt

PREPARATION TIME: 10 MINUTES

MARINATING TIME: 30 MINUTES OR MORE

In a large bowl, combine the corn, onions, green peppers, peas, pimentos, chili peppers, parsley and cilantro. Toss well.

In a small bowl, whisk together the oil, lime juice, vinegar, garlic powder, basil, cumin and black pepper and salt to taste.

Stir the oil mixture into the vegetables and marinate in the refrigerator until ready to serve. Taste to adjust seasonings.

Per serving: 187 calories, 5.1 g. total fat (18% of calories), 3.4 g. monounsaturated fat, 0.6 g. polyunsaturated fat, 0.7 g. saturated fat, 6.9 g. protein, 32.6 g. carbohydrate, 2.5 g. dietary fiber, 0 mg. cholesterol, 450 mg. sodium

Serves 6

Low-Fat Lunches

Gingerbread Muffins

These are moist and aromatic muffins with an old-fashioned flavor. Just the warm fragrance of baking gingerbread builds anticipation. They're always a favorite.

PREPARATION TIME: 10 MINUTES

BAKING TIME: 20 MINUTES

1¼	cups whole-grain flour
¼	cup nonfat dry milk
1½	teaspoons ground ginger
¾	teaspoon ground cinnamon
½	teaspoon baking soda
½	teaspoon baking powder
¼	teaspoon ground nutmeg
¼	teaspoon ground cloves
¼	cup skim milk
6	tablespoons applesauce
¼	cup molasses
3	tablespoons maple syrup
1	tablespoon canola oil
1	egg white, lightly beaten

Preheat the oven to 350°. Line 12 muffin cups with paper liners.

In a large bowl, sift together the flour, dry milk, ginger, cinnamon, baking soda, baking powder, nutmeg and cloves.

In a small bowl, combine the skim milk, applesauce, molasses, maple syrup, oil and egg white.

Pour over the flour mixture.

Mix until the dry ingredients are moistened, but be sure that you don't overmix.

Spoon the batter into the prepared muffin cups.

Bake for 20 minutes, or until a toothpick inserted in the center of a muffin comes out clean.

Remove the muffins from the tin and cool on a wire rack.

> **FRESH-START COOKING TIP**
> In many recipes for muffins and quick breads, you can reduce fat by substituting an equal amount of unsweetened applesauce for half of the butter or oil. In fact, you can usually replace as much as 75 percent of the butter or oil with applesauce or prune butter.

Per muffin: 93 calories, 1.4 g. total fat (13% of calories), 0.7 g. monounsaturated fat, 0.4 g. polyunsaturated fat, 0.2 g. saturated fat, 2.7 g. protein, 18.2 g. carbohydrate, 1.7 g. dietary fiber, 0 mg. cholesterol, 70 mg. sodium

Makes 12

Day 12

Oriental Noodles
Wonton Chips

I was surprised to learn that this is one meal my young kids will always eat. The mild flavor of soy sauce and peanut butter interests them. And the crunchy wonton chips are a real treat.

NUTRITIONAL ANALYSIS FOR LUNCH

Per serving: 540 calories, 10.8 g. total fat (18% of calories), 3.8 g. monounsaturated fat, 4.2 g. polyunsaturated fat, 1.6 g. saturated fat, 17.6 g. protein, 94.5 g. carbohydrate, 7.2 g. dietary fiber, 61 mg. cholesterol, 331 mg. sodium

---

Oriental Noodles

When buying Chinese noodles, look for some that have little or no added oil or eggs. You'll find roasted sesame oil and rice-wine vinegar in the Asian foods section of your grocery store.

PREPARATION AND COOKING TIME: 30 MINUTES

10	ounces Chinese noodles
¼	cup + 2 tablespoons nonfat chicken or vegetable broth
2	tablespoons roasted sesame oil
¼	cup rice-wine vinegar
1½	tablespoons low-sodium soy sauce
1½	teaspoons natural peanut butter
1½	teaspoons ground ginger
1	teaspoon garlic powder
¾	teaspoon sugar
½	teaspoon freshly ground black pepper
1–3	teaspoons minced fresh cilantro
⅛	teaspoon red-pepper flakes (optional)
2	carrots, julienned
1½	cups small broccoli florets
1	zucchini, cubed
1	can (8 ounces) water chestnuts, drained and sliced
4	ounces pimentos, chopped
3	scallions, sliced
½	tomato, chopped (optional)

Cook the noodles in a large pot of boiling water for 2 to 3 minutes, or until al dente. Drain and rinse the noodles under cool water. Toss with ¼ cup of the broth. Set aside.

In a small bowl, combine the oil, vinegar, soy sauce, peanut butter, ginger, garlic powder, sugar, black pepper, cilantro and red-pepper flakes (if using). Pour over the noodles and toss. Set aside.

In a no-stick frying pan over medium heat, cook the carrots and broccoli with the remaining 2 tablespoons broth for a few minutes, or until crisp-tender. Add the zucchini and cook for a few minutes more.

Combine the broccoli mixture, water chestnuts, pimentos, scallions and noodles. Taste to adjust the seasonings. Serve at room temperature and garnish with the tomatoes (if using).

Per serving: 494 calories, 10.8 g. total fat (17% of calories), 3.8 g. monounsaturated fat, 4.2 g. polyunsaturated fat, 1.6 g. saturated fat, 15.6 g. protein, 85.5 g. carbohydrate, 7.2 g. dietary fiber, 61 mg. cholesterol, 293 mg. sodium

Serves 4

Wonton Chips

Wonton chips are a breeze to make, and kids especially love their crunchy texture. Try sprinkling spices over the wontons before baking them to vary the flavor. The chips keep well and taste great with a variety of dips. Look for wonton wraps in the produce section of grocery stores.

PREPARATION TIME: 5 MINUTES

BAKING TIME: 5–7 MINUTES

8 fresh wonton wraps
   Salt (optional)

Preheat the oven to 350°. Lightly coat a baking sheet with no-stick spray.

Cut the wonton wraps into triangles and place in a single layer on the prepared baking sheet. Sprinkle with the salt (if using) to taste.

Bake for 5 to 7 minutes, or until the wontons just begin to brown.

Per serving: 46 calories, 0 g. total fat (0% of calories), 0 g. monounsaturated fat, 0 g. polyunsaturated fat, 0 g. saturated fat, 2 g. protein, 9 g. carbohydrate, 0 g. dietary fiber, 0 mg. cholesterol, 38 mg. sodium

Serves 4

Day 13

Thick and Hearty Vegetable Chili or Southwestern Chicken Chili Old-Fashioned Cornbread

There are so many variations of chili—with beans or without, hot or not, with meat or vegetables—each with its own special qualities. And what's better to make a bowl of chili complete than a thick chunk of cornbread?

Below are two unique chili recipes. If you have a favorite chili recipe of your own, you can easily make some healthful substitutions.

Start by replacing the beef with ground turkey breast (make sure all the fat and skin have been removed before it's ground). If oil or another fat is called for, use only one to three tablespoons of olive or canola oil.

Cut back on or eliminate salt. Add some of the seasonings called for in my recipes and use a tomato sauce that has no added fat. Be sure to serve your chili with a salad if your recipe doesn't call for vegetables.

NUTRITIONAL ANALYSIS FOR LUNCH

Per serving (with Thick and Hearty Vegetable Chili): 450 calories, 8.1 g. total fat (16% of calories), 3.7 g. monounsaturated fat, 2.1 g. polyunsaturated fat, 0.8 g. saturated fat, 20.4 g. protein, 80.7 g. carbohydrate, 9.2 g. dietary fiber, 0 mg. cholesterol, 829 mg. sodium

Per serving (with Southwestern Chicken Chili): 510 calories, 13.8 g. total fat (24% of calories), 5.1 g. monounsaturated fat, 3.3 g. polyunsaturated fat, 2.8 g. saturated fat, 42.6 g. protein, 72.1 g. carbohydrate, 16.5 g. dietary fiber, 56 mg. cholesterol, 1,295 mg. sodium

Thick and Hearty Vegetable Chili

For many of us, a steaming bowl of chili brings back memories of cold, snowy days. I've created a new version of this old favorite, with vegetables replacing the beef. For something a little different, serve the chili over brown rice or another whole grain, a baked potato or a pizza crust. Or use it in lasagna—use your imagination. This chili freezes well and reheats nicely.

PREPARATION TIME: 25 MINUTES

COOKING TIME: 30 MINUTES OR MORE

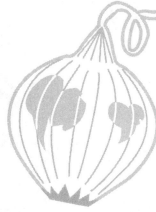

1	tablespoon olive oil
1	onion, chopped
1	carrot, thinly sliced
1	green pepper, chopped
8	ounces mushrooms, sliced
1	small zucchini, sliced
12	black olives (optional)
4	large cloves garlic, minced
1	can (28 ounces) tomatoes (with juice), chopped
2	cups nonfat low-sodium tomato sauce
1	can (4 ounces) green chili peppers, diced
4	cups cooked kidney, pinto, black or adzuki beans
3	tablespoons chili powder
1	tablespoon dried oregano
2	teaspoons ground cumin
2	teaspoons paprika
	Red-pepper flakes (optional)
	Ground red pepper (optional)
1	tablespoon white-wine vinegar
	Chopped fresh cilantro (optional)
	Nonfat sour cream or yogurt (optional)

Warm the oil in a large pot over medium heat.

Add the onions, carrots, green peppers, mushrooms, zucchini, olives (if using) and garlic.

Sauté for 20 minutes.

Add the tomatoes (with juice), tomato sauce, chili peppers, beans, chili powder, oregano, cumin, paprika and red-pepper flakes (if using) and red pepper (if using) to taste.

Simmer for at least 30 minutes; stir often to prevent burning.

Add the vinegar and cilantro (if using) to taste. Simmer briefly.

Serve garnished with the sour cream or yogurt (if using).

Per serving: 285 calories, 4.4 g. total fat (13% of calories), 1.8 g. monounsaturated fat, 0.9 g. polyunsaturated fat, 0.5 g. saturated fat, 15.5 g. protein, 50.6 g. carbohydrate, 5.6 g. dietary fiber, 0 mg. cholesterol, 510 mg. sodium

Serves 6

Southwestern Chicken Chili

This chili recipe uses boneless, skinless chicken breasts and white beans. It gets its mildly spicy flavor from green chili peppers.

This is a quick, easy and very tasty recipe as is, but it adapts well to the addition of just about anything else you might like to add.

You can easily adjust this recipe to achieve your favorite level of spiciness. For a milder flavor, reduce the amount of green chili peppers; for a little extra heat, add the optional red-pepper flakes.

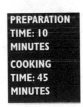

PREPARATION TIME: 10 MINUTES

COOKING TIME: 45 MINUTES

1	tablespoon olive oil
1	pound boneless, skinless chicken breasts, cut into bite-size pieces
1	onion, chopped
8	ounces mushrooms, thickly sliced
4	large cloves garlic, minced
1	can (4 ounces) green chili peppers, chopped
1	teaspoon ground cumin
½	teaspoon dried oregano
⅛	teaspoon red-pepper flakes (optional)
1½	cups nonfat chicken broth
2	cans (15 ounces each) cannellini, navy, Great Northern or other beans, rinsed and drained
½–1	teaspoon chopped fresh cilantro
2	ounces part-skim Monterey Jack cheese, shredded

Warm the oil in a large pot over medium heat. Add the chicken and sauté for 5 minutes, or until the pieces are browned. Remove the chicken and set aside.

Add the onions to the pot and sauté for several minutes. Stir in the mushrooms and garlic; cook for several minutes more. Add the chili peppers, cumin, oregano, red-pepper flakes (if using) and broth. Cover and simmer for 30 minutes, stirring occasionally.

Add the chicken, beans and cilantro; stir gently to mix well. Simmer on low heat for 15 minutes. Taste to adjust the seasonings, adding more red-pepper flakes, if desired. Sprinkle the Monterey Jack over each serving.

Per serving: 345 calories, 10.1 g. total fat (22% of calories), 3.2 g. monounsaturated fat, 2.1 g. polyunsaturated fat, 2.5 g. saturated fat, 37.7 g. protein, 42 g. carbohydrate, 12.9 g. dietary fiber, 56 mg. cholesterol, 976 mg. sodium

Serves 4

Old-Fashioned Cornbread

This is a light, subtly sweet, cakelike whole-grain corn-bread with corn kernels throughout. Leftovers make excellent snacks, warm or cold.

**PREPARATION
TIME: 10
MINUTES

BAKING TIME:
20 MINUTES**

1	cup whole-wheat pastry flour or other whole-grain flour
¾	cup coarse yellow cornmeal
⅓	cup sugar
3	teaspoons baking powder
¾	teaspoon salt
1	cup skim milk
2	egg whites, lightly beaten
2	tablespoons canola oil or melted unsalted butter
1	cup frozen corn, thawed

Preheat the oven to 425°. Lightly coat an 8″ × 8″ baking dish with no-stick spray.

In a large bowl, combine the flour, cornmeal, sugar, baking powder and salt.

In a small bowl, combine the milk, egg whites and oil or

butter. Pour over the flour mixture. Mix until the dry ingredients are moistened; do not overmix. Fold in the corn.

Pour into the prepared baking dish. Bake for 20 minutes, or until a toothpick inserted into the center of the bread comes out clean.

Cool the cornbread on a wire rack. Cut into 9 squares.

Per square: 165 calories, 3.7 g. total fat (19% of calories), 1.9 g. monounsaturated fat, 1.2 g. polyunsaturated fat, 0.3 g. saturated fat, 4.9 g. protein, 30.1 g. carbohydrate, 3.6 g. dietary fiber, 0 mg. cholesterol, 319 mg. sodium

Makes 9 squares

Day 14

Lentil Spread in Pita Pockets
Citrus-Season Salad
with Ginger-Horseradish Dressing

The lentil spread is easy to prepare but needs about 45 minutes of virtually unattended cooking time. It is delicious reheated in the microwave, so you can prepare it ahead of time for excellent leftovers. If you'd like, you can also cut the recipe in half to make three servings.

NUTRITIONAL ANALYSIS FOR LUNCH

Per serving: 447 calories, 8.9 g. total fat (18% of calories), 5.1 g. monounsaturated fat, 1.2 g. polyunsaturated fat, 1.2 g. saturated fat, 24.5 g. protein, 70.9 g. carbohydrate, 4.2 g. dietary fiber, 0 mg. cholesterol, 589 mg. sodium

Lentil Spread in Pita Pockets

Lentils are an excellent source of fiber. Unlike most other legumes, they don't have to be soaked before cooking. In this recipe, lentils are cooked to a consistency similar to that of refried beans and can serve as a flavorful alternative to them in Mexican dishes. You can serve lentil spread on bread or in pita pockets with low-fat fillings.

Low-Fat Lunches

PREPARATION TIME: 10 MINUTES

COOKING TIME: 45 MINUTES

1	tablespoon olive oil
½	cup chopped onions
2	large cloves garlic, minced
½	red or green pepper, chopped
1½	cups dried lentils, sorted and rinsed
4	cups nonfat chicken or vegetable broth
1	carrot, shredded
1	tablespoon molasses
1	tablespoon sherry wine vinegar
1	teaspoon ground cumin
1	teaspoon ground coriander
1	teaspoon dried marjoram
1–3	teaspoons minced fresh cilantro
	Salt
	Freshly ground black pepper
	Hot-pepper sauce (optional)
6	pita breads

In a large saucepan, combine the oil, onions, garlic and red or green peppers. Cook and stir over medium heat for 3 minutes.

Add the lentils and broth. Bring to a boil.

Reduce the heat to medium low and cover the pan.

Cook, stirring occasionally, for 30 minutes.

Stir in the carrots, molasses, vinegar, cumin, coriander, marjoram, cilantro and salt and black pepper to taste.

Add the hot-pepper sauce (if using) to taste.

Cover the pan and simmer for about 15 minutes, or until the liquid is absorbed and the flavors are blended.

Remove from the heat and keep covered until serving time.

Cut the pitas in half and stuff with the lentil mixture. Add fillings such as lettuce, tomatoes, sprouts, thin avocado slices, salsa, grated low-fat cheese and nonfat sour cream.

Per serving: 349 calories, 3.6 g. total fat (9% of calories), 1.8 g. monounsaturated fat, 0.5 g. polyunsaturated fat, 0.4 g. saturated fat, 21.2 g. protein, 59.7 g. carbohydrate, 1.3 g. dietary fiber, 0 mg. cholesterol, 540 mg. sodium

Serves 6

Citrus-Season Salad
with Ginger-Horseradish Dressing

Most of the fat in this salad comes from the avocado, but the remainder of the meal is low in fat. The ginger-horseradish dressing is a perfect topping for the salad.

Citrus-Season Salad

PREPARATION TIME: 15 MINUTES

- 6 cups mixed greens (Bibb, romaine and red-leaf or green-leaf lettuce) torn into bite-size pieces
- 2 tangerines, peeled and sectioned
- 1 cup sliced mushrooms
- 6 radishes, thinly sliced
- 1 avocado, sliced
  Alfalfa sprouts (optional)

Ginger-Horseradish Dressing

- ¼ cup nonfat yogurt or mayonnaise
- ¼ cup nonfat sour cream
- ¼ cup orange juice or tangerine juice
- 2 teaspoons prepared horseradish
- 1 teaspoon ground ginger
- ¼ teaspoon honey

To make the citrus-season salad: Divide the greens among 6 salad bowls.

Top each portion with equal amounts of the tangerines, mushrooms, radishes, avocado and sprouts (if using). Set aside.

To make the ginger-horseradish dressing: In a blender, combine the yogurt or mayonnaise, sour cream, orange juice or tangerine juice, horseradish, ginger and honey. Mix until smooth. Spoon over the salad or store in the refrigerator until ready to serve.

Per serving: 98 calories, 5.3 g. total fat (45% of calories), 3.3 g. monounsaturated fat, 0.7 g. polyunsaturated fat, 0.8 g. saturated fat, 3.3 g. protein, 11.2 g. carbohydrate, 2.9 g. dietary fiber, 0 mg. cholesterol, 49 mg. sodium

Serves 6

Low-Fat Lunches

Chapter Nineteen

Fresh-Start Recipes for Low-Fat Dinners

If you're following the Low-Fat Living Program, it's imperative to put aside the high-risk, high-fat recipes for meat loaf, fried chicken and creamy casseroles that so many Americans are used to and replace them with the kinds of recipes you'll find in this chapter.

There's no reason to rely on traditional American dinners when a whole world of culinary choices is at your doorstep. In this chapter you'll find recipes that originated in Italy, Spain, India, Thailand, Mexico and the Middle East. And these menus include some quick, low-fat versions of fast-food favorites like fajitas, pizza, burgers, tacos and french fries. In just a couple of weeks, you can discover a fascinating array of flavors, yet all the ingredients are easy to find in most supermarkets and natural foods stores.

Here are our favorite menus for two weeks of low-fat dinners, with page numbers to help you quickly find the recipes.

Low-Fat Dinners

Day 1

Chicken Cutlets with Raspberry Vinaigrette (page 312)
Lemon Linguine Parmesan (page 313)
Salad Nouveau (page 314)
Creamy Garlic Dressing (page 314)

Day 2

Tacos (page 315)

Day 3

Picante Seafood Veracruz (page 317)
Baked Yams with Nutmeg Cream (page 318)
Brown Basmati Rice with Lemon (page 318)

Day 4

Angel Hair Pasta with Fresh Tomato Sauce (page 320)
Mixed Green Salad
with Creamy Fresh Basil Dressing (page 321)

Day 5

Santa Fe Chicken Fajitas (page 322)
Southwestern Black Beans (page 323)
Mexicali Rice (page 324)

Day 6

White Pizza (page 325)
Mesclun Greens
with Italian Parmesan Vinaigrette (page 327)

Day 7

Turkey Burgers (page 329)
Spicy French Potatoes (page 330)
Fresh Green Bean Salad (page 330)

Day 8

Chicken Baked with Sherry-Peach Sauce (page 332)
Couscous Pilaf (page 333)
Honey-Glazed Baby Carrots (page 334)
Spinach Salad with Pears, Walnuts and Warm Mustard
Vinaigrette (page 334)

Day 9

Pepper-Seared Sea Scallops (page 336)
Fettuccine with Roasted Red Pepper Sauce (page 336)
Specialty Green Beans (page 337)
Red-Leaf Lettuce with Pine Nuts, Cherries and Dried-Tomato
Vinaigrette (page 338)

Day 10

Thai Stir-Fry (page 339)
Hot-and-Sour Soup (page 341)

Day 11

Pasta Rustica (page 342)
Caesar-Style Salad (page 344)

Day 12

Swiss Dijon Chicken Rolls (page 345)
Mashed Potatoes with a Difference (page 346)
Broccoli Lemon Amandine (page 347)
European Mixed Vegetable Salad (page 347)
Balsamic Splash (page 348)

Day 13

Village Paella (page 349)
Red- and Green-Leaf Lettuce
with Maple-Walnut Dressing (page 351)

Day 14

Old-Fashioned Chicken and Vegetable Stew (page 352)
Greens with Baby Beets, Toasted Walnuts
and Maple-Raspberry Vinaigrette (page 354)

Day 1

Chicken Cutlets with Raspberry Vinaigrette
Lemon Linguine Parmesan
Salad Nouveau
Creamy Garlic Dressing

This menu is appropriate for both fast family-style dining and elegant entertaining. Its origin is the light and flavorful California cuisine. A loaf of crispy Whole-Wheat French Bread (page 399) is always a nice addition to a meal such as this.

NUTRITIONAL ANALYSIS FOR DINNER

Per serving: 628 calories, 13.4 g. total fat (19% of calories), 6.1 g. monounsaturated fat, 2.7 g. polyunsaturated fat, 3.2 g. saturated fat, 38.1 g. protein, 87.3 g. carbohydrate, 3.2 g. dietary fiber, 53 mg. cholesterol, 459 mg. sodium

Chicken Cutlets
with Raspberry Vinaigrette

Raspberries, raspberry vinegar and white wine combine to make an incredibly delicious sauce to pour over lightly sautéed chicken breasts. For a vegetarian alternative, sauté 4 ounces of tempeh or tofu per person and double the amount of sauce. This dish is fast and simple and will please a variety of tastes.

PREPARATION AND COOKING TIME: 35 MINUTES

4	boneless, skinless chicken breast halves
	Freshly ground black pepper
	Salt
1	tablespoon canola oil or unsalted butter
¼	cup dry white wine
2	tablespoons raspberry vinegar
1	cup fresh or frozen raspberries

Place the chicken between pieces of wax paper or plastic wrap. Using a meat mallet, pound slightly to an even thickness. Season with the pepper and salt.

Warm the oil or butter in a large no-stick frying pan over medium heat. Add the chicken and cook for 5 to 10 minutes, or until lightly browned on each side and cooked throughout.

Remove the chicken to a platter and keep warm.

Add the wine, vinegar and raspberries to the pan. Raise the heat to high and cook until the sauce thickens slightly.

Pour the sauce over the warm chicken and serve immediately.

> Per serving: 145 calories, 5.5 g. total fat (35% of calories), 2.7 g. monounsaturated fat, 1.5 g. polyunsaturated fat, 0.8 g. saturated fat, 17 g. protein, 4 g. carbohydrate, 1.4 g. dietary fiber, 46 mg. cholesterol, 40 mg. sodium

Serves 4

> **FRESH-START COOKING TIP**
> In recipes where the taste of a small amount of butter is essential, you can get more flavor with less butter if you heat the butter until it turns light brown. The French call this beurre noisette.

Lemon Linguine Parmesan

The flavor of this pasta is simple and delicate.

> **PREPARATION AND COOKING TIME: 10–20 MINUTES**

1	tablespoon olive oil
2	cloves garlic, minced
½	cup skim milk or evaporated skim milk
12	ounces linguine
½	cup lemon juice
⅓	cup grated Parmesan cheese
¼	cup minced fresh parsley
	Freshly ground black pepper

In a small saucepan over medium heat, cook the oil and garlic for 1 minute. Add the milk. Reduce the heat to low and heat gently.

Meanwhile, cook the linguine in a large pot of boiling water for 8 to 10 minutes, or until al dente. Drain well and transfer to a large bowl. Add the lemon juice and toss well.

Pour the garlic mixture over the pasta and toss. Add the Parmesan, parsley and pepper to taste. Toss well again. Serve immediately.

> Per serving: 405 calories, 7.3 g. total fat (16% of calories), 3.4 g. monounsaturated fat, 0.9 g. polyunsaturated fat, 2.3 g. saturated fat, 15.7 g. protein, 68.7 g. carbohydrate, 0.3 g. dietary fiber, 7 mg. cholesterol, 179 mg. sodium

Serves 4

Low-Fat Dinners

Salad Nouveau

Here's a true gourmet salad. Add whatever other ingredients you like best.

To top it off, serve Salad Nouveau with the Creamy Garlic Dressing below.

**PREPARATION
TIME: 10
MINUTES**

4   cups mixed greens (such as radicchio, arugula, endive and leaf lettuce) torn into bite-size pieces
4   shallots, chopped
12 spears asparagus, cooked
4   tablespoons sliced pimentos
    Hearts of palm, sliced (optional)
    Sun-dried tomatoes, finely chopped (optional)

Divide the greens among 4 individual bowls. Top with the shallots, asparagus, pimentos, hearts of palm (if using) and tomatoes (if using).

Per serving: 46 calories, 0.5 g. total fat (5% of calories), 0.01 g. monounsaturated fat, 0.2 g. polyunsaturated fat, 0.09 g. saturated fat, 4 g. protein, 8.4 g. carbohydrate, 1.5 g. dietary fiber, 0 mg. cholesterol, 17 mg. sodium

Serves 4

Creamy Garlic Dressing

Nonfat mayonnaise and nonfat sour cream form the base for this low-fat dressing with a mild garlic flavor. Nonfat yogurt and low-fat cottage cheese would also work well in this recipe.

**PREPARATION
TIME:
5 MINUTES**

¼   cup nonfat mayonnaise
¼   cup nonfat sour cream
1   small clove garlic, minced
½   teaspoon Dijon mustard
½   teaspoon minced fresh parsley
⅛   teaspoon onion powder
2   tablespoons skim milk
    Freshly ground black pepper
    Salt (optional)

In a blender or food processor, combine the mayonnaise, sour cream, garlic, mustard, parsley, onion powder, milk and pepper and salt (if using) to taste. Blend until smooth.

Refrigerate before serving. Thin with more skim milk, if desired.

Per serving: 32 calories, 0.06 g. total fat (2% of calories), 0.02 g. monounsaturated fat, 0.1 g. polyunsaturated fat, 0.01 g. saturated fat, 1.4 g. protein, 6.2 g. carbohydrate, 0.01 g. dietary fiber, 0.1 mg. cholesterol, 223 mg. sodium

Serves 4

Day 2

3 Tacos

When I need a quick, easy meal I'm sure my kids will eat, I make these tacos. The ingredients are ones I keep stocked, so I can produce a meal that pleases all in 15 minutes.

Two or three tacos is a meal in itself. For a heartier dinner, add some Mexicali Rice (page 324).

For just a little something extra, try a light dessert from chapter 20.

NUTRITIONAL ANALYSIS FOR DINNER

Per serving: 456 calories, 11 g. total fat (22% of calories), 0.03 g. monounsaturated fat, 0.2 g. polyunsaturated fat, 2.4 g. saturated fat, 25.8 g. protein, 68.7 g. carbohydrate, 3.9 g. dietary fiber, 12 mg. cholesterol, 1,302 mg. sodium

Tacos

This meal can please a variety of taste preferences and is almost a night off for the cook. You can make these tacos with either hard taco shells or soft tortillas made from flour or even whole wheat.

Try adding ground turkey breast cooked with taco seasoning. Add extra vegetables such as onions, peppers or cucumbers to the topping mixture.

If you want to prepare nachos, place the filling ingredients on top of a layer of baked tortilla chips and pop them under the broiler to melt the cheese.

FRESH-START COOKING TIP
Canned evaporated skim milk can be whipped into a light and frothy mock whipped cream that makes a nice topping for fresh fruit. Place a can of evaporated skim milk, a stainless steel or glass bowl and beaters from an electric mixer in the freezer for an hour. Pour the milk and one teaspoon of pure vanilla extract into the chilled bowl. Beat on high speed just until peaks form. Serve immediately. You can add ¼ cup of sugar and a tablespoon of brandy or Grand Marnier once the peaks form, if desired

PREPARATION
AND COOKING
TIME: 15
MINUTES

12   taco shells or tortillas
1   can (16 ounces) fat-free refried beans
2   tomatoes, chopped
2   cups shredded romaine lettuce
4   ounces low-fat Cheddar cheese, shredded
    Nonfat sour cream
    Salsa or picante sauce

Preheat the oven to 350°. If using taco shells, place on a baking sheet and bake for 6 minutes, or the amount of time recommended on the package. If using tortillas, microwave or warm slightly.

Heat the beans in the microwave or on top of the stove.

In a medium bowl, combine the tomatoes and lettuce.

Place the taco shells or tortillas on a plate and the beans, tomato-lettuce mixture, Cheddar, sour cream and salsa or picante sauce in bowls, so everyone can make his own taco.

Per taco: 152 calories, 3.6 g. total fat (20% of calories), 0.01 g. monounsaturated fat, 0.07 g. polyunsaturated fat, 0.8 g. saturated fat, 8.6 g. protein, 22.9 g. carbohydrate, 1.3 g. dietary fiber, 4 mg. cholesterol, 434 mg. sodium

Makes 12

Day 3

**Picante Seafood Veracruz
Baked Yams with Nutmeg Cream
Brown Basmati Rice with Lemon**

For variety, you can replace the seafood in the Picante Seafood Veracruz with chicken. Or for a vegetarian entrée, use tempeh or tofu.

Yams are a nice change of pace from baked potatoes. Here I top them with nonfat sour cream lightly spiced with nutmeg.

NUTRITIONAL
ANALYSIS
FOR DINNER

Per serving: 587 calories, 11.3 g. total fat (17% of calories), 5.8 g. monounsaturated fat, 2.7 g. polyunsaturated fat, 1.5 g. saturated fat, 34.1 g. protein, 87.1 g. carbohydrate, 8.3 g. dietary fiber, 36 mg. cholesterol, 532 mg. sodium

Picante Seafood Veracruz

A mildly spicy tomato-based sauce cooks the seafood until tender. If you enjoy a more pronounced bite, add a little hot-pepper sauce or use hot picante sauce or salsa instead of mild.

The seafood servings may seem small compared with restaurant portions, but the nutritional analysis shows that 4 ounces of seafood per person is the most healthful amount. Serve this dish over the Brown Basmati Rice with Lemon (page 318).

(page 318)

1	tablespoon olive oil
1	small onion, chopped
½	green pepper, sliced
1	can (14 ounces) tomato puree or crushed tomatoes
3	tablespoons dry red wine
½	cup mild picante sauce or salsa
1	pound halibut, snapper, salmon, swordfish or sea scallops
2	tablespoons minced fresh parsley
1	teaspoon chopped fresh cilantro (optional)

PREPARATION AND COOKING TIME: 40 MINUTES

Warm the oil in a large no-stick frying pan over medium heat. Add the onions and peppers; cook for 5 minutes.

Stir in the tomato puree or tomatoes, wine and picante sauce or salsa. Reduce the heat to medium low, cover and simmer for 20 minutes.

Place the seafood, parsley and cilantro (if using) in the pan. Spoon some of the sauce over the seafood.

Cover the pan and cook for about 10 minutes, or until the fish flakes apart easily with a fork or the scallops are cooked through.

Baste the seafood with the sauce several times during cooking. Serve the fish and sauce over rice.

Per serving: 222 calories, 6.6 g. total fat (26% of calories), 3.4 g. monounsaturated fat, 1.2 g. polyunsaturated fat, 0.8 g. saturated fat, 25.9 g. protein, 14.5 g. carbohydrate, 2.8 g. dietary fiber, 36 mg. cholesterol, 301 mg. sodium

Serves 4

Low-Fat Dinners

Baked Yams with Nutmeg Cream

Sweet potatoes and true yams actually come from different types of plants. True yams grow in Africa. Two types of sweet potato grow in the United States. I prefer those with sweet orange flesh—commonly sold as yams in supermarkets. Another type of sweet potato has firm, yellow flesh and is less sweet.

PREPARATION TIME: 5 MINUTES

BAKING TIME: 35–45 MINUTES

4   yams
½   cup nonfat sour cream
½   teaspoon ground nutmeg

Preheat the oven to 425°. Wash the yams and place them on a baking sheet. Bake for 35 to 45 minutes, or until tender.

In a small bowl, combine the sour cream and nutmeg. Chill until ready to serve.

Using a sharp knife, cut a large X in each baked yam. Push into the yam on all 4 sides to squeeze the flesh up and out of the opening. Top each yam with the nutmeg cream.

Per serving: 190 calories, 0.3 g. total fat (1% of calories), 0.02 g. monounsaturated fat, 0.08 g. polyunsaturated fat, 0.3 g. saturated fat, 4 g. protein, 42.6 g. carbohydrate, 3.4 g. dietary fiber, 0 mg. cholesterol, 51 mg. sodium

Serves 4

Brown Basmati Rice with Lemon

Basmati rice has a wonderful aroma and flavor. It can be found in many grocery stores, specialty shops and natural foods stores. If you can't find it, substitute long-grain brown rice.

PREPARATION AND COOKING TIME: 45–50 MINUTES

1   tablespoon canola oil or unsalted butter
2   shallots, chopped
2   cloves garlic, minced
2   tablespoons lemon juice
1   tablespoon grated lemon rind
1   tablespoon minced fresh parsley
½   teaspoon sugar

Salt

Freshly ground black pepper

1½ cups nonfat chicken or vegetable broth

¾ cup brown basmati rice

Warm the oil or butter in a medium saucepan over medium heat.

Add the shallots and garlic. Sauté for 3 minutes.

Add the lemon juice, lemon rind, parsley, sugar and salt and pepper to taste.

Stir in the broth and bring to a boil.

Add the rice. Reduce the heat to medium low.

Cover and simmer for 35 to 45 minutes, or until the water is absorbed.

Remove the rice from the heat.

Fluff lightly with a fork and keep covered until serving time.

Per serving: 175 calories, 4.4 g. total fat (23% of calories), 2.4 g. monounsaturated fat, 1.4 g. polyunsaturated fat, 0.4 g. saturated fat, 4.2 g. protein, 30 g. carbohydrate, 2.1 g. dietary fiber, 0 mg. cholesterol, 180 mg. sodium

Serves 4

Day 4

Angel Hair Pasta with Fresh Tomato Sauce
Mixed Green Salad
with Creamy Fresh Basil Dressing

This is fast and simple to prepare with very little cooking. The pasta is filling, yet the meal is light.

Make the dressing ahead of time, if possible, since the fresh basil flavor improves as it stands. If desired, serve the meal with crusty whole-grain bread.

NUTRITIONAL ANALYSIS FOR DINNER

Per serving: 510 calories, 13.8 g. total fat (24% of calories), 7.1 g. monounsaturated fat, 1.6 g. polyunsaturated fat, 3.8 g. saturated fat, 19.9 g. protein, 75 g. carbohydrate, 4.1 g. dietary fiber, 10 mg. cholesterol, 324 mg. sodium

Angel Hair Pasta
with Fresh Tomato Sauce

Angel hair pasta (also called vermicelli or capellini) is a very thin spaghetti. It is a big favorite with my family. Because its texture is so fine, the pasta needs a light and fresh-tasting sauce like the one in this recipe, made from garden-fresh red tomatoes.

You can serve this meal warm, straight from the stove. Or you can let the sauce come to room temperature and serve it over cooled pasta.

PREPARATION TIME: 35 MINUTES

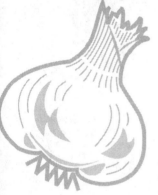

2	tablespoons olive oil
6	cloves garlic, minced
8	large ripe tomatoes, chopped (about 7 cups)
½	cup dry white wine
1	tablespoon chopped fresh oregano or 1 teaspoon dried
1	tablespoon chopped fresh basil or 1 teaspoon dried
	Freshly ground black pepper
	Salt (optional)
1	pound angel hair pasta
¾	cup grated Parmesan cheese

Warm the oil in a large saucepan over medium heat. Add the garlic and cook for 2 minutes. Stir in 5½ cups of the tomatoes and the wine, oregano, basil and pepper and salt (if using) to taste. Bring the sauce to a boil. Reduce the heat to low and simmer for 20 minutes.

Add the remaining tomatoes and remove the sauce from the heat.

Cook the pasta in a large pot of boiling water for 2 to 3 minutes, or until al dente. Drain well and toss with half of the Parmesan. Pour the sauce over the pasta and toss again. Top with the remaining Parmesan and serve.

Per serving: 438 calories, 10.1 g. total fat (21% of calories), 4.6 g. monounsaturated fat, 1.2 g. polyunsaturated fat, 3.3 g. saturated fat, 16.8 g. protein, 67.6 g. carbohydrate, 2.6 g. dietary fiber, 10 mg. cholesterol, 258 mg. sodium

Serves 6

Mixed Green Salad
with Creamy Fresh Basil Dressing

Many varieties of delicious salad greens are not yet very popular in America but are commonly eaten in Europe. The flavors and textures vary from sweet, juicy and crunchy to pleasantly bitter and soft. Add small amounts of new varieties to your current favorites. Try some of these in combination: romaine, leaf, Boston, Bibb and buttercrunch lettuce, Belgian endive, curly endive (chicory), escarole, radicchio, arugula and mache. Depending on the type of greens you choose, usually 1 large head, 2 medium heads or 9 to 12 cups of leaves yields about 6 servings.

The creamy low-fat dressing is deliciously scented and flavored with fresh basil. Don't try to use dried basil; the flavor is not nearly the same.

1	clove garlic, minced
½	cup nonfat sour cream
3	tablespoons chopped fresh basil
2	tablespoons white-wine vinegar or champagne vinegar
1½	tablespoons olive oil
1½	teaspoons Dijon mustard
½	teaspoon freshly ground black pepper
	Salt (optional)
9–12	cups mixed greens torn into bite-size pieces

In a blender or food processor, combine the garlic, sour cream, basil, vinegar, oil, mustard and pepper and salt (if using) to taste. Puree until very smooth and creamy.

Refrigerate in a covered jar or container for several hours. For best flavor, chill overnight.

Divide the greens among 6 individual salad plates and drizzle with the dressing.

Per serving: 72 calories, 3.7 g. total fat (44% of calories), 2.5 g. monounsaturated fat, 0.4 g. polyunsaturated fat, 0.5 g. saturated fat, 3.1 g. protein, 7.4 g. carbohydrate, 1.5 g. dietary fiber, 0 mg. cholesterol, 66 mg. sodium

Serves 6

FRESH-START COOKING TIP
The best croutons for a salad are home-made rather than store-bought, since homemade croutons have no extra fat, sodium or artificial ingredients. To make your own low-fat croutons, place bread cubes in a bowl and coat them very lightly with cooking spray. Sprinkle the bread cubes with garlic powder and fresh or dried herbs, then toss well. Place the cubes on a baking sheet and bake at 350° for 10 to 15 minutes, or until crisp.

PREPARATION TIME: 10 MINUTES

CHILLING TIME: SEVERAL HOURS

Low-Fat Dinners

Day 5

Sante Fe Chicken Fajitas
Southwestern Black Beans
Mexicali Rice

The preparation for this meal can be started the night before, making the next day's dinner a breeze. The beans and fajita mixture taste even better when they have marinated overnight, although that step is not necessary.

To shorten the cooking time, prepare the chicken first, so it can marinate while you fix the remainder of the meal. For variety, try using shrimp, tofu or tempeh instead of chicken.

NUTRITIONAL ANALYSIS FOR DINNER

Per serving: 576 calories, 13.8 g. total fat (22% of calories), 4.5 g. monounsaturated fat, 2.7 g. polyunsaturated fat, 1 g. saturated fat, 30.5 g. protein, 90.5 g. carbohydrate, 11 g. dietary fiber, 37 mg. cholesterol, 595 mg. sodium

Santa Fe Chicken Fajitas

PREPARATION AND COOKING TIME: 25 MINUTES

You can make these fajitas as spicy as you like by using anything from mild to extra-hot salsa. Any of these toppings can be rolled inside the tortillas with the chicken: nonfat sour cream, shredded part-skim Monterey Jack or Cheddar cheese, hot peppers and chopped tomatoes.

FRESH-START COOKING TIP
Liquid smoke can be found in the condiment section of your grocery store or supermarket. It is a good substitute for the flavor of bacon and ham in soups, stews, casseroles and other dishes. Use it sparingly, though—a little goes a very long way.

1	pound boneless, skinless chicken breasts
1	red onion, thickly sliced
1	green pepper, sliced
¾	cup salsa or picante sauce
6	tablespoons lime juice
3	cloves garlic, minced
2	teaspoons chili powder
1	teaspoon dried oregano
½	teaspoon ground cumin
¼	teaspoon natural smoke flavoring
	Salt
	Freshly ground black pepper
	Pinch of sugar
1	tablespoon canola or olive oil
10	tortillas

Cut the chicken into thin strips. In a large bowl, combine the chicken, onions and green peppers. In a medium bowl, combine the salsa or picante sauce, lime juice, garlic, chili powder, oregano, cumin, smoke flavoring, salt and pepper to taste and sugar. Pour over the chicken mixture. Marinate in the refrigerator for at least 1 hour, until ready to cook.

Warm the oil in a large no-stick frying pan over medium-high heat. Add the chicken and vegetables. Raise the heat to high and cook, stirring frequently, until the chicken is cooked through.

To serve, divide the filling evenly among the tortillas. Add the desired toppings and roll up the tortillas. Serve immediately.

Per serving: 325 calories, 8.2 g. total fat (23% of calories), 2.1 g. monounsaturated fat, 1.2 g. polyunsaturated fat, 0.6 g. saturated fat, 19.3 g. protein, 43.9 g. carbohydrate, 2.7 g. dietary fiber, 37 mg. cholesterol, 47 mg. sodium

Serves 5

Southwestern Black Beans

This bean dish is similar to a salad or relish. It has quite a few ingredients, yet is fast and easy to put together. As the beans marinate, the flavors intensify.

1	can (15 ounces) black beans, rinsed and drained
½	green pepper, chopped
¼	cup frozen corn, thawed
1	tomato, chopped
¼	cup finely chopped red onions
3	tablespoons lime juice
1	tablespoon canola oil
1	tablespoon white-wine vinegar
1	tablespoon reduced-sodium soy sauce
1	teaspoon sugar or honey
2	teaspoons chili powder
1	teaspoon garlic powder
	Freshly ground black pepper
	Hot-pepper sauce

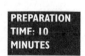

PREPARATION TIME: 10 MINUTES

In a large bowl, combine the beans, green peppers, corn, tomatoes and onions. Set aside.

In a small bowl or cup, mix the lime juice, oil, vinegar, soy sauce, sugar or honey, chili powder, garlic powder and black pepper and hot-pepper sauce to taste. Pour over the bean mixture and marinate at room temperature until ready to serve.

Per serving: 121 calories, 3.8 g. total fat (22% of calories), 1.6 g. monounsaturated fat, 0.9 g. polyunsaturated fat, 0.2 g. saturated fat, 7.8 g. protein, 21.2 g. carbohydrate, 6 g. dietary fiber, 0 mg. cholesterol, 381 mg. sodium

Serves 5

Mexicali Rice

For this dish, rice is cooked in a tomato-based sauce, giving it a Mexican flair. For milder-tasting rice, use less green chili peppers.

PREPARATION TIME: 10 MINUTES

COOKING TIME: 45–60 MINUTES

1	teaspoon canola oil
¼	cup chopped onions
¼	cup chopped green peppers
1	tablespoon canned chopped green chili peppers
1	cup nonfat chicken or vegetable broth
½	cup tomato juice or vegetable juice cocktail
2	teaspoons Worcestershire sauce
1	teaspoon chili powder
1	teaspoon sugar
¼	teaspoon dried oregano
¼	teaspoon garlic powder
	Freshly ground black pepper
¾	cup long-grain brown rice

Warm the oil in a large saucepan over medium heat. Add the onions and green peppers. Sauté for 3 minutes. Stir in the chili peppers. Cook for 3 minutes, stirring often.

Add the broth, tomato juice or vegetable juice cocktail, Worcestershire sauce, chili powder, sugar, oregano, garlic powder and black pepper to taste. Bring the mixture to a boil. Add the rice and return to a boil. Reduce the heat to low, cover and simmer for 45 to 60 minutes, or until the liquid is absorbed and the rice is soft.

Remove the pan from the heat and keep covered until ready to serve. Toss the rice gently with a fork.

Per serving: 130 calories, 1.8 g. total fat (13% of calories), 0.8 g. monounsaturated fat, 0.6 g. polyunsaturated fat, 0.2 g. saturated fat, 3.4 g. protein, 25.4 g. carbohydrate, 2.3 g. dietary fiber, 0 mg. cholesterol, 167 mg. sodium

Serves 5

Day 6

White Pizza
Mesclun Greens
with Italian Parmesan Vinaigrette

Pizza is a favorite food in America. It can be made in dozens of ways, with any number and combination of ingredients, to please just about everyone. In this white pizza, a blend of nonfat cream cheese, cottage cheese, herbs and spices takes the place of the usual tomato sauce. You can add any of the traditional pizza toppings to these individual pizzas.

The salad contains mesclun, a traditional European mixture of lettuces, chicories, mustards, cresses, once-wild greens and culinary herbs. It's a popular salad served in many fine resturants.

NUTRITIONAL ANALYSIS FOR DINNER

Per serving: 486 calories, 11.5 g. total fat (21% of calories), 4.4 g. monounsaturated fat, 0.9 g. polyunsaturated fat, 4.6 g. saturated fat, 25.9 g. protein, 71.8 g. carbohydrate, 5.2 g. dietary fiber, 25 mg. cholesterol, 1,033 mg. sodium

White Pizza

This recipe gives directions for making your own pizza crust, but for a fast-meal option, you can use a store-bought crust or focaccia. Try toasting pita bread and using it for fast pita pizzas. Tomato sauce may be substituted for the creamy topping, too. Reheated leftovers make a delicious lunch.

Semolina flour is also referred to as pasta flour. It adds a delicious quality to the crust. If semolina is not available, you can substitute half whole-wheat and half unbleached flour; for a heartier whole-grain crust, use all whole-wheat flour. You can also flavor the dough by adding garlic powder, oregano, basil and black pepper before kneading it.

If you need only 2, 3 or 4 pizzas, make the whole recipe for the dough and freeze what you don't use. To use the frozen dough, let it thaw overnight or all day.

PREPARATION AND RISING TIME: 55 MINUTES

BAKING TIME: 15 MINUTES

Crust
2 cups warm water (110°–115°)
1 teaspoon honey or sugar
2 tablespoons active dry yeast
2 teaspoons salt
2 cups semolina flour
1 cup whole-wheat flour
1⅓–1¾ cups unbleached flour

Sauce
¾ cup nonfat cream cheese
¼ cup nonfat cottage cheese
¼ teaspoon garlic powder
¼ teaspoon dried basil
⅛ teaspoon dried oregano
Freshly ground black pepper

Toppings
¾ cup chopped red onions
1 green pepper, chopped
½ cup sliced roasted red peppers
1½ cups sliced mushrooms
3 tomatoes, sliced
8 ounces mozzarella cheese, shredded

To make the crust: Coat a large bowl with a small amount of olive oil.

In a small bowl, combine the water, honey or sugar and yeast. Let stand for 5 to 10 minutes.

Meanwhile, in a food processor fitted with a plastic or steel blade, combine the salt, semolina flour and whole-wheat flour. Add the yeast mixture and 1 cup of the unbleached flour. Process until a ball forms in the bowl.

Gradually add the remaining flour until the dough feels smooth to the touch and not too sticky.

Transfer the dough to the oiled bowl and turn it so that it is entirely coated with oil.

Cover loosely with plastic wrap and set in a warm place—about 80° to 85°—for 30 to 45 minutes. (An oven with the light on is about the right temperature for warming.)

To make the sauce: In a blender or food processor, combine the cream cheese, cottage cheese, garlic powder, basil, oregano and pepper to taste. Set aside.

To assemble the pizzas: Preheat the oven to 450°. Lightly coat 2 baking sheets with no-stick spray. Sprinkle with a little flour.

Divide the dough into 8 pieces.

Place the pieces on the prepared baking sheet and press into 6″ circles.

Spread the sauce over the dough.

Top with the onions, green peppers, red peppers, mushrooms, tomatoes and mozzarella.

Bake on the bottom rack of the oven for 15 minutes, or until the mozzarella is melted and the crust is golden.

Per pizza: 367 calories, 5.5 g. total fat (14% of calories), 1.4 g. monounsaturated fat, 0.6 g. polyunsaturated fat, 3 g. saturated fat, 20 g. protein, 59 g. carbohydrate, 5.1 g. dietary fiber, 20 mg. cholesterol, 801 mg. sodium

Makes 8

Mesclun Greens with Italian Parmesan Vinaigrette

Mesclun greens can be found in many groceries, specialty shops and natural foods stores. They come prewashed, so you can just add dressing and serve. The tastes range from sweet to pleasantly bitter. This salad is one of my family's favorites.

PREPARATION TIME: 5 MINUTES

½ cup nonfat chicken broth or water
3 tablespoons red-wine vinegar
3 tablespoons balsamic vinegar
2 tablespoons olive oil
3 tablespoons chopped fresh parsley
2 tablespoons finely chopped shallots
1 large clove garlic, minced
½ teaspoon dried basil, finely crushed
¼ teaspoon dried oregano, finely crushed
⅛ teaspoon freshly ground black pepper
8 tablespoons grated Parmesan cheese
16 cups mesclun greens

In a medium bowl or jar, combine the broth or water, red-wine vinegar, balsamic vinegar, oil, parsley, shallots, garlic, basil, oregano, pepper and Parmesan. Whisk or shake until well-blended.

Place the greens in a large bowl and toss with the dressing. For a single serving, place 2 cups of the greens on a plate and top with 2 tablespoons of the dressing.

Per serving: 119 calories, 6 g. total fat (42% of calories), 3 g. monounsaturated fat, 0.3 g. polyunsaturated fat, 1.6 g. saturated fat, 5.9 g. protein, 12.8 g. carbohydrate, 0.07 g. dietary fiber, 5 mg. cholesterol, 232 mg. sodium

Serves 8

Day 7

Turkey Burgers
Spicy French Potatoes
Fresh Green Bean Salad

A burger and fries is an American favorite. Here is a low-fat, low-cholesterol version of this popular meal—ground turkey breast replaces beef, and oven-baked potatoes substitute for traditional french fries.

Served with the Fresh Green Bean Salad, Turkey Burgers and Spicy French Potatoes make a great summer meal.

NUTRITIONAL ANALYSIS FOR DINNER

Per serving: 592 calories, 10.8 g. total fat (16% of calories), 4.6 g. monounsaturated fat, 1.5 g. polyunsaturated fat, 1.7 g. saturated fat, 34.9 g. protein, 93.3 g. carbohydrate, 8.5 g. dietary fiber, 49 mg. cholesterol, 703 mg. sodium

Turkey Burgers

Unlike beef burgers, those made from ground turkey breast are low in fat and cholesterol. They have a mild flavor, so you can add a number of spices to create the burger that best suits your family's tastes. For a vegetarian alternative, try one of the meatless burgers that uses vegetables, beans and grains. For a great fast-meal option, make extra burgers, wrap them individually and freeze until needed.

1 pound ground turkey breast, skin and fat removed before grinding
½ onion, fincly chopped
½ green pepper, finely chopped
3 tablespoons steak sauce
  Freshly ground black pepper
4 whole-grain buns
4 leaves lettuce
1 tomato, cut into 4 slices
4 tablespoons ketchup
4 teaspoons mustard

PREPARATION AND COOKING TIME: 20–30 MINUTES

In a large bowl, combine the turkey, onions, green peppers, steak sauce and black pepper to taste. Mix well and form into 4 patties.

Grill or broil the patties for 15 to 20 minutes, or until lightly browned on both sides; be careful not to undercook or overcook. Serve each burger on a bun with 1 leaf of the lettuce, 1 slice of the tomato, 1 tablespoon of the ketchup and 1 teaspoon of the mustard.

> **FRESH-START COOKING TIP**
> Be wary when buying ground turkey and chicken. Skin and dark meat are often included, which drives up the fat content. Ask the butcher to grind skinless breast meat only.

Per serving: 253 calories, 3.8 g. total fat (13% of calories), 0.4 g. monounsaturated fat, 0.7 g. polyunsaturated fat, 0.8 g. saturated fat, 26.1 g. protein, 28.9 g. carbohydrate, 3 g. dietary fiber, 49 mg. cholesterol, 668 mg. sodium

Serves 4

Spicy French Potatoes

French fries were the inspiration for these potatoes. They are cut thick, coated with olive oil and herbs and baked, not fried. Although they don't get very crispy, they are a real taste treat and go well with burgers.

PREPARATION TIME: 10 MINUTES

BAKING TIME: 20 MINUTES

3 potatoes, cut into thin wedges
2 medium yams or sweet potatoes, cut into thin wedges
1 tablespoon olive oil or canola oil
1 teaspoon garlic powder
1 teaspoon paprika
1 teaspoon dried basil
  Salt
  Freshly ground black pepper

Preheat the oven to 475°. Lightly coat a baking sheet with no-stick spray.

In a very large bowl, combine the potatoes, yams or sweet potatoes, oil, garlic powder, paprika, basil and salt and pepper to taste. Mix well.

Spread the potatoes in a single layer on the prepared baking sheet and bake for 20 minutes, or until lightly browned.

Line a large bowl with several layers of paper towels. Spoon the potatoes into the bowl and serve warm.

Per serving: 222 calories, 3.7 g. total fat (15% of calories), 2.5 g. monounsaturated fat, 0.4 g. polyunsaturated fat, 0.5 g. saturated fat, 3.5 g. protein, 45 g. carbohydrate, 2.8 g. dietary fiber, 0 mg. cholesterol, 12 mg. sodium

Serves 4

Fresh Green Bean Salad

This marinated salad tastes best with fresh green beans, although you may use frozen beans. The longer the salad marinates, the more flavor it will have.

PREPARATION AND COOKING TIME: 20–25 MINUTES

MARINATING TIME: I HOUR OR MORE

4 cups green beans, cut into bite-size pieces
2 tablespoons olive oil
2 tablespoons red-wine vinegar

2 tablespoons nonfat chicken or vegetable broth
1 clove garlic, minced
1 tablespoon snipped fresh chives
½ teaspoon sugar or honey
½ teaspoon paprika
½ teaspoon reduced-sodium soy sauce
¼ teaspoon Dijon mustard
  Freshly ground black pepper
1 large tomato, diced
½ cup cooked chick-peas or ½ cup canned chick-peas, rinsed and drained

Steam the beans for 10 minutes, or until tender but still bright green. Set aside.

In a small cup or bowl, mix the oil, vinegar, broth, garlic, chives, sugar or honey, paprika, soy sauce, mustard and pepper to taste.

In a large bowl, combine the beans, tomatoes, chick-peas and oil mixture. Toss gently. Cover and marinate for at least 1 hour; stir occasionally.

Per serving: 117 calories, 3.3 g. total fat (23% of calories), 1.7 g. monounsaturated fat, 0.4 g. polyunsaturated fat, 0.4 g. saturated fat, 5.3 g. protein, 19.4 g. carbohydrate, 2.7 g. dietary fiber, 0 mg. cholesterol, 23 mg. sodium

Serves 4

Day 8

Chicken Baked with Sherry-Peach Sauce
Couscous Pilaf
Honey-Glazed Baby Carrots
Spinach Salad with Pears, Walnuts and Warm Mustard Vinaigrette

This meal is great for a special family dinner or for entertaining. The recipes serve eight but can be cut in half to serve four. Leftovers are easily reheated. It is an impressive meal that's quite simple to prepare.

NUTRITIONAL ANALYSIS FOR DINNER

Per serving: 566 calories, 12.5 g. total fat (20% of calories), 3.9 g. monounsaturated fat, 3.9 g. polyunsaturated fat, 3.1 g. saturated fat, 29.5 g. protein, 83.5 g. carbohydrate, 14.3 g. dietary fiber, 54 mg. cholesterol, 419 mg. sodium

Chicken Baked with Sherry-Peach Sauce

The chicken in this recipe is baked on the bone in a sweet and savory sauce, then finished off with sherry and peaches. Try using any other fruits—either fresh or frozen—that sound tasty.

PREPARATION AND COOKING TIME:
20 MINUTES
BAKING TIME:
1 HOUR

8	bone-in, skinless chicken breast halves
	Garlic powder
	Salt
	Freshly ground black pepper
2	onions, sliced
1	cup nonfat chicken broth
½	cup brown sugar
2	tablespoons arrowroot
1	cup chili sauce
1	cup sherry
1½	cups sliced peaches

FRESH-START COOKING TIP

Cooking sprays are useful for coating both no-stick and regular saucepans, frying pans, grill rings, baking sheets and even food. But don't go overboard. Most manufacturers recommend a one- to two-second spray. Choose sprays made with olive oil and canola oil whenever possible.

Cut any excess fat from the chicken. Place the chicken, bone side down, in a single layer in a large baking dish. Season with the garlic powder, salt and pepper. Broil for several minutes, until the chicken is slightly browned. Set aside.

Coat a medium saucepan with no-stick spray. Cook the onions over medium heat for 5 minutes. Add the broth, brown sugar, arrowroot and chili sauce. Raise the heat to high and bring the sauce to a boil, stirring constantly. Remove the pan from the heat and pour the sauce over the chicken.

Cover the chicken with a piece of foil. Refrigerate until ready to bake or continue with the next step.

Preheat the oven to 350°. Bake the chicken for 30 minutes. Remove the foil, and pour the sherry and peaches over the chicken. Bake uncovered, basting occasionally, for 30 minutes more, or until the chicken is cooked through and the sauce is bubbling.

Per serving: 162 calories, 2 g. total fat (11% of calories), 0.7 g. monounsaturated fat, 0.4 g. polyunsaturated fat, 0.6 g. saturated fat, 17.8 g. protein, 15.3 g. carbohydrate, 1.2 g. dietary fiber, 46 mg. cholesterol, 196 mg. sodium

Serves 8

Couscous Pilaf

Couscous (pronounced KOOS-koos) is actually a form of pasta made from semolina flour. The little grains are popular in Moroccan cuisine.

Couscous is commonly packaged in a box and can be found near the rice in most grocery stores. Couscous is quick to make and can be ready in 10 minutes, start to finish. For variety in flavor and texture, you can add other vegetables and herbs to the saucepan before adding the couscous.

1	tablespoon unsalted butter or canola oil
1	tablespoon minced shallots
1	tablespoon minced fresh parsley
3⅓	cups water
½	teaspoon salt (optional)
	Freshly ground black pepper
1½	boxes (10 ounces each) couscous

PREPARATION AND COOKING TIME: 10 MINUTES

Warm the butter or oil in a large saucepan over medium heat.

Add the shallots and parsley; cook for several minutes.

Add the water, salt (if using) and pepper to taste.

Bring the mixture to a boil.

Pour in the couscous, cover and remove from the heat. Let stand for 5 minutes.

Before serving, fluff the couscous lightly with a fork.

Per serving: 214 calories, 1.9 g. total fat (8% of calories), 0.5 g. monounsaturated fat, 0.2 g. polyunsaturated fat, 1 g. saturated fat, 6.8 g. protein, 41.3 g. carbohydrate, 8.3 g. dietary fiber, 4 mg. cholesterol, 6 mg. sodium

Serves 8

Low-Fat Dinners

Honey-Glazed Baby Carrots

Simple and slightly sweet, these carrots are sure to be loved by all.

PREPARATION AND COOKING TIME: 25 MINUTES

1	tablespoon unsalted butter or margarine
2	tablespoons minced shallots or onions
4	cups baby carrots (1¼ pounds)
1	cup nonfat chicken or vegetable broth
2½	tablespoons honey
¼	teaspoon ground nutmeg
1	tablespoon chopped fresh parsley
	Salt (optional)
	Freshly ground black pepper

Melt the butter or margarine in a large saucepan over medium heat. Add the shallots or onions. Cook for 2 minutes.

Stir in the carrots and broth. Bring to a boil. Reduce the heat to low and cook, covered, for 15 minutes, or until the carrots are just tender.

Raise the heat to medium high. Add the honey, nutmeg, parsley and salt (if using) and pepper to taste. Stir until the sauce becomes syrupy.

Per serving: 69 calories, 1.7 g. total fat (21% of calories), 0.4 g. monounsaturated fat, 0.1 g. polyunsaturated fat, 1 g. saturated fat, 1.2 g. protein, 13.1 g. carbohydrate, 2.3 g. dietary fiber, 4 mg. cholesterol, 84 mg. sodium

Serves 8

Spinach Salad with Pears, Walnuts and Warm Mustard Vinaigrette

For this easy salad, I combine spinach with fresh pears and walnuts and then toss them with a warm mustard dressing.

PREPARATION AND COOKING TIME: 10 MINUTES

10	ounces fresh spinach torn into bite-size pieces
1	tablespoon olive oil
1	large shallot, minced

2   tablespoons white-wine vinegar
4   tablespoons coarse mustard
2   tablespoons honey
1   tablespoon nonfat sour cream
     Salt
     Freshly ground black pepper
2   large pears, quartered and sliced lengthwise
½   cup walnut pieces

Put the spinach in a large salad bowl.

Warm the oil in a small saucepan over medium heat. Add the shallots and cook for several minutes.

Whisk in the vinegar, mustard, honey, sour cream and salt and pepper to taste. Cook and mix until heated through.

Toss the warm dressing with the spinach and quickly divide it among 8 individual plates. Top each salad with the pears and walnuts and serve immediately.

Per serving: 121 calories, 6.9 g. total fat (47% of calories), 2.3 g. monounsaturated fat, 3.2 g. polyunsaturated fat, 0.5 g. saturated fat, 3.7 g. protein, 13.8 g. carbohydrate, 2.5 g. dietary fiber, 0 mg. cholesterol, 133 mg. sodium

Serves 8

Day 9

Pepper-Seared Sea Scallops
Fettuccine with Roasted Red Pepper Sauce
Specialty Green Beans
Red-Leaf Lettuce with Pine Nuts, Cherries
and Dried-Tomato Vinaigrette

When preparing a meal from a number of recipes, as in this case, it's best to organize your cooking time. Start by making the vinaigrette, cooking the pasta sauce and steaming the beans. Set up the salad, then finish making the Specialty Green Beans, which can be left on very low heat, along with the pasta sauce, while you complete the remainder of the meal. Right before you are ready to serve, cook the pasta and scallops.

NUTRITIONAL
ANALYSIS
FOR DINNER
Per serving: 578 calories, 13.4 g. total fat (21% of calories), 6.8 g. monounsaturated fat, 2.3 g. polyunsaturated fat, 1.4 g. saturated fat, 28.1 g. protein, 88.8 g. carbohydrate, 2.8 g. dietary fiber, 23 mg. cholesterol, 307 mg. sodium

Pepper-Seared Sea Scallops

This recipe is fast and simple to make yet is quite elegant.

PREPARATION AND COOKING TIME: 15 MINUTES

20 sea scallops
 1 teaspoon canola oil
    Coarsely cracked black pepper
    Salt

Rinse the scallops and pat dry between paper towels.

Warm the oil in a large no-stick frying pan over medium-high heat.

Coat the scallops with the pepper and salt to taste.

Add to the pan and cook for 3 to 5 minutes on each side, being careful to neither overcook nor undercook. Serve immediately.

Per serving: 72 calories, 1.7 g. total fat (22% of calories), 0.7 g. monounsaturated fat, 0.5 g. polyunsaturated fat, 0.1 g. saturated fat, 11.9 g. protein, 1.7 g. carbohydrate, 0 g. dietary fiber, 23 mg. cholesterol, 114 mg. sodium

Serves 4

Fettuccine
with Roasted Red Pepper Sauce

This is a fast and easy pasta sauce with a uniquely sweet flavor. Spicy red-pepper flakes add a nice bite and can be added individually at the table.

PREPARATION AND COOKING TIME: 15 MINUTES

 1   teaspoon olive oil
¼   cup chopped onions
 1   large clove garlic, minced
¾   cup sliced roasted red peppers

  4   pecan halves
  1   teaspoon balsamic vinegar
  ¼   cup nonfat chicken or vegetable broth
      Salt
      Freshly ground black pepper
      Red-pepper flakes (optional)
 12   ounces fettuccine

Warm the oil in a small saucepan over medium heat.

Add the onions and garlic. Cook for several minutes, still on medium heat.

In a blender or food processor, combine the onion mixture, roasted peppers and pecans.

Puree until smooth. Pour the puree back into the saucepan.

Stir in the vinegar, broth and salt, black pepper and red-pepper flakes (if using) to taste. Taste and adjust the seasoning. Keep warm on the lowest heat.

Cook the fettuccine in a large pot of boiling water for 8 to 10 minutes, or until al dente.

Drain and rinse the pasta.

Toss with the sauce and serve immediately.

> *Per serving: 351 calories, 4 g. total fat (10% of calories), 1.9 g. monounsaturated fat, 1 g. polyunsaturated fat, 0.5 g. saturated fat, 11.5 g. protein, 66.3 g. carbohydrate, 0.5 g. dietary fiber, 0 mg. cholesterol, 37 mg. sodium*

Serves 4

Specialty Green Beans

The inspiration for this recipe was a dish served at one of my favorite restaurants, which specialized in grilled foods.

  1   pound whole green beans
  2   teaspoons olive oil
  4   cloves garlic, thinly sliced
  ½   tablespoon reduced-sodium soy sauce
      Freshly ground black pepper
      Red-pepper flakes
  1   teaspoon sugar

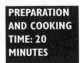

PREPARATION AND COOKING TIME: 20 MINUTES

Steam the beans for 5 minutes, or until bright green and partially cooked. Drain well.

Warm the oil in a large no-stick frying pan over medium heat.

Add the garlic and cook for 3 minutes. Stir in the beans, soy sauce, black pepper to taste, red-pepper flakes to taste and sugar. Toss until the beans are well-coated. Cook for about 10 minutes, stirring often, until the beans are tender.

Per serving: 64 calories, 2.4 g. total fat (30% of calories), 1.7 g. monounsaturated fat, 0.3 g. polyunsaturated fat, 0.3 g. saturated fat, 2.4 g. protein, 10.2 g. carbohydrate, 0.5 g. dietary fiber, 0 mg. cholesterol, 73 mg. sodium

Serves 4

Red-Leaf Lettuce with Pine Nuts, Cherries and Dried-Tomato Vinaigrette

The rich and tangy dried-tomato dressing complements the pine nuts and cherries of the salad. If you can't get dried cherries, substitute raisins.

PREPARATION TIME: 10 MINUTES

¼ cup boiling water
4 sun-dried tomatoes
8 cups red-leaf lettuce torn into bite-size pieces
4 tablespoons dried cherries
4 teaspoons pine nuts
¼ cup cold water
1 tablespoon red-wine vinegar
1 tablespoon balsamic vinegar
1 tablespoon olive oil
1 teaspoon sugar
½ teaspoon dried basil
¼ teaspoon garlic powder
⅛ teaspoon salt
   Freshly ground black pepper

Pour the boiling water over the tomatoes and soak for several minutes.

Divide the lettuce among 4 individual plates. Sprinkle with the cherries and pine nuts.

In a medium bowl, whisk together the cold water, red-wine vinegar, balsamic vinegar, oil, sugar, basil, garlic powder, salt and pepper to taste. Set aside.

In a blender or food processor, puree the tomatoes with the soaking water. Stir the puree into the oil mixture.

Serve the salads drizzled with 1 or 2 tablespoons of the dressing.

Per serving: 91 calories, 5.3 g. total fat (48% of calories), 2.5 g. monounsaturated fat, 0.5 g. polyunsaturated fat, 0.5 g. saturated fat, 2.3 g. protein, 10.6 g. carbohydrate, 1.8 g. dietary fiber, 0 mg. cholesterol, 83 mg. sodium

Serves 4

Day 10

Thai Stir-Fry
Hot-and-Sour Soup

Thai food is traditionally quite spicy, yet the "hotness" doesn't mask the flavor of the food. In the recipes below, I use chili puree with garlic to create the spiciness. Use more or less to suit your own taste. Look for ingredients such as the chili puree, rice wine and rice vinegar in the Asian foods section of grocery or specialty stores.

NUTRITIONAL ANALYSIS FOR DINNER

Per serving: 602 calories, 13.9 g. total fat (21% of calories), 5.4 g. monounsaturated fat, 5.3 g. polyunsaturated fat, 2.1 g. saturated fat, 32.8 g. protein, 88.2 g. carbohydrate, 10.1 g. dietary fiber, 139 mg. cholesterol, 1,436 mg. sodium

Thai Stir-Fry

This recipe has a lot of ingredients and quite a few steps, but it's actually easy to make. Just follow the steps. Let the shrimp marinate and the rice cook while you cut the veg-

etables and get the remaining ingredients together.

For variety, replace the shrimp with boneless, skinless chicken breast pieces, scallops, tofu, tempeh or just other vegetables, such as broccoli, Chinese cabbage, celery or bok choy. You can also use any other type of rice or cooked whole grain. Remember to adjust the spiciness to your taste by adding or subtracting from the amount of chili puree with garlic.

PREPARATION AND COOKING TIME: 45 MINUTES

4	cups nonfat chicken broth or water
1¾	cups brown rice
1	pound medium shrimp, peeled and deveined
1	tablespoon reduced-sodium soy sauce
1	tablespoon rice wine or dry white wine
1	clove garlic, minced
1	teaspoon + 1 tablespoon roasted sesame oil
1	tablespoon arrowroot
1	tablespoon chili puree with garlic
½	teaspoon sugar
	Salt (optional)
1	teaspoon rice vinegar
1	red onion, quartered and thickly sliced
1	green pepper, cut into ½" squares
2	carrots, sliced
1	tablespoon minced fresh cilantro
1	can (20 ounces) pineapple chunks (with juice)
4	scallions, sliced
4	tablespoons peanuts

Bring 3½ cups of the broth or water to a boil in a medium saucepan over high heat. Add the rice and reduce the heat to medium low. Cover and cook for 35 to 45 minutes, or until the water is absorbed. Remove from the heat and fluff gently with a fork. Cover and set aside.

Using a sharp knife, butterfly the shrimp by cutting halfway through down the entire length of the back.

In a medium bowl, mix the soy sauce, wine, garlic and 1 teaspoon of the oil. Add the shrimp and marinate until ready to use.

In a small bowl, combine the arrowroot, chili puree, sugar, salt (if using) to taste, vinegar and remaining ½ cup broth or water. Mix well and set aside.

In a large no-stick frying pan or wok, cook the shrimp and marinade over medium heat for 1 to 2 minutes on each side, or until the shrimp turn pink. Do not overcook. Remove from the pan and set aside.

In the same pan, heat the remaining 1 tablespoon oil over medium-high heat.

Add the onions, peppers and carrots. Cook for 5 to 10 minutes, stirring often. Pour the chili puree mixture over the vegetables. Reduce the heat to low and cook for several minutes more.

Add the shrimp, cilantro and pineapple (with juice).

Reduce the heat to medium and stir-fry for several minutes, until the shrimp is cooked through. Taste and adjust seasoning.

To serve, place the rice on individual plates and top with the stir-fry. Garnish with the scallions and peanuts.

Per serving: 508 calories, 10.1 g. total fat (18% of calories), 4 g. monounsaturated fat, 3.7 g. polyunsaturated fat, 1.6 g. saturated fat, 26.1 g. protein, 79.5 g. carbohydrate, 7.2 g. dietary fiber, 139 mg. cholesterol, 660 mg. sodium

Serves 5

Hot-and-Sour Soup

The "hot-and-sour" in this soup refers to a slightly spicy sweet-and-sour flavor that comes from a few staple ingredients. To create a more filling soup, add extra vegetables, sliced chicken breast, cubed tofu or Chinese noodles.

1	tablespoon roasted sesame oil
1	clove garlic, minced
4	ounces mushrooms, sliced
4	cups nonfat chicken or vegetable broth
3	tablespoons rice wine or dry white wine
2	tablespoons rice vinegar
2	tablespoons reduced-sodium soy sauce
½–1	teaspoon chili puree with garlic
1	carrot, shredded
2	cups chopped bok choy or spinach
2	cups broccoli florets

PREPARATION AND COOKING TIME: 25 MINUTES

Warm the oil in a large saucepan over medium heat. Cook the garlic and mushrooms for several minutes, until soft.

Stir in the broth, wine, vinegar, soy sauce, chili puree, carrots, bok choy or spinach and broccoli.

Bring to a boil.

Reduce the heat to low and cook for 5 minutes, or until the vegetables are cooked.

Taste and adjust the seasoning, adding more wine, vinegar, soy sauce or chili puree if desired.

Per serving: 94 calories, 3.8 g. total fat (33% of calories), 1.4 g. monounsaturated fat, 1.6 g. polyunsaturated fat, 0.5 g. saturated fat, 6.7 g. protein, 8.7 g. carbohydrate, 2.9 g. dietary fiber, 0 mg. cholesterol, 776 mg. sodium

Serves 4

Day 11

Pasta Rustica
Caesar-Style Salad

FRESH-START COOKING TIP
Leftovers from last night's dinner can be wonderful brown-bag lunches. You can reheat casseroles, soups, stews, grain and legume dishes, even pasta in the microwave. If cooking isn't feasible, use a Thermos to keep cold foods cool and hot foods warm. A minicooler works well if there's no refrigerator available.

This meal is fast and hearty, with a European country flair. The recipes can be divided in half to make three servings instead of six. But I like to make the full recipes and save the leftovers to reheat for lunch. I use yogurt instead of oil in the salad to create a surprisingly similar feel to traditional Caesar salad.

NUTRITIONAL ANALYSIS FOR DINNER

Per serving: 535 calories, 10.8 g. total fat (18% of calories), 5 g. monounsaturated fat, 1.3 g. polyunsaturated fat, 2.9 g. saturated fat, 22.5 g. protein, 91.2 g. carbohydrate, 7 g. dietary fiber, 9 mg. cholesterol, 589 mg. sodium

Pasta Rustica

The chunky tomato-based sauce for this dish has the warmth and feeling of the country yet is anything but plain and simple. Try adding other vegetables, such as sun-dried tomatoes or peperoncini, for variety.

1	tablespoon olive oil
7	cloves garlic, sliced
1	onion, cut into strips
1	green pepper, sliced
1	can (28 ounces) tomato puree
1	can (6 ounces) tomato paste
½	cup dry red wine
1½	teaspoons dried basil
1½	teaspoons dried oregano
18	small black olives, pitted
16	small green olives, pitted
¼	cup sliced roasted red peppers or pimentos
1	can (14 ounces) artichoke hearts packed in water, drained and sliced
¼	cup chopped fresh parsley
	Freshly ground black pepper
1	pound pasta shells, gnocci or other pasta
6	tablespoons grated Parmesan cheese

PREPARATION AND COOKING TIME: 30 MINUTES

Warm the oil in a large saucepan over medium heat.

Add the garlic, onions and green peppers. Cook for 5 to 10 minutes.

Stir in the tomato puree, tomato paste, wine, basil, oregano, black olives, green olives, red peppers or pimentos, artichoke hearts, parsley and black pepper to taste.

Reduce the heat to medium low.

Cover and simmer, stirring occasionally. Allow to simmer for about 15 minutes.

Cook the pasta in a large pot of boiling water for 8 to 10 minutes, or until al dente.

Drain well and transfer to a large bowl. Pour the sauce over the pasta and toss well.

Serve the pasta in individual bowls; sprinkle each serving with 1 tablespoon of the Parmesan.

Per serving: 489 calories, 9.4 g. total fat (16% of calories), 4.6 g. monounsaturated fat, 1.2 g. polyunsaturated fat, 2.1 g. saturated fat, 18.3 g. protein, 86.8 g. carbohydrate, 5.6 g. dietary fiber, 5 mg. cholesterol, 482 mg. sodium

Serves 6

Low-Fat Dinners

Caesar-Style Salad

This variation of Caesar salad is dramatically lower in fat and calories than the traditional recipe. And it doesn't use a lot of oil or raw egg, as the original does.

PREPARATION TIME: 5 MINUTES

9   cups romaine lettuce torn into bite-size pieces
½   cup nonfat yogurt
2   teaspoons lemon juice
2   teaspoons balsamic vinegar
1   teaspoon Worcestershire sauce
1   small clove garlic, minced
½   teaspoon anchovy paste
½   cup grated Parmesan cheese

Place the lettuce in a large salad bowl.

In a blender or food processor, puree the yogurt, lemon juice, vinegar, Worcestershire sauce, garlic, anchovy paste and ¼ cup of the Parmesan until smooth. Pour the mixture over the lettuce and toss well. Sprinkle with the remaining ¼ cup Parmesan and toss again. Serve on individual plates.

Per serving: 46 calories, 1.4 g. total fat (37% of calories), 0.4 g. monounsaturated fat, 0.1 g. polyunsaturated fat, 0.8 g. saturated fat, 4.2 g. protein, 4.4 g. carbohydrate, 1.4 g. dietary fiber, 4 mg. cholesterol, 107 mg. sodium

Serves 6

Day 12

Swiss Dijon Chicken Rolls
Mashed Potatoes with a Difference
Broccoli Lemon Amandine
European Mixed Vegetable Salad
Balsamic Splash

You can use this menu for a casual family supper or garnish it decoratively for a more elegant dinner. If you'd like, you may serve a simple sauce of your choosing over the chicken.

NUTRITIONAL ANALYSIS FOR DINNER

Per serving: 564 calories, 15.4 g. total fat (25% of calories), 5.1 g. monounsaturated fat, 1.6 g. polyunsaturated fat, 7.2 g. saturated fat, 41.3 g. protein, 68 g. carbohydrate, 9.1 g. dietary fiber, 64 mg. cholesterol, 757 mg. sodium

Swiss Dijon Chicken Rolls

I make these rolls by sprinkling shredded Jarlsberg light Swiss cheese (or other part-skim Swiss) on chicken breasts, rolling them up to enclose the cheese and dipping them sequentially in a Dijon sauce and then in bread crumbs.

1   pound boneless, skinless chicken breast halves
¾   cup shredded Jarlsberg light Swiss cheese
6   tablespoons evaporated skim milk
4   tablespoons Dijon mustard
¾   cup bread crumbs
4   tablespoons grated Parmesan cheese
2   teaspoons dried tarragon
     Freshly ground black pepper

PREPARATION TIME: 25 MINUTES

BAKING TIME: 45 MINUTES

Preheat the oven to 375°. Lightly coat an 8″ × 8″ baking dish with no-stick spray. Place the chicken between pieces of wax paper or plastic wrap. With a meat mallet, pound to about ¼″ thickness. Place an equal amount of the Swiss cheese in the center of each breast. Set aside.

In a small bowl, mix the milk and mustard. Set aside.

In a medium bowl, combine the bread crumbs, Parmesan, tarragon and pepper to taste.

Roll up each chicken breast, beginning with the smaller end. Dip each roll into the milk mixture and then into the bread crumb mixture to coat completely. Place in the prepared baking dish with the rolled end down. Cover and bake for 30 minutes. Uncover and bake for 15 minutes more, or until golden.

Per serving: 243 calories, 9 g. total fat (34% of calories), 1.3 g. monounsaturated fat, 0.5 g. polyunsaturated fat, 4.1 g. saturated fat, 30.4 g. protein, 8.3 g. carbohydrate, 0.2 g. dietary fiber, 64 mg. cholesterol, 476 mg. sodium

Serves 4

FRESH-START COOKING TIP
Evaporated skim milk can be substituted for heavy cream, half-and-half or whole milk in many recipes. It can help turn a potentially high-fat disaster into a low-fat pleasure.

Mashed Potatoes with a Difference

My husband has fond memories of mashed potatoes and likes them in their simplest form. But there are many variations, and each family has its favorite. You can beat the potatoes until they're smooth or leave them chunky. You can also choose to remove the peels from the potatoes or leave them on.

Here's our family favorite, which has a mild flavor twist. I cook sweet potatoes and a clove of garlic with regular potatoes. The resulting potatoes have a light texture and are much lower in fat than most recipes, especially since I don't add egg yolks or butter and I use nonfat sour cream and mayonnaise.

PREPARATION AND COOKING TIME: 20–25 MINUTES

2   large baking potatoes, peeled and cubed
2   yams or sweet potatoes, peeled and cubed
1   large clove garlic, minced
2   tablespoons nonfat sour cream
1   tablespoon nonfat mayonnaise
2   tablespoons nonfat milk
   Freshly ground black pepper
   Salt (optional)

Place the potatoes, yams or sweet potatoes and garlic in a large saucepan.

Add cold water to cover. Bring to a boil. Turn the heat to medium and cook for 15 to 20 minutes, or until the potatoes are tender. Drain well.

Add the sour cream, mayonnaise, milk and pepper and salt (if using) to taste.

Beat or mash the potatoes to the desired texture, adding more milk if necessary.

Taste and adjust the seasoning; serve immediately.

Per serving: 166 calories, 0.2 g. total fat (1% of calories), 0.01 g. monounsaturated fat, 0.08 g. polyunsaturated fat, 0.2 g. saturated fat, 3.3 g. protein, 38.2 g. carbohydrate, 1.9 g. dietary fiber, 0.1 mg. cholesterol, 71 mg. sodium

Serves 4

Broccoli Lemon Amandine

In this recipe, broccoli spears are dressed with a lemon-mayonnaise sauce and sprinkled with sliced almonds.

1	bunch broccoli
3	tablespoons nonfat sour cream
2	tablespoons skim milk
1	tablespoon nonfat or low-fat mayonnaise
2	teaspoons lemon juice
1	teaspoon grated lemon rind
¼	teaspoon sugar
⅛	teaspoon salt
⅛	teaspoon dried tarragon
	Freshly ground black pepper
2	tablespoons sliced almonds, lightly toasted

PREPARATION AND COOKING TIME: 15 MINUTES

Cut the broccoli into spears, peel the tough skin from the stalks and rinse. Steam for 10 minutes, or until tender.

In a blender or food processor, combine the sour cream, milk, mayonnaise, lemon juice, lemon rind, sugar, salt, tarragon and pepper to taste. Blend until smooth.

Place the broccoli in a serving dish and pour the sauce on top. Sprinkle with the almonds and serve.

Per serving: 77 calories, 2.4 g. total fat (24% of calories), 1.2 g. monounsaturated fat, 0.6 g. polyunsaturated fat, 2.4 g. saturated fat, 5.7 g. protein, 11.2 g. carbohydrate, 4 g. dietary fiber, 0.1 mg. cholesterol, 169 mg. sodium

Serves 4

European Mixed Vegetable Salad

This is a decorative salad that you compose right in individual bowls. I've given you one combination of ingredients below, but you can also use other vegetables, such as cooked corn kernels (fresh or frozen), chopped red or green peppers, cherry tomatoes, sliced cucumbers, cooked green beans and sliced artichoke hearts.

Top the salad with your favorite dressing or Balsamic Splash (page 348).

Low-Fat Dinners

PREPARATION TIME: 10 MINUTES

4   cups lettuce torn into bite-size pieces
1   cup shredded carrots
1   cup shredded raw or canned beets
1   cup shredded zucchini
    Sliced pimentos (optional)

Divide the lettuce among 4 individual bowls. Add the carrots, beets, zucchini and pimentos (if using) in separate piles on top of the lettuce.

Per serving: 39 calories, 0.3 g. total fat (6% of calories), 0.02 g. monounsaturated fat, 0.1 g. polyunsaturated fat, 0.04 g. saturated fat, 1.8 g. protein, 8.5 g. carbohydrate, 3 g. dietary fiber, 0 mg. cholesterol, 36 mg. sodium

Serves 4

Balsamic Splash

Balsamic vinegar is a dark, sweet, syrupy vinegar made in Italy and aged in wooden casks. The unique flavor quickly becomes a favorite of those who try it.

PREPARATION TIME: 5 MINUTES

3   tablespoons balsamic vinegar
2   tablespoons olive oil
1   tablespoon nonfat chicken broth or water
1   clove garlic, minced
1   teaspoon mustard seeds
½   teaspoon mustard powder
¼   teaspoon honey
    Freshly ground black pepper

In a jar or small bowl, combine the vinegar, oil, broth or water, garlic, mustard seeds, mustard powder, honey and pepper to taste. Shake or whisk well.

Per tablespoon: 39 calories, 3.5 g. total fat (80% of calories), 2.6 g. monounsaturated fat, 0.3 g. polyunsaturated fat, 0.5 g. saturated fat, 0.1 g. protein, 1.8 g. carbohydrate, 0 g. dietary fiber, 0 mg. cholesterol, 5 mg. sodium

Makes ½ cup

Day 13

Village Paella
Red- and Green-Leaf Lettuce
with Maple-Walnut Dressing

One of the key ingredients in paella (*pie-AY-a*), a Spanish rice dish, is saffron—the world's most expensive spice. It takes 75,000 crocus blossoms to make one pound of dried saffron.

Saffron is most often sold in a small, one-gram vial, which gives you more than enough for this paella recipe. Be sure to buy the true saffron threads; there's a much less costly saffron that comes from Mexican safflowers, but its flavor isn't as good.

Many grocery stores, gourmet shops and natural foods stores carry saffron. Serve the meal with crusty whole-grain bread, if desired.

NUTRITIONAL ANALYSIS FOR DINNER

Per serving: 536 calories, 12.7 g. total fat (21% of calories), 5.4 g. monounsaturated fat, 4.3 g. polyunsaturated fat, 1.7 g. saturated fat, 39.6 g. protein, 56.9 g. carbohydrate, 5.4 g. dietary fiber, 107 mg. cholesterol, 567 mg. sodium

Village Paella

Paella is a combination of rice, seafood, poultry and vegetables traditionally cooked in a special shallow iron pan with double handles. (Indeed, the dish gets its name from the Latin patella, *meaning "pan." But you can make a very successful paella in a large frying pan.)*

Paella is one of those dishes that have a few basic ingredients, with additions of the chef's choosing, so you may use any type of seafood or poultry. (Just a reminder if you're using seafood: Remember to presoak clams or mussels in the shell and to rinse them very well to remove sand.)

You could also create a vegetarian paella with tempeh, tofu and vegetables such as asparagus and artichoke hearts.

In this recipe, I've used halibut, a chicken breast, shrimp and scallops. Leftovers reheat very well.

PREPARATION TIME: 20 MINUTES
COOKING TIME: 1 HOUR

2 tablespoons olive oil
1 whole boneless, skinless chicken breast, cut into bite-size pieces
1 onion, chopped
1 green pepper, thinly sliced
4 cloves garlic, thinly sliced
1½ cups brown rice
1 cup canned Italian tomatoes, drained and quartered
1½ cups dry white wine
4 cups nonfat chicken broth or clam juice
1 teaspoon dried oregano
½ teaspoon saffron threads
¼ cup hot water
2 tablespoons minced fresh parsley
8 ounces halibut, cut into bite-size pieces
8 ounces scallops
8 ounces shrimp, peeled and deveined
1 cup green peas
Freshly ground black pepper
Salt

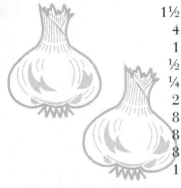

Warm 1 tablespoon oil in a paella pan or large no-stick frying pan over medium heat.

Add the chicken and cook for 5 minutes. Remove from the pan and set aside.

In the same pan, cook the onions, peppers and garlic in the remaining 1 tablespoon oil for 5 minutes.

Stir in the rice and cook for 3 minutes, or until slightly browned.

Add the tomatoes, wine, broth or clam juice and oregano. Raise the heat to high and bring to a boil. Cover and reduce the heat to low.

Meanwhile, soak the saffron in the water until needed.

After the rice has cooked for 30 minutes, add the saffron and soaking water and the parsley to the pan (do not stir the rice). Let the rice cook for another 5 to 10 minutes.

Add the halibut, scallops, shrimp and chicken to the rice. Cook for 7 to 10 minutes longer.

Add the peas. Cook for 3 minutes. The rice should be soft and most of the water absorbed. Season with the salt and pepper.

Remove the paella from the heat and keep it covered until ready to serve.

This dish looks beautiful when set in the center of the table and served right from the pan into individual bowls.

> *Per serving: 461 calories, 8.6 g. total fat (17% of calories), 4.5 g. monounsaturated fat, 1.7 g. polyunsaturated fat, 1.4 g. saturated fat, 37.5 g. protein, 47.7 g. carbohydrate, 3.7 g. dietary fiber, 107 mg. cholesterol, 556 mg. sodium*

Serves 6

Red- and Green-Leaf Lettuce with Maple-Walnut Dressing

This simple salad is complemented by a light, sweet dressing. It's one of my children's favorites.

6	cups green-leaf lettuce torn into bite-size pieces
6	cups red-leaf lettuce torn into bite-size pieces
6	walnut halves
2	tablespoons maple syrup
2	tablespoons apple juice
1	tablespoon walnut oil
1	tablespoon white-wine vinegar
	Salt
	Freshly ground black pepper

PREPARATION TIME: 10 MINUTES

Place the green-leaf lettuce and red-leaf lettuce in a large salad bowl. Set aside.

In a blender or food processor, combine the walnuts, maple syrup, juice, oil, vinegar and salt and pepper to taste.

Mix until well-blended.

Pour the dressing over the lettuce and serve on individual plates.

> *Per serving: 75 calories, 4.1 g. total fat (45% of calories), 0.9 g. monounsaturated fat, 2.6 g. polyunsaturated fat, 0.3 g. saturated fat, 2.1 g. protein, 9.2 g. carbohydrate, 1.7 g. dietary fiber, 0 mg. cholesterol, 11 mg. sodium*

Serves 6

Day 14

Old-Fashioned Chicken and Vegetable Stew
Greens with Baby Beets, Toasted Walnuts
and Maple-Raspberry Vinaigrette

I've made a switch here, transforming traditional beef stew into a creamy chicken stew. It's loaded with vegetables and served over yolk-free egg noodles. The stew has a hearty, old-fashioned feeling with a surprisingly gourmet flavor. The unique salad completes the meal, although a slice of whole-grain bread is good with it, too.

NUTRITIONAL ANALYSIS FOR DINNER

Per serving: 596 calories, 14.3 g. total fat (22% of calories), 4.9 g. monounsaturated fat, 6.7 g. polyunsaturated fat, 1.5 g. saturated fat, 28.9 g. protein, 89.6 g. carbohydrate, 7 g. dietary fiber, 30 mg. cholesterol, 597 mg. sodium

Old-Fashioned Chicken
and Vegetable Stew

This stew adapts well to a variety of substitutions. You can use seafood instead of chicken (add the seafood during the last few minutes of cooking). For a vegetarian option, just add a larger assortment of vegetables and use vegetable broth. It's also good served over rice.

PREPARATION AND COOKING TIME: 45 MINUTES

1	pound boneless, skinless chicken breasts
	Salt
	Freshly ground black pepper
	Garlic powder
2	tablespoons canola oil
20	pearl onions
3	cloves garlic, minced
1	red pepper, cut into large squares
8	ounces mushrooms, thickly sliced
4	cups nonfat chicken broth
½	cup chopped fresh parsley
½	teaspoon dried marjoram
½	teaspoon dried thyme
1	bay leaf

1   cup baby carrots
1   parsnip, peeled and sliced
2   potatoes, cubed
1   yam or sweet potato, cubed
1   cup green beans, cut into 1" pieces
12 ounces yolk-free egg noodles
2   tablespoons arrowroot
2   tablespoons whole-grain flour
4   tablespoons water
½   cup nonfat sour cream

Cut the chicken into chunks and season well with the salt, black pepper and garlic powder.

Warm 1 tablespoon of the oil in a large soup pot over medium heat. Add the chicken and brown for about 5 minutes. Remove from the pot and set aside.

In the same pot, heat the remaining 1 tablespoon oil. Add the onions, garlic, red peppers and mushrooms. Cook for 5 minutes.

Add the broth, parsley, marjoram, thyme and bay leaf. Bring to a boil, reduce the heat to low and cook for 5 minutes.

Stir in the carrots, parsnips, potatoes, yams or sweet potatoes, green beans and chicken. Bring to a boil, then reduce the heat to medium low. Cover and cook for 15 minutes.

Meanwhile, cook the noodles in a large pot of boiling water for 5 to 8 minutes, or until al dente. Drain and rinse. Set aside.

In a small cup, mix the arrowroot, flour, water and a few tablespoons of the hot broth from the stew. Stirring continuously, slowly pour the arrowroot mixture into the stew. Cook for a few more minutes.

Remove the stew from the heat and remove the bay leaf. Slowly stir in the sour cream. Season with a little extra pepper and salt, if desired.

Serve the stew over the noodles in individual bowls.

Per serving: 464 calories, 7.1 g. total fat (14% of calories), 3.3 g. monounsaturated fat, 2.1 g. polyunsaturated fat, 0.9 g. saturated fat, 25.9 g. protein, 73.1 g. carbohydrate, 4 g. dietary fiber, 30 mg. cholesterol, 392 mg. sodium

Serves 6

Low-Fat Dinners

Greens with Baby Beets, Toasted Walnuts and Maple-Raspberry Vinaigrette

This salad is a combination of bright and lively flavors.

PREPARATION TIME: 10 MINUTES

3	tablespoons chopped walnuts
12	cups green-leaf lettuce torn into bite-size pieces
2	tablespoons walnut oil or other nut oil
5	tablespoons raspberry vinegar
3	tablespoons maple syrup
3	tablespoons water
½	teaspoon dried basil
	Freshly ground black pepper
	Salt
1	can (15 ounces) baby beets packed in water, drained and sliced

Preheat the oven to 350°. Place the walnuts on a baking sheet and bake for 5 minutes. Watch carefully so that they don't burn. Remove from the oven and set aside.

Divide the lettuce among 6 individual plates and sprinkle each serving with 1½ teaspoons of the walnuts.

In a small bowl, whisk together the oil, vinegar, maple syrup, water, basil and pepper and salt to taste. Stir in the beets. Pour over the lettuce and serve.

Per serving: 132 calories, 7.2 g. total fat (45% of calories), 1.6 g. monounsaturated fat, 4.6 g. polyunsaturated fat, 0.6 g. saturated fat, 3 g. protein, 16.5 g. carbohydrate, 3 g. dietary fiber, 0 mg. cholesterol, 205 mg. sodium

Serves 6

Chapter Twenty

Fresh-Start Recipes for Low-Fat Snacks and Desserts

There are many delicious low-fat, high-fiber snacks and desserts available these days in grocery stores and natural foods stores. The new nutritional labeling makes it easier than ever before to know what you're getting in a product. Be sure to look for snacks and desserts that are made from whole grains and that get less than 25 percent of their calories from fat. And don't forget fresh fruit in season as a perfect ending to a meal.

When you want to enjoy some homemade snacks and desserts, turn to the recipes in this chapter. They include our favorite cookies—Chewy Oatmeal-Raisin and Old-Fashioned Molasses—as well as cakes, fruit breads and surprising low-fat treats such as Whole-Grain Cocoa Angel Food Cake and Chocolate Cream Cheese Delight. Use these recipes as a starting point for your own creations and as an example of how you can transform your own recipes, making healthier versions of the ones you love the best.

Chewy Oatmeal-Raisin Cookies

These cookies are low in fat yet are moist and chewy. They're always a favorite with those who try them. To keep them moist, store on a plate covered with plastic wrap. Try using currants in place of raisins.

PREPARATION TIME: 10 MINUTES

BAKING TIME: 10–15 MINUTES

¼	cup unsalted butter or margarine, melted
¼	cup honey or maple syrup
3–4	tablespoons skim milk
1	egg, 2 egg whites or ¼ cup fat-free egg substitute
2	tablespoons vanilla
1¼	cups rolled oats
1½	cups whole-wheat pastry flour
½	cup brown sugar
1	teaspoon baking powder
½	teaspoon baking soda
½	teaspoon ground cinnamon
½	teaspoon ground nutmeg
¾	cup raisins

Preheat the oven to 375°. Lightly coat 2 baking sheets with no-stick spray.

In a small bowl, mix the butter or margarine, honey or maple syrup, milk, egg, egg whites or egg substitute and vanilla. Set aside.

In a large bowl, mix the oats, flour, brown sugar, baking powder, baking soda, cinnamon, nutmeg and raisins.

Pour the egg mixture into the oat mixture.

Stir just enough to incorporate the ingredients.

Drop the batter by rounded teaspoons onto the prepared baking sheets. Leave at least 1″ or so between cookies.

Bake for 10 to 15 minutes, or until lightly browned. (Watch them carefully, because they burn easily.) Remove the cookies and cool on a rack.

Per cookie: 69 calories, 1.8 g. total fat (22% of calories), 0.5 g. monounsaturated fat, 0.2 g. polyunsaturated fat, 0.9 g. saturated fat, 1.3 g. protein, 12.4 g. carbohydrate, 0.7 g. dietary fiber, 10 mg. cholesterol, 28 mg. sodium

Makes 36

Old-Fashioned Molasses Cookies

Traditionally, molasses cookies are drizzled with a sugar syrup, which you may add if you like. To make the syrup, use a fork to stir a very small amount of warm skim milk into about 1 cup powdered sugar until it's smooth and very thick. Once the cookies have cooled, drizzle a small amount of the syrup onto each cookie with the fork.

¼	cup unsalted butter or margarine, softened
¾	cup honey
½	cup molasses
1	egg, 2 egg whites or ¼ cup fat-free egg substitute
2½	cups whole-wheat pastry flour
1	teaspoon ground cinnamon
1	teaspoon ground ginger
1	teaspoon baking soda
¼	teaspoon ground cloves
½	cup currants (optional)
½	cup nonfat buttermilk

PREPARATION TIME: 15–20 MINUTES

BAKING TIME: 12–15 MINUTES

Preheat the oven to 350°. Lightly coat 2 baking sheets with no-stick spray.

In a large bowl, using an electric mixer, cream the butter or margarine until smooth. Beat in the honey, molasses and egg, egg whites or egg substitute. Set aside.

In another large bowl, combine the flour, cinnamon, ginger, baking soda and cloves. Stir in the currants (if using).

Beat the flour mixture and buttermilk into the egg mixture. Stir until well-mixed.

Drop the batter by teaspoons onto the prepared baking sheets. Bake for 12 to 15 minutes. Remove the cookies and cool on a rack.

Per cookie: 68 calories, 1.5 g. total fat (19% of calories), 0.4 g. monounsaturated fat, 0.1 g. polyunsaturated fat, 0.8 g. saturated fat, 1.3 g. protein, 13.1 g. carbohydrate, 1 g. dietary fiber, 9 mg. cholesterol, 40 mg. sodium

Makes 40

Low-Fat Snacks and Desserts

Almond and Hazelnut Biscotti

The mildly nutty flavor and crunchy texture of these Italian cookies make them a perfect after-dinner treat or midday snack.

PREPARATION TIME: 20 MINUTES

BAKING TIME: 25–30 MINUTES

SECOND BAKING TIME: 15 MINUTES

2	ounces almonds (about ¼ cup)
1	ounce hazelnuts (about 26 nuts)
3½	cups whole-wheat pastry flour
½	teaspoon baking powder
½	teaspoon baking soda
½	teaspoon ground cinnamon
⅛	teaspoon ground allspice
2	tablespoons unsalted butter or margarine, softened
1½	cups sugar
3	egg whites
1	egg, 2 egg whites or ¼ cup fat-free egg substitute
1	teaspoon vanilla
1	teaspoon finely grated orange rind or lemon rind

Preheat the oven to 375°. Position the oven rack so that the biscotti bake in the top third of the oven. Lightly coat a baking sheet with no-stick spray.

Chop the almonds and hazelnuts in a food processor or by hand until finely ground. In a large bowl, mix the ground nuts, flour, baking powder, baking soda, cinnamon and allspice.

In another large bowl, using an electric mixer, beat the butter or margarine until smooth. Add the sugar, 3 egg whites, egg, 2 egg whites or egg substitute, vanilla and orange rind or lemon rind. Mix until blended.

Stir the nut mixture into the egg mixture. Knead the dough inside the bowl until the mixture is well-combined. Divide the dough in half. With floured hands, form each half into a rough 5″ × 12″ rectangle on the prepared baking sheet. Bake for 25 to 30 minutes, or until a toothpick inserted into the center comes out dry.

Remove the biscotti from the oven and reduce the heat to 325°. Slice each rectangle crosswise into 20 pieces. Arrange the biscotti on the baking sheet, cut sides up, and bake for 15 minutes more.

Remove from the oven and cool completely on a wire rack.

The biscotti will harden as they cool. Store in an airtight container.

> *Per biscotti: 86 calories, 2 g. total fat (20% of calories), 0.9 g. monounsaturated fat, 0.3 g. polyunsaturated fat, 0.5 g. saturated fat, 2.3 g. protein, 15.6 g. carbohydrate, 1.5 g. dietary fiber, 7 mg. cholesterol, 25 mg. sodium*

Makes 40

Whole-Grain Mandelbrot

Mandelbrot is a slightly sweet, crisp cookie similar to biscotti. It is a perfect snack with a cup of warm tea or a glass of cold skim milk to dunk them in. Traditionally, they are made with additional butter, eggs, candied fruit and nuts. My version is much lower in fat. Before baking, sprinkle the mandelbrot with some cinnamon and sugar if desired.

3	cups whole-wheat pastry flour
¾	cup sugar
1	tablespoon baking powder
1	teaspoon ground cinnamon
½	cup raisins
½	cup currants
½	cup chopped dates
¼	cup melted unsalted butter or canola oil
2	teaspoons vanilla
½	teaspoon almond extract
⅓	cup skim milk
2	eggs, 4 egg whites or ½ cup fat-free egg substitute

PREPARATION TIME: 10 MINUTES

BAKING TIME: 30 MINUTES

SECOND BAKING TIME: 5 MINUTES

Preheat the oven to 350°. Lightly coat a baking sheet with no-stick spray.

In a large bowl, combine the flour, sugar, baking powder and cinnamon. Stir in the raisins, currants and dates.

In a small bowl, mix the butter or oil, vanilla, almond extract, milk and eggs, egg whites or egg substitute. Pour into the flour mixture and stir just enough to incorporate the ingredients.

Turn the dough out onto a counter and knead a few times. Separate the dough into 3 pieces and shape into flat, oblong loaves. Place the loaves several inches apart on the prepared baking sheet. Bake for 30 minutes, or until lightly browned.

Remove the loaves from the oven. While they are still hot, slice each horizontally into 8 pieces. Turn each piece on its side and return the baking sheet to the oven for 5 minutes more. Remove the mandelbrot from the oven and cool on the baking sheet. Store in a covered container.

Per mandelbrot: 123 calories, 2.7 g. total fat (19% of calories), 0.6 g. monounsaturated fat, 0.2 g. polyunsaturated fat, 1.4 g. saturated fat, 2.9 g. protein, 23.2 g. carbohydrate, 2.5 g. dietary fiber, 23 mg. cholesterol, 45 mg. sodium

Makes 24

Raspberry-Currant Scones

Scones are originally from Britain and are commonly eaten there at teatime. These have a cookielike crust surrounding raspberry jam—but you can use any flavor.

PREPARATION TIME: 15 MINUTES

BAKING TIME: 20 MINUTES

3	cups whole-wheat pastry flour
5	teaspoons baking powder
½	teaspoon ground nutmeg
5	tablespoons unsalted butter or margarine
¼	cup sugar
⅓	cup currants
½	cup skim milk
16	teaspoons unsweetened raspberry jam, fruit spread, conserves or jelly

Preheat the oven to 350°. Lightly coat a baking sheet with no-stick spray. In a medium bowl, mix the flour, baking powder and nutmeg. Using a food processor, pastry blender or 2 knives, cut in the butter or margarine to form fine crumbs. Stir in the sugar and currants. Mix in enough of the milk to form a stiff dough.

Roll the dough into 16 balls. Place the balls on the prepared baking sheet. Use your thumb to make a deep well in the center of each ball. Smooth out the edges and fill each hole with 1 teaspoon of the jam, fruit spread, conserves or jelly.

Bake for 20 minutes, or until golden brown. Remove from the oven and cool on a wire rack.

Per scone: 146 calories, 4.2 g. total fat (25% of calories), 1.2 g. monounsaturated fat, 0.3 g. polyunsaturated fat, 2.5 g. saturated fat, 3.5 g. protein, 25.2 g. carbohydrate, 3.1 g. dietary fiber, 10 mg. cholesterol, 109 mg. sodium

Makes 16

Zucchini Spice Bread

The zucchini in this bread adds a nice texture without a lot of zucchini taste. The bread is moist and has a fabulous aroma.

Zucchini spice bread stores well in the freezer. If you want separate slices ready to thaw at any time, cut and wrap individual pieces in plastic wrap before putting them in the freezer.

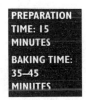

PREPARATION TIME: 15 MINUTES
BAKING TIME: 35–45 MINUTES

3	cups whole-wheat pastry flour
½	cup sugar
1	tablespoon ground cinnamon
1½	teaspoons baking powder
1½	teaspoons baking soda
1	teaspoon ground nutmeg
2	eggs, 4 egg whites or ½ cup fat-free egg substitute
2	cups shredded unpeeled zucchini
1	cup honey
2	tablespoons melted unsalted butter or canola oil
¼	cup unsweetened applesauce
1	tablespoon vanilla

Preheat the oven to 350°.

Lightly coat two 8″ × 4″ loaf pans with no-stick spray.

In a large bowl, mix the flour, sugar, cinnamon, baking powder, baking soda and nutmeg.

In a medium bowl, beat the eggs, egg whites or egg substitute, zucchini, honey, butter or oil, applesauce and vanilla.

(continued)

Low-Fat Snacks and Desserts

Pour into the flour mixture and mix just enough to incorporate the ingredients.

Pour the batter into the prepared pans. Bake for 35 to 45 minutes, or until a toothpick inserted into the center comes out slightly moist but not wet.

Cool the bread slightly in the pans, then remove and cool on a rack.

Per slice: 157 calories, 2.1 g. total fat (11% of calories), 0.4 g. monounsaturated fat, 0.2 g. polyunsaturated fat, 1 g. saturated fat, 3.3 g. protein, 33.1 g. carbohydrate, 2.5 g. dietary fiber, 25 mg. cholesterol, 122 mg. sodium

Makes 20 slices

Pumpkin-Cranberry Bread

Enjoy this autumn treat year-round by using canned pumpkin. You can double the recipe to make use of a full 16-ounce can. If you wish, you can substitute raisins for the cranberries.

PREPARATION TIME: 15 MINUTES

BAKING TIME: 1 HOUR

1½	cups whole-wheat pastry flour
1	teaspoon ground cinnamon
1	teaspoon baking soda
½	teaspoon baking powder
½	teaspoon ground cloves
½	teaspoon ground nutmeg
½	cup dried cranberries
1	cup unsweetened canned pumpkin
¾	cup honey
1	egg, 2 egg whites or ¼ cup fat-free egg substitute
2	tablespoons unsweetened applesauce
1	tablespoon melted unsalted butter or canola oil
1	tablespoon vanilla

Preheat the oven to 350°. Lightly coat an 8" × 4" loaf pan with no-stick spray.

In a large bowl, mix the flour, cinnamon, baking soda, baking powder, cloves and nutmeg. Toss in the cranberries.

In a medium bowl, combine the pumpkin, honey, egg, egg whites or egg substitute, applesauce, butter or oil and vanilla.

Stir into the flour mixture and mix just enough to incorporate the ingredients.

Pour the batter into the prepared pan and bake for 1 hour, or until a toothpick inserted into the center comes out moist but not wet.

Cool the bread slightly in the pan, then remove and cool on a rack.

Per slice: 178 calories, 2.2 g. total fat (11% of calories), 0.4 g. monounsaturated fat, 0.2 g. polyunsaturated fat, 1 g. saturated fat, 3.4 g. protein, 38.1 g. carbohydrate, 3.6 g. dietary fiber, 25 mg. cholesterol, 146 mg. sodium

Makes 10 slices

Apple Spice Cake

This light cake is filled with bits of fresh apple and has a very special topping. The recipe also makes great muffins (divide the batter among muffin tins lined with paper baking cups and bake for 30 minutes).

1	tablespoon softened unsalted butter or canola oil
1	cup + 1 tablespoon sugar
1	egg, 2 egg whites or ¼ cup fat-free egg substitute
2	tablespoons unsweetened applesauce
¾	cup skim milk
1½	tablespoons vanilla
2	cups whole-wheat pastry flour
1	teaspoon baking powder
1	teaspoon baking soda
2½	teaspoons ground cinnamon
½	teaspoon ground nutmeg
¼	teaspoon ground cloves
¼	teaspoon ground allspice
2	cups diced apples
2	tablespoons finely ground pecans

PREPARATION TIME: 10 MINUTES

BAKING TIME: 45 MINUTES

Low-Fat Snacks and Desserts

Preheat the oven to 350°. Lightly coat an 8″ × 4″ loaf pan with no-stick spray.

In a medium bowl, beat the butter or oil, 1 cup of the sugar, egg, egg whites or egg substitute, applesauce, milk and vanilla.

In a large bowl, combine the flour, baking powder, baking soda, 2 teaspoons of the cinnamon, nutmeg, cloves, allspice and apples.

Stir into the oil mixture and combine just enough to incorporate the ingredients.

Pour the batter into the prepared pan.

In a small bowl, mix the pecans, the remaining 1 tablespoon sugar and the remaining ½ teaspoon cinnamon. Sprinkle the mixture on top of the batter.

Bake for 45 minutes, or until a toothpick inserted into the center comes out moist but not wet.

Cool the bread slightly in the pan, then remove and cool on a rack.

Per serving: 220 calories, 3.2 g. total fat (13% of calories), 1 g. monounsaturated fat, 0.5 g. polyunsaturated fat, 1.1 g. saturated fat, 4.7 g. protein, 44.9 g. carbohydrate, 3.7 g. dietary fiber, 25 mg. cholesterol, 170 mg. sodium

Serves 10

Banana Bread

In this recipe I've reduced the fat yet kept the very moist, rich taste and texture of the original family recipe.

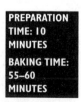

PREPARATION TIME: 10 MINUTES

BAKING TIME: 55–60 MINUTES

2	tablespoons unsalted butter, softened, or canola oil
¾	cup unsweetened applesauce
¼	teaspoon salt
2½	cups sugar
4	eggs or 1 cup fat-free egg substitute
½	cup nonfat sour cream
1	tablespoon vanilla
3½	cups whole-wheat pastry flour
2½	teaspoons baking soda
5	very ripe bananas, well-mashed

Preheat the oven to 350°. Lightly coat two 8″ × 4″ loaf pans with no-stick spray.

In a large bowl, using an electric mixer, beat the butter or oil, applesauce, salt, sugar, eggs or egg substitute, sour cream and vanilla. In a small bowl, mix the flour and baking soda. Pour into the egg mixture. Add the bananas. Stir just enough to incorporate the ingredients. Pour the batter into the prepared pans. Bake for 55 to 60 minutes, or until a toothpick inserted into the center comes out moist but not wet.

Cool the bread slightly in the pans, then remove and cool on a rack.

Per slice: 228 calories, 2.7 g. total fat (10% of calories), 0.4 g. monounsaturated fat, 0.2 g. polyunsaturated fat, 1.2 g. saturated fat, 5 g. protein, 48.6 g. carbohydrate, 3.3 g. dietary fiber, 46 mg. cholesterol, 189 mg. sodium

Makes 20 slices

Carrot-Pineapple Cake

The little chunks of pineapple make this recipe unique. If desired, you can bake the batter in muffin cups or a bundt pan, but you'll have to adjust the baking time accordingly.

3	cups whole-wheat pastry flour
¼	cup sugar
2	teaspoons baking powder
1	teaspoon ground cinnamon
1	teaspoon ground nutmeg
2	teaspoons baking soda
¼	teaspoon ground cloves
¼	teaspoon ground allspice
½	cup currants
2	tablespoons melted unsalted butter or canola oil
1	cup honey
1	tablespoon vanilla
3	eggs, 6 egg whites or ¾ cup fat-free egg substitute
¾	cup unsweetened applesauce
½	cup nonfat sour cream

PREPARATION TIME: 15 MINUTES

BAKING TIME: 45–60 MINUTES

(continued)

Low-Fat Snacks and Desserts

1   can (8 ounces) unsweetened crushed pineapple (with juice)
2   cups shredded, loosely packed carrots

Preheat the oven to 350°.

Lightly coat two 8″ × 4″ loaf pans with no-stick spray.

In a large bowl, combine the flour, sugar, baking powder, cinnamon, nutmeg, baking soda, cloves and allspice.

Stir in the currants.

In a small bowl, mix the butter or oil, honey, vanilla, eggs, egg whites or egg substitute, applesauce and sour cream. Pour into the flour mixture.

Add the pineapple (with juice) and carrots. Mix just enough to incorporate the ingredients.

Pour the batter into the prepared pans.

Bake for 45 to 60 minutes, or until a toothpick inserted into the center comes out moist but not wet.

If you're using muffin cups, the baking time will be slightly less.

Allow more time if you're using a bundt pan.

Per serving: 168 calories, 2.3 g. total fat (12% of calories), 0.4 g. monounsaturated fat, 0.2 g. polyunsaturated fat, 1.1 g. saturated fat, 4.2 g. protein, 34.3 g. carbohydrate, 3 g. dietary fiber, 36 mg. cholesterol, 168 mg. sodium

Serves 20

Whole-Grain Cocoa Angel Food Cake

In this recipe, whole-grain flour makes a slightly heartier cake than the traditional white flour does. Although the ingredient list is quite short, there are quite a few steps to follow because of the cake's delicate nature. For a fancy nonfat treat, serve a slice of the cake with fresh berries and a little nonfat frozen yogurt.

Angel food cake is special because it's made without added fat. Egg whites create the airy, delicate texture.

¾	cup whole-wheat pastry flour
¼	cup unsweetened cocoa powder
1¼	cups sugar
10	egg whites
1	teaspoon cream of tartar
1	teaspoon vanilla
½	teaspoon lemon extract

PREPARATION TIME: 20 MINUTES

BAKING TIME: 45 MINUTES

COOLING TIME: 1½ HOURS

Preheat the oven to 350°.

Place the flour, cocoa and ¼ cup of the sugar in a sifter; sift into a medium bowl. Repeat the sifting 5 times. Set aside.

Sift the remaining 1 cup sugar into a separate bowl. Set aside.

Place the egg whites in a large bowl. Using an electric mixer, beat until foamy. Add the cream of tartar and beat until the egg whites form stiff peaks but are not dry.

Fold in the 1 cup sifted sugar, 1 tablespoon at a time. Add the vanilla and lemon extract.

Slowly sift small amounts of the flour mixture over the batter and fold it in until all the flour is incorporated.

Pour the batter into an ungreased 10″ straight-sided tube pan. Bake for 45 minutes.

Remove the pan from the oven and turn it upside down to cool. Let stand for 1½ hours. (I like to invert the pan over the neck of a sturdy bottle to prevent the cake from shrinking as it cools.)

When the cake is fully cooled, run a knife around the edges of the pan to remove the cake.

Per serving: 126 calories, 0.3 g. total fat (2% of calories), 0.04 g. monounsaturated fat, 0.06 g. polyunsaturated fat, 0.07 g. saturated fat, 4.3 g. protein, 27.9 g. carbohydrate, 1 g. dietary fiber, 0 mg. cholesterol, 48 mg. sodium

Serves 12

Chocolate Cream Cheese Delight

The rich-tasting creaminess of this low-fat, easy-to-make, no-bake cheesecake comes from a combination of nonfat cream cheese, reduced-fat (or light) cream cheese

Low-Fat Snacks and Desserts

and unflavored gelatin. Unsweetened cocoa—use Dutch process or regular—and sugar create the chocolate flavor.

This is a real warm-weather treat. For a larger cake, double the filling recipe and use the same amount of crust in a 9" or 10" springform pan.

PREPARATION TIME: 15 MINUTES

CHILLING TIME: ABOUT 4 HOURS

Crust

¾	cup low-fat graham cracker crumbs
2	tablespoons unsalted butter or margarine, melted

Filling

1	envelope unfavored gelatin
¼	cup skim milk, well-chilled
¾	cup skim milk, boiling
4	ounces light cream cheese, softened
4	ounces nonfat cream cheese, softened
½	cup nonfat sour cream
½	cup nonfat cottage cheese
⅔	cup sugar
1	tablespoon vanilla
5	tablespoons unsweetened cocoa powder, regular or Dutch process

Preheat the oven to 350°. Lightly coat a 9″ springform pan or pie plate with no-stick spray.

To make the crust: In a small bowl, combine the cracker crumbs and butter or margarine. Press into the prepared pan and bake for 5 minutes. Cool on a rack.

To make the filling: In a blender, sprinkle the gelatin over the cold milk. Let stand for 2 minutes.

Add the hot milk and blend on low speed for 2 minutes.

Add the light cream cheese, nonfat cream cheese, sour cream, cottage cheese, sugar, vanilla and cocoa. Blend on high speed for several minutes, until smooth.

Pour the filling into the baked crust and chill for about 4 hours, or until firm.

Per serving: 171 calories, 5.1 g. total fat (26% of calories), 1.8 g. monounsaturated fat, 0.2 g. polyunsaturated fat, 2.8 g. saturated fat, 8.2 g. protein, 23.9 g. carbohydrate, 0.2 g. dietary fiber, 13 mg. cholesterol, 221 mg. sodium

Serves 10

Sour Cream Coffee Cake

This is one of Robert's favorite cakes. It's basic, simple and filled with whole-grain goodness. For variety, try adding chopped fruit to the batter before baking it.

Cake

1½	cups whole-wheat pastry flour
1	cup sugar
2	teaspoons baking powder
1	teaspoon baking soda
1	cup nonfat sour cream
2	eggs, lightly beaten
½	teaspoon vanilla
¼	teaspoon orange extract

Topping

2	tablespoons whole-wheat pastry flour
5	tablespoons brown sugar
2	tablespoons chopped pecans
1	tablespoon unsalted butter or margarine

PREPARATION TIME: 10 MINUTES

BAKING TIME: 35 MINUTES

Preheat the oven to 350°. Lightly coat an 8″ × 8″ baking pan with no-stick spray.

To make the cake: In a large bowl, combine the flour, sugar, baking powder and baking soda.

In a medium bowl, whisk together the sour cream, eggs, vanilla and orange extract. Pour into the flour mixture and stir until combined. Pour the batter into the prepared pan and set aside.

To make the topping: In a blender or food processor, combine the flour, brown sugar, pecans and butter or margarine. Blend until the mixture forms fine crumbs. Sprinkle over the batter.

Bake for 35 minutes, or until the center looks set and a toothpick inserted into the center comes out moist but not wet. Cool on a rack before slicing.

Per serving: 136 calories, 2.1 g. total fat (14% of calories), 0.6 g. monounsaturated fat, 0.3 g. polyunsaturated fat, 0.7 g. saturated fat, 4 g. protein, 26.5 g. carbohydrate, 1.6 g. dietary fiber, 29 mg. cholesterol, 130 mg. sodium

Serves 16

Low-Fat Snacks and Desserts

Sweet Potato–Cherry Squares
with Orange Icing

Moist and cakelike, these whole-grain squares are topped with an orange icing that complements the cake. You can replace the sweet potatoes with carrots, using the same quantity specified in this recipe.

Raisins, currants or dried cranberries can be substituted for the dried cherries. These squares are a big hit with our kids and their friends.

PREPARATION TIME: 15 MINUTES

BAKING TIME: 30–40 MINUTES

Cake

2	tablespoons unsalted butter, softened, or canola oil
1½	cups brown sugar
1	cup unsweetened applesauce
2	eggs, 4 egg whites or ½ cup fat-free egg substitute
1	tablespoon vanilla
1	teaspoon orange extract
3	cups whole-wheat pastry flour
2	teaspoons ground cinnamon
1	teaspoon baking soda
½	teaspoon ground nutmeg
½	teaspoon baking powder
¼	teaspoon salt (optional)
3	cups shredded, firmly packed sweet potatoes
1½	cups dried cherries

Icing

2	cups confectioners' sugar
3	tablespoons orange juice
1	teaspoon orange extract or grated rind of 1 orange

Preheat the oven to 350°.

Lightly coat a 13″ × 9″ baking pan with no-stick spray.

To make the cake: In a large bowl, beat the butter or oil, brown sugar, applesauce, eggs, egg whites or egg substitute, vanilla and orange extract.

In a small bowl, combine the flour, cinnamon, baking soda, nutmeg, baking powder and salt (if using). Stir the flour mixture into the egg mixture just until mixed. Stir in the sweet potatoes and cherries.

Pour the batter into the prepared pan and bake for 30 to 40 minutes, or until a toothpick inserted into the center comes out moist but not wet. Cool completely on a rack.

To make the icing: Place the confectioners' sugar in a medium bowl. Add the orange juice and orange extract or orange rind. Mix until smooth. Spread on the top of the cooled cake. Let the icing set before cutting into squares.

Per square: 192 calories, 1.8 g. total fat (8% of calories), 0.3 g. monounsaturated fat, 0.2 g. polyunsaturated fat, 0.8 g. saturated fat, 3.1 g. protein, 42.5 g. carbohydrate, 2.3 g. dietary fiber, 21 mg. cholesterol, 69 mg. sodium

Makes 24

Lemon Delicacy Bars

A fluffy layer of lemon tops a moist granola-type crust on these light yet flavorful bars.

Crust

¾	cup rolled oats
2	tablespoons whole-wheat pastry flour
¼	cup brown sugar
1	teaspoon ground cinnamon
1	tablespoon canola oil

Topping

1	tablespoon unsalted butter or margarine, softened
½	cup sugar
2	egg yolks
	Grated rind of 1 lemon
	Juice of 1 lemon
6	tablespoons whole-wheat pastry flour
1	cup evaporated skim milk
3	egg whites

PREPARATION TIME: 15 MINUTES

BAKING TIME: 50 MINUTES

Preheat the oven to 350°.

Lightly coat an 8″ × 8″ baking pan with no-stick spray.

To make the crust: In a medium bowl, combine the oats, flour, brown sugar, cinnamon and oil.

(continued)

Mix well and press into the prepared pan.

Bake for 15 minutes, or until lightly browned.

Set aside.

To make the topping: In a large bowl, cream the butter or margarine with an electric mixer. Beat in the sugar, egg yolks, lemon rind, lemon juice, flour and milk.

In a separate bowl, using an electric mixer with clean beaters, beat the egg whites until stiff peaks form. Fold the egg whites into the lemon mixture until well-combined.

Pour the lemon mixture onto the crust and bake for 35 minutes, or until the top just begins to brown.

Remove from the oven and cool on a rack. Let cool completely before cutting into bars.

> *Per bar: 103 calories, 2.5 g. total fat (22% of calories), 0.8 g. monounsaturated fat, 0.4 g. polyunsaturated fat, 0.8 g. saturated fat, 3.3 g. protein, 17.3 g. carbohydrates, 0.5 g. dietary fiber, 29 mg. cholesterol, 24 mg. sodium*

Makes 16

Dutch Cocoa Fudge Brownies

These low-fat brownies will surprise you with their rich chocolate flavor and fudgelike texture. They're a fast, simple treat.

PREPARATION TIME: 5 MINUTES

BAKING TIME: 25 MINUTES

2	tablespoons unsalted butter or margarine, softened
1	cup sugar
½	cup unsweetened applesauce
1	egg or 2 egg whites
2	teaspoons vanilla
½	cup unsweetened cocoa powder, regular or Dutch process
¾	cup whole-wheat pastry flour

Preheat the oven to 350°.

Lightly coat an 8″ × 8″ baking pan with no-stick spray.

In a medium bowl, using an electric mixer, beat the butter or margarine, sugar, applesauce, egg or egg whites and vanilla. Then slowly beat in the cocoa and flour.

Pour the batter into the prepared pan and bake for 25 minutes, or until a toothpick inserted into the center of the brownies comes out moist but not wet.

Cool on a rack before cutting.

Per brownie: 96 calories, 2.2 g. total fat (19% of calories), 0.5 g. monounsaturated fat, 0.1 g. polyunsaturated fat, 1.1 g. saturated fat, 1.7 g. protein, 19.2 g. carbohydrate, 0.9 g. dietary fiber, 18 mg. cholesterol, 2 mg. sodium

Makes 16

Apple Crumb Pie

This apple pie has a special crumb crust and topping that combine wonderfully with the spicy filling. Almost any kind of apples will do, but as with most baked-apple recipes, tart ones are best. Try it à la mode with nonfat frozen yogurt.

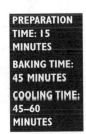

PREPARATION TIME: 15 MINUTES

BAKING TIME: 45 MINUTES

COOLING TIME: 45–60 MINUTES

Crust
2½	cups whole-wheat pastry flour
½	cup sugar
1	teaspoon ground cinnamon
¼	cup unsalted butter or margarine
2	tablespoons honey

Filling
8–9	tart apples, thinly sliced (peel if desired)
½	cup sugar
¼	cup whole-wheat pastry flour
2	tablespoons vanilla
3	teaspoons ground cinnamon
1	teaspoon ground nutmeg

Preheat the oven to 425°. Oil a 9″ or 10″ springform pan.

To make the crust: In a large bowl, mix the flour, sugar and cinnamon.

Using a pastry blender, food processor or 2 knives, cut in the butter or margarine and honey to form fine crumbs.

(continued)

Pat two-thirds of the mixture on the bottom and up the sides of the prepared pan.

To make the filling: Place the apples in a large bowl.

Add the sugar, flour, vanilla, cinnamon and nutmeg. Toss to coat the apples.

Spoon the filling into the crust.

Bake for 25 minutes.

Remove the pie from the oven and top with the remaining crust crumbs.

Pat the crust down gently and sprinkle lightly with more cinnamon.

Return the pie to the oven and bake for another 20 minutes, or until golden.

Cool for 45 to 60 minutes before removing the sides of the pan and slicing.

> *Per serving: 268 calories, 5 g. total fat (16% of calories), 1.3 g. monounsaturated fat, 0.5 g. polyunsaturated fat, 2.7 g. saturated fat, 4 g. protein, 55 g. carbohydrates, 5.6 g. dietary fiber, 11 mg. cholesterol, 3 mg. sodium*

Serves 12

Cherry Pie

Though rolled piecrusts can be difficult to make low-fat and with whole-grain flour, this recipe gives excellent results. For a nonfat variation, bake the filling in cups and serve "baked cherries."

PREPARATION TIME: 20 MINUTES

BAKING TIME: 50 MINUTES

Filling

2	cans (16 ounces each) pitted unsweetened tart red cherries
½	cup arrowroot
⅔	cup sugar
3	drops almond extract

Crust

1	cup whole-wheat pastry flour
2	tablespoons sugar
¼	cup unsalted butter or margarine
4–8	tablespoons ice water

Preheat the oven to 375°.

To make the filling: Drain the cherries and reserve the liquid. Set aside. In a small saucepan, combine the arrowroot and ⅓ cup of the sugar. Pour in the reserved cherry juice. Cook over medium heat, stirring often, until the mixture is thick and bubbly. Stir in the remaining ⅓ cup sugar, cherries and almond extract. Cook and stir for another 3 minutes.

To make the crust: In a large bowl, combine the flour and sugar. Using a pastry blender, food processor or 2 knives, cut the butter or margarine into the flour mixture until the mixture resembles coarse meal. Slowly stir in the water, 1 tablespoon at a time, to form a stiff dough. Roll out the dough to fit a 9″ pie plate. Place the dough in the plate and flute the edges. Pour the filling into the crust.

Place a baking sheet under the pie to catch any juices that overflow. Bake for 50 minutes. Remove from the oven and cool on a rack.

> *Per serving: 251 calories, 6.5 g. total fat (22% of calories), 1.8 g. monounsaturated fat, 0.4 g. polyunsaturated fat, 3.9 g. saturated fat, 3 g. protein, 48 g. carbohydrate, 3.3 g. dietary fiber, 17 mg. cholesterol, 10 mg. sodium*

Serves 8

Apple Crisp

In this version of apple crisp, apples, cinnamon and raisins are surrounded by a granola-like crust. Try substituting pears or peaches for the apples and dried cherries, cranberries or currants for the raisins.

Filling

8	tart apples, sliced (peel if desired)
	Juice of 1 lemon
¾	cup raisins
½	cup sugar
2	tablespoons whole-wheat pastry flour
1	teaspoon ground cinnamon

PREPARATION TIME: 20 MINUTES

BAKING TIME: I HOUR

(continued)

1	teaspoon ground nutmeg
1	teaspoon vanilla
¼	teaspoon ground cloves
¼	teaspoon ground allspice

Crust

2	cups rolled oats
¾	cup oat bran or other bran
¼	cup unsalted butter or margarine, melted
½	cup whole-wheat pastry flour
½	cup sugar
2	tablespoons honey
2	teaspoons ground cinnamon

Preheat the oven to 350°. Lightly coat a 13″ × 9″ baking pan with no-stick spray.

To make the filling: In a very large bowl, mix the apples, lemon juice, raisins, sugar, flour, cinnamon, nutmeg, vanilla, cloves and allspice. Set aside.

To make the crust: In a medium bowl, mix the oats, bran, butter or margarine, flour, sugar, honey and cinnamon. Firmly pat half of the crust on the bottom of the prepared baking pan. Place the filling evenly over the crust, making sure to fill the corners.

Firmly pat the remaining crust on top of the filling.

Cover the pan with aluminum foil and bake for 45 minutes. Uncover and bake for another 15 minutes, or until the top is lightly browned. Let cool slightly before serving.

Per serving: 190 calories, 3.9 g. total fat (17% of calories), 1.1 g. monounsaturated fat, 0.5 g. polyunsaturated fat, 1.9 g. saturated fat, 3.1 g. protein, 39.6 g. carbohydrate, 2.7 g. dietary fiber, 7 mg. cholesterol, 3 mg. sodium

Serves 18

Lemon Tapioca Pudding

A family favorite in our house, this cool, refreshing, low-fat dessert or snack is easy to make. You can substitute any flavor extract for lemon.

PREPARATION AND COOKING TIME: 10 MINUTES

CHILLING TIME: 2 HOURS OR MORE

2¾   cups skim milk
3   tablespoons quick-cooking tapioca
5   tablespoons maple syrup, honey or sugar
1   egg or 1 egg white
1   teaspoon vanilla
½   teaspoon lemon extract
    Pinch of ground nutmeg

In a medium saucepan, combine the milk, tapioca, maple syrup, honey or sugar, egg or egg white, vanilla, lemon extract and nutmeg. Let stand for 5 minutes.

Cook over medium heat, whisking until the mixture comes to a boil. Boil for 3 minutes, stirring constantly.

Remove the pudding from the heat and pour into 4 serving cups. Refrigerate for 2 hours or more, until well-chilled.

Per serving: 153 calories, 0.3 g. total fat (2% of calories), 0.1 g. monounsaturated fat, 0 g. polyunsaturated fat, 0.2 g. saturated fat, 6.6 g. protein, 30.1 g. carbohydrate, 0 g. dietary fiber, 3 mg. cholesterol, 103 mg. sodium

Serves 4

Perfect Pumpkin Pudding

This is really a recipe for pumpkin pie but without the crust, to keep the fat content low. The whole eggs help to create the creamy texture.

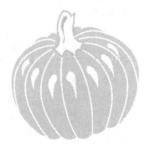

PREPARATION TIME: 5 MINUTES

BAKING TIME: 45–50 MINUTES

2   eggs
¾   cup sugar
2   cups pumpkin puree
1   tablespoon molasses
1   teaspoon ground cinnamon
½   teaspoon ground ginger
¼   teaspoon ground nutmeg
¼   teaspoon ground cloves
1½   cups evaporated skim milk

Preheat the oven to 425°. Lightly coat 8 small oven-safe dishes with no-stick spray.

(continued)

Low-Fat Snacks and Desserts

Place the eggs in a large bowl. Using an electric mixer, beat in the sugar, pumpkin, molasses, cinnamon, ginger, nutmeg and cloves. Then beat in the milk.

Pour the mixture into the prepared dishes and bake for 10 minutes. Reduce the heat to 350° and bake for 35 to 40 minutes more, or until the top is lightly browned and the pudding has set. Serve warm or chilled.

Per serving: 156 calories, 1.4 g. total fat (8% of calories), 0.1 g. monounsaturated fat, 0 g. polyunsaturated fat, 0.5 g. saturated fat, 5.8 g. protein, 31.1 g. carbohydrate, 1.7 g. dietary fiber, 55 mg. cholesterol, 62 mg. sodium

Serves 8

Raspberry Coulis

Coulis (koo-LEE) is the French name for a thick puree or sauce. Fresh-tasting and mildly sweet, this coulis can be spooned over frozen or plain yogurt, pudding, cakes, pancakes or French toast. Try other fruit as well as raspberries.

COOKING TIME: 20 MINUTES

3   cups packed fresh or unsweetened frozen raspberries
¼   cup sugar

Place the raspberries and sugar in a heavy saucepan. Cook over medium heat for 20 minutes, stirring often.

Let the sauce cool. Store in a covered jar in the refrigerator until ready to use.

Per serving: 62 calories, 0.3 g. total fat (5% of calories), 0 g. monounsaturated fat, 0.2 g. polyunsaturated fat, 0 g. saturated fat, 0.6 g. protein, 15.4 g. carbohydrate, 2.8 g. dietary fiber, 0 mg. cholesterol, 0 mg. sodium

Serves 6

Pita Chips

To make these chips, the pita is cut into triangles and baked until crisp. Use these chips as you would fried corn or tortilla chips: as a snack (with or without spreads), for nachos and with soups or salads.

PREPARATION
TIME: 5
MINUTES
BAKING TIME:
8–10 MINUTES

4   whole-wheat pita breads

Preheat the oven to 350°.

With a sharp knife, cut the pitas in half to form 2 pockets. Then cut each half into 3 triangles.

Cut each triangle piece at the bottom fold to form 2 single-layer triangles.

Place the bread on a baking sheet without overlapping the triangles.

Bake for 8 to 10 minutes, or until the chips are crisp and lightly browned.

Per 6 chips: 85 calories, 0.9 g. total fat (8% of calories), 0.1 g. monounsaturated fat, 0.3 g. polyunsaturated fat, 0.1 g. saturated fat, 3.2 g. protein, 17.6 g. carbohydrate, 1.9 g. dietary fiber, 0 mg. cholesterol, 170 mg. sodium

Makes 48

Black Olive and Pimento Spread

This creamy spread is a delicious substitute for high-fat cream cheese spreads. Though the olives are high in fat, you're getting only a small amount if you limit a serving to 2 tablespoons. Try it on bagels, crackers or celery sticks. It's great used for hors d'oeuvres.

1   cup nonfat cream cheese
½   teaspoon dried basil
¼   teaspoon garlic powder
15   black olives, chopped
¼   cup diced pimentos
1   tablespoon chopped fresh chives

PREPARATION
TIME: 5
MINUTES

In a medium bowl, mix the cream cheese, basil and garlic powder until well-blended.

(continued)

Low-Fat Snacks and Desserts

Stir in the olives, pimentos and chives.
Refrigerate in a covered container until ready to serve.

*Per 2 tablespoons: 24 calories, 0.9 g. total fat
(22% of calories), 0.5 g. monounsaturated fat,
0.1 g. polyunsaturated fat, 0.1 g. saturated
fat, 2.9 g. protein, 1.1 g. carbohydrate, 0.1 g.
dietary fiber, 3 mg. cholesterol, 138 mg. sodium*

Makes 1½ cups

Cinnamon, Raisin and Nut Spread

*This is our favorite spread to take on car trips. We serve
it with whole-grain Pita Chips (page 378).*

**PREPARATION
TIME: 5
MINUTES**

1	cup nonfat cream cheese
1	teaspoon maple syrup
¼	teaspoon finely grated lemon rind
¼	teaspoon ground cinnamon
⅛	teaspoon ground nutmeg
¼	cup raisins or currants
¼	cup finely chopped walnuts or almonds

In a medium bowl, mix the cream cheese, maple syrup,
lemon rind, cinnamon and nutmeg until smooth and creamy.
Stir in the raisins or currants and walnuts or almonds. Refrigerate in a covered container until ready to serve.

*Per 2 tablespoons: 37 calories, 1 g. total fat
(24% of calories), 0.2 g. monounsaturated fat,
0.6 g. polyunsaturated fat, 0.1 g. saturated
fat, 3.2 g. protein, 3.7 g. carbohydrate, 0.2 g.
dietary fiber, 3 mg. cholesterol, 114 mg. sodium*

Makes 1½ cups

Baba Ghanoush

*There are as many spellings for this Mediterranean
spread as there are ways to make it. Traditional recipes include eggplant, garlic and large amounts of olive oil. Here's*

my lower-fat interpretation. Serve it with thick slices of whole-grain bread.

2 medium eggplants, sliced
2 cloves garlic, unpeeled
2 tablespoons lemon juice
2 tablespoons olive oil
2 tablespoons minced fresh parsley
  Salt
  Freshly ground black pepper

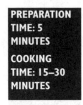

PREPARATION TIME: 5 MINUTES

COOKING TIME: 15–30 MINUTES

Place the eggplant and garlic on a lightly oiled broiler pan or grill. Coat the eggplant very lightly with olive oil cooking spray. Cook for several minutes, until the garlic peel is browned. Turn the garlic and cook for a few minutes more, until browned. Remove the garlic.

Continue cooking the eggplant until lightly browned on one side. Turn the slices and cook until browned. Remove the skin from the garlic and eggplant.

In a blender or food processor, puree the garlic and eggplant until smooth. As the mixture blends, add the lemon juice, olive oil, parsley and salt and pepper to taste.

Taste to adjust the seasoning and serve at room temperature.

Per 2 tablespoons: 25 calories, 1.5 g. total fat (48% of calories), 1 g. monounsaturated fat, 0.2 g. polyunsaturated fat, 0.2 g. saturated fat, 0.4 g. protein, 3.1 g. carbohydrate, 0 g. dietary fiber, 0 mg. cholesterol, 2 mg. sodium

Makes 2½ cups

Cucumber and Yogurt Spread

The first time I tasted this refreshing nonfat spread was in a fabulous Greek restaurant. As soon as we were seated, tzatziki (the Greek name for the spread) and thick slices of hearty bread were placed on the table. I found the spread addictive and can't even remember the other dishes I ate that afternoon. The spread's thickness comes from draining

the yogurt—an important step. Be sure to serve the spread
with thick slices of whole-grain bread.

**PREPARATION
TIME: 20
MINUTES**

**DRAINING
TIME: SEVERAL
HOURS OR
OVERNIGHT**

2   cups nonfat plain yogurt
1   large cucumber, peeled
½   teaspoon salt
2   small cloves garlic, minced

Place the yogurt in a yogurt funnel or a strainer lined with cheesecloth. Place over a bowl and refrigerate; allow to drain for several hours or overnight.

Grate or finely chop the cucumber. Place in a colander, sprinkle with the salt and allow to drain for 20 minutes. Rinse and drain the cucumbers again, if desired.

In a deep bowl, mix a small amount of the yogurt with the garlic. Stir in the remaining yogurt and fold in the cucumbers. Chill.

Per serving: 55 calories, 0.2 g. total fat (3% of calories), 0 g. monounsaturated fat, 0 g. polyunsaturated fat, 0.1 g. saturated fat, 5.4 g. protein, 7.9 g. carbohydrate, 0 g. dietary fiber, 2 mg. cholesterol, 283 mg. sodium

Serves 5

Chapter Twenty-One

Fresh-Start Recipes for Homemade Yeast Breads

Throughout this book, we've often recommended whole-grain bread for your Low-Fat Living Program. It's tasty, filling and more nutritious than bread that's made with refined flour. Toasted whole-grain bread with a tangy spread of fruit preserves is the cornerstone of a high-nutrition, high-fiber breakfast. And for anyone who loves the grainy flavor and texture of fresh-baked bread, it's the best part of lunches and snacks.

You have a choice, of course. You can buy whole-grain bread at many supermarkets and most natural foods stores. But there's a wonderful alternative: baking it yourself.

The sight and scent of freshly baked bread have a timeless romantic appeal—which may be one of the reasons that more Americans than ever are reclaiming the lost art of bread-baking. The question is, why did we ever stop baking bread in the first place?

Many of us grew up believing that you have to spend all

day in the kitchen if you're going to bake fresh bread. Obviously, we can't do that. With our busy schedules and heavy reliance on convenience foods, many of us have just never tried it. But it's a fallacy to assume that bread-baking is time-consuming.

To bake a yeast bread that requires some kneading and then needs to rise, you do have to be home over a period of several hours. But the most time you'll need at one stretch is 20 minutes. Otherwise, you're just dropping by the kitchen for 2 to 5 minutes each hour or so. Once you get into the rhythm of bread-baking, you'll find that you do it almost automatically, without setting a timer or glancing at the clock.

And it's not something you have to do every day, either. Baking a double recipe—which usually means four loaves of bread—doesn't take any longer than making a single one, so you can make enough in one batch to last several days. When you're done, you'll have one moist, warm, freshly baked loaf to eat immediately and several more to refrigerate or freeze for future use.

The whole-grain bread you bake at home will usually be more nutritious and taste much better than store-bought varieties. You can eat it with breakfast, lunch and dinner or have a slice for a snack. You and your family will appreciate the extra-special taste.

If this is your first time baking fresh, yeast-risen bread, you can start with any one of the whole-grain bread recipes in this book. These are family favorites, but you should know that you can substitute whole-wheat flour in many traditional yeast-bread recipes that call for white all-purpose flour. That's because whole-wheat flour, like white flour, contains gluten, the all-important component that reacts with active yeast and helps make the bread rise. Apart from wheat flour, most other whole-grain flours have either very little or no gluten and are rarely used alone in yeast breads. But they can always be mixed with whole-wheat flour to produce delicious multigrain breads.

Before you begin, have a look at the general procedures that follow under "Basic Ingredients," "Proofing the Yeast" and "Baking Methods." Though the principles are the same for all yeast breads, you'll find you have lots of latitude about the method you use. After a while, every experienced baker develops his own way of doing things.

Basic Ingredients

When you've selected the bread recipe you want to try, assemble the ingredients. The dry ingredients need to be at room temperature before you begin, and liquids must be warmed slightly. Here's an overview of the basic ingredients and how they're used.

Active dry yeast. This must be kept refrigerated. Compressed or cake yeast may also be used. There's also a quick-rising form of dry yeast, which can speed up bread-making time. Because yeast becomes inactive as it ages—even if refrigerated—you should buy only as much as you will use before the expiration date on the pacakage.

Liquids. Recipes may call for water, skim milk, potato water or other liquids. For active dry yeast, the liquid must be warmed to between 100° and 115°. (I generally aim for a temperature of 110° to 115°, which is what I specify in the recipes that follow.) This range is important, and you may need a thermometer to make sure it's right. If yeast is exposed to a temperature much higher than 115°, the "active" element in the yeast (which is actually a tiny fungus) will die. When the temperature falls below about 100°, it takes longer to get the reaction that will make the bread rise. For compressed yeast, the temperature should be between 80° and 95°.

Flour. Since flour needs to have a significant gluten content and whole-wheat flour and unbleached flour are high in gluten, these are the flours of choice for most yeast breads. The gluten traps the carbon dioxide bubbles given off by the yeast. Then the gluten stretches as the bubbles expand, so it holds the dough together while the bread is rising.

Yeast-bread recipes include other grains, of course. Rye, corn, oat, millet, buckwheat, barley, rice, soy, potato, triticale, amaranth, quinoa and sorghum flour can be mixed with wheat flour, but by themselves, they have little or no gluten. The less gluten the flour has, the more dense the bread will be.

Sweeteners. You don't need sweeteners in yeast breads, but small amounts may be used for flavor. They also act as natural preservatives. And you can use sweeteners to start the action of the yeast at the beginning of a recipe.

Salt. Since it's not a necessary ingredient in bread-making, salt can be decreased or eliminated from a recipe if desired.

Salt does help control the rate at which the dough rises, however, so if you're making a dough without salt, be sure to watch it carefully and adjust the timing to prevent overrising.

Fats. To provide some flavor and help create a moist loaf that resists drying out during storage, some recipes use very small amounts of fat. But you can make bread with no fat at all and still get great results. To oil the pans, you can use a little unsalted butter or margarine or an oil like canola or safflower that's low in saturated fat and high in monounsaturated and polyunsaturated fats. You'll probably use the least oil if you spray the pans with no-stick cooking spray, which is my preference when I'm baking.

Proofing the Yeast

Since all methods of making yeast breads depend on the live action of the yeast, you can first "proof" the yeast, which is the process that tests the activity of the live culture. If you proof the yeast and don't get a reaction, there's no point in using it, since the dough won't rise.

The reaction begins when you add a warm liquid to the yeast. As mentioned, for active dry yeast you need to heat the liquid to 100° to 115°, while compressed or cake yeast takes a liquid temperature in the range of 80° to 95°. Five to ten minutes after you add the liquid, the yeast mixture should begin to froth. If it doesn't, chances are (1) the liquid was too hot and killed the active culture, (2) the liquid was too cold and didn't provide an environment warm enough for the yeast to grow quickly or (3) the yeast was too old. Check the expiration date on the package, then buy some yeast that has a long storage life.

If the yeast mixture does not activate after five to ten minutes, you can give it a second try by adding a teaspoon of sweetener. Let it proof for another five minutes. If the mixture still does not react, pour it out and begin again with new yeast.

Baking Methods

There are six basic steps to the baking process: mixing the ingredients, kneading the dough, letting the dough rise, punching down the dough, shaping the dough and letting it rise again, then baking the dough. I've used a variety of methods for the first step, and all work well.

Step 1: Mixing the Ingredients

Since there are a number of different ways to do this step, the choice is up to you. Each time you make bread, you can try a different method and then choose your favorite. Or if your first trial goes well, just stick with it every time.

The fast-and-simple method. Heat the liquid to 100° to 115° and pour it into a large bowl. Add sweetener if desired and sprinkle the yeast on top. Let proof for five to ten minutes.

Pour in the remaining ingredients slowly, adding only enough flour to form a stiff dough. Then proceed with Step 2.

The sponge method. Proof the yeast as described above.

To the proofed yeast, slowly add approximately one-quarter of the flour that's called for in the recipe. Mix with an electric mixer on low speed.

When the flour is mixed in, switch to high speed and beat for three minutes. Or use a wooden spoon, beating for 300 strokes. The resulting mixture is called a sponge.

By hand, stir in half of the original quantity of flour (you'll still have one-quarter left) and the other ingredients. Then go on to Step 2.

Alternatively, you might want to give the sponge a chance to rise before you add more flour and knead it. Cover the sponge with a damp cloth, wax paper or plastic wrap and put it in a warm area (preferably 80° to 85°). Let the dough rise for approximately an hour. (This extra step may improve the texture of the loaf and is sometimes well-worth the extra time required, but it's certainly not necessary.) Stir in as much flour as necessary (the amount will vary) and the other ingredients before you proceed with Step 2.

The wet-and-dry method. This is probably my least favorite method. Mix one-quarter of the flour with the salt, the yeast and any other dry ingredients in a large bowl. Heat all the liquid ingredients in a saucepan until the temperature is between 100° and 115°.

Pour the liquid into the dry ingredients and beat with an electric mixer (or vigorously by hand) for three minutes.

Slowly add half of the original quantity of flour, mixing by hand. Then proceed with Step 2.

Step 2: Kneading the Dough

Turn the dough out onto a floured counter or another surface. It will be crumbly, lumpy and sticky at this point.

Begin kneading by pulling the top of the dough toward you with your right hand, then pushing the heel of that hand into the center of the dough. With your left hand, push the dough in a clockwise direction. Repeat with the right hand, then the left again and so on, in a steady, rhythmic motion.

As you go, knead in enough of the remaining flour to form dough that is soft yet firm. Do this by sprinkling flour on the counter and kneading the dough on top of it.

The process of kneading and adding flour is not an exact science. Just work out some type of rhythmic movement similar to the one I've described here, and you're sure to succeed.

If the dough is still sticky, you can always knead in more flour. You don't want to add too much, though, since this will result in a heavier, denser loaf. But don't worry: Whatever you do the first time, your bread will still turn out fine. And you can make adjustments next time, after you've experimented with your first loaf and learned how much flour to knead in. It takes some practice. Also, the amount of flour needed for yeast breads varies, depending on the temperature and humidity inside and outside your home as well as the age and type of flour used.

Knead the dough for approximately ten minutes. When it has been kneaded enough, it will have a smooth, elastic texture and a cool feeling. Dough made with whole-grain flours other than wheat will tend to stay slightly sticky.

After you've kneaded the dough, you can wrap it and freeze it for several months. This is a convenient way to have ready-made dough available for future use. When you're ready to use it, just remove the frozen dough from the freezer, unwrap it and place it in a lightly oiled bowl. Cover the bowl and put it in a warm place to thaw and rise overnight. Then you can skip Step 3 and go to Step 4.

Step 3: Letting the Dough Rise

Lightly oil the inside of a very large bowl. Place the dough in the bowl and turn it over once to coat the top and bottom with oil. Lightly cover the dough with wax paper, plastic wrap or a damp cloth. Now you need to keep the rising dough in a warm, draft-free place. A gas oven with a pilot light is about the right temperature. If you have an electric oven, you can heat it slightly for just a minute, then turn the heat off and place the bread inside. Have a thermometer available to check the temperature periodically. I like to switch on the oven light to help keep the oven warm.

Remember, if the temperature is too high, the yeast will die. But if it's too cool, the dough will take much longer to rise. It usually takes between 45 and 60 minutes for the dough to fully rise. When it's about double its original size, it's ready.

Step 4: Punching Down the Dough

Once the dough has doubled in size, remove it from the bowl and punch it down. This means you literally hit the dough to flatten it, redistributing the gluten and air bubbles. Then you can either proceed with Step 5 or, for a finer-textured bread, knead the dough for 2 minutes and put it aside to rise for about 45 minutes more. This extra rise is not necessary for most breads, but it's recommended in some recipes.

Note: If you're putting some dough aside to freeze, this is another point where you can stop the process, wrap the remaining dough in wax paper and put it in the freezer. When you take it out to use later on, start with Step 5.

Step 5: Shaping the Dough

Bread dough can be shaped almost any way you can imagine. Here are instructions for making three common shapes. For others, see specific recipes in this book or refer to other bread cookbooks.

The traditional pan loaf. Divide the dough into the number of loaves indicated in your recipe. Flatten each loaf into a rectangle that's approximately seven by ten inches.

Beginning with the seven-inch side of the rectangle, roll the dough tightly into a log shape. Pinch all the seams and ends closed with your thumb and forefinger, then roll the dough gently on the counter to smooth over the seams.

When you've formed the loaves, place them seam side down in lightly greased loaf pans. Cover again and set in a warm place to rise for about 45 minutes, or until they've almost doubled in size.

The round loaf. Divide the dough into the number of

loaves indicated in your recipe. Cupping the dough with your hands, shape each piece into a smooth circle.

Lightly oil a baking sheet and sprinkle cornmeal or flour on it. Place the loaves far enough apart on the baking sheet that when they rise and spread, they will not touch.

Cover, move to a warm area and let rise for about 45 minutes. The round loaves should almost double in size.

Rolls. Divide the dough into the number of rolls desired. The rolls can be shaped into rounds and spaced close together in a baking dish, so they touch when baked. Or they can be set apart a few inches. First, let them rise until almost doubled in size. Then:

■ Shape each piece of dough into a small round loaf for individual buns.

■ Roll each piece of dough into a six-inch strand and tie it into a knot.

■ Divide each piece of dough into three pieces and shape each piece into a small ball. Place all three pieces in one muffin cup. When they bake, they'll form a single clover-leaf-shaped roll.

Step 6: Baking

Many breads—but not all—are baked at 350°. Follow the directions in each recipe for oven temperature and cooking time.

Sometimes, because of variables in your oven or baking pan or other factors, the bread might not be fully baked in the length of time the recipe states. So you should test it to make sure it's done.

Remove the bread from the oven. If it's in a pan, carefully invert the loaf onto a wire rack to remove it. If it's done, the crust will be brown and the bread will sound hollow when you tap the bottom with your fingers.

If it needs to bake longer, put it back in the pan or on the baking sheet and pop it in the oven for a few more minutes.

When the bread has finished baking, remove it from the pan and place it on a rack. The bread should cool slightly before you slice and eat it—although it's hard to keep my family from sneaking a piece right away. The trouble is, if the bread is cut before it has cooled enough, the center will be too moist and taste uncooked.

Note: Baking at high altitudes requires special considerations. Yeast doughs rise more rapidly at high altitudes, but using less yeast than the recipe calls for will slow the rising time.

For baking bread at higher altitudes, you may need to use more liquid and less yeast than indicated in the recipe. And you'll find that you probably need longer baking times and somewhat higher temperatures. So you'll need to experiment a bit, and be sure to make revisions in your recipes when you get the combination that works.

Yeast Bread Recipes

Many of these yeast breads contain a significant amount of whole-wheat flour, which creates a denser, less fluffy bread than white flour.

You may substitute unbleached flour for some of the whole-wheat flour in all the recipes until you and your family become accustomed to a whole-grain loaf. Similarly, you can use all whole-wheat flour in the recipes that call for unbleached flour.

Remember, baking bread is not an exact science. Use these recipes as a starting point and have fun with them, substituting ingredients where desired to create your own favorite recipes.

Country Farmhouse Bread

This is a true European country bread with a crispy flour-dusted crust and hearty whole-grain flavor.

2	cups skim milk
½	cup water
2	tablespoons unsalted butter or margarine
1	tablespoon honey
1	tablespoon active dry yeast
2	teaspoons salt
5–6	cups whole-wheat flour

BAKING TIME: 35–40 MINUTES

In a small saucepan, heat the milk, water, butter or margarine and honey to 110° to 115°. Pour the liquid into a large bowl and sprinkle the yeast on top. Set aside to proof for 5 to 10 minutes.

Add the salt, then stir in 2½ cups of the flour. Beat well for 3 minutes with an electric mixer (or beat vigorously by hand).

Turn the mixture out onto a floured counter and knead in enough of the remaining flour to form a soft, unsticky dough. Knead for 10 minutes, or until it is smooth and elastic. Form into a ball.

Lightly coat a very large bowl with a little oil. Add the dough and turn the ball to coat with the oil. Cover the bowl and set aside in a warm place (80° to 85°), allowing the dough to rise for 1 hour, or until doubled in size.

Lightly oil a large baking sheet and sprinkle it with flour.

Punch down the dough and shape it into a round loaf. Place the loaf on the prepared baking sheet.

Brush the top with water, dust with flour and make a few ¼"-deep slashes on the top from end to end. Cover lightly and let rise in a warm place for 45 minutes, or until about doubled in size.

Preheat the oven to 375°. Bake the loaf for 35 to 40 minutes, or until the loaf is browned and sounds hollow when tapped on the bottom. Remove the bread from the baking sheet and cool on a wire rack.

Per slice: 158 calories, 2.3 g. total fat (12% of calories), 0.6 g. monounsaturated fat, 0.4 g. polyunsaturated fat, 1.1 g. saturated fat, 6.5 g. protein, 30.1 g. carbohydrate, 4.7 g. dietary fiber, 5 mg. cholesterol, 284 mg. sodium

Makes 1 large loaf; 16 slices

Honey Cracked-Wheat Bread

The addition of cracked wheat gives this mildly sweet bread a crunchy texture. The hearty loaves make great sandwich bread as well as toast. By varying the ingredients you can create a number of different flavors and textures. Try rolled oats instead of bran or substitute sunflower seeds for sesame seeds, for instance.

2 cups warm water (110°–115°)
2 tablespoons active dry yeast
4½–5½ cups whole-wheat flour
1 cup cracked wheat
½ cup oat bran or wheat bran
⅓ cup sesame seeds
⅓ cup honey
2 tablespoons molasses
1 tablespoon canola oil
2 teaspoons salt

Pour the water into a large bowl and sprinkle the yeast on top. Set aside to proof for 5 to 10 minutes.

Stir in 2 cups of the flour. Beat for 3 minutes with an electric mixer (or beat vigorously by hand).

Stir in the cracked wheat, bran, sesame seeds, honey, molasses, oil and salt.

Turn out onto a floured counter and knead in enough of the remaining flour to form a workable dough. Knead for 10 minutes, or until smooth and elastic. Form into a ball.

Lightly coat a large bowl with a little oil. Add the dough and turn the ball to coat with the oil.

Cover the bowl and set aside in a warm place (80° to 85°), allowing the dough to rise for 1 hour, or until doubled in size.

Lightly oil two 9" × 5" loaf pans or coat them with no-stick cooking spray.

Punch down the dough and divide it in half.

Shape each piece into a loaf and place in the prepared pans. Cover and let rise in a warm place for 30 to 45 minutes.

Preheat the oven to 375°. Bake for 30 to 45 minutes, or until the loaves sound hollow when tapped on the bottom. Remove the bread from the pans and cool on a wire rack.

Per slice: 136 calories, 2.3 g. total fat (14% of calories), 0.8 g. monounsaturated fat, 0.8 g. polyunsaturated fat, 0.3 g. saturated fat, 4.9 g. protein, 26.5 g. carbohydrate, 3.4 g. dietary fiber, 0 mg. cholesterol, 182 mg. sodium

Makes 2 loaves; 24 slices

Honey Dinner Rolls

These little rolls are very tasty and quite light for a whole-grain bread.

**BAKING TIME:
20–30
MINUTES**

1 cup warm water (110°–115°)
1 tablespoon active dry yeast
¼ cup honey
3 cups whole-wheat flour
¼ cup nonfat dry milk
1 egg
2 tablespoons unsalted butter or margarine, melted
1 teaspoon salt

Pour the water into a large bowl and sprinkle the yeast on top. Set aside to proof for 5 to 10 minutes.

Slowly add the honey and 1 cup of the flour. Beat well for 3 minutes with an electric mixer (or beat vigorously by hand). Beat in the milk, egg, butter or margarine and salt.

Turn out onto a floured counter and knead in enough of the remaining flour to form a soft, unsticky dough. Knead for 10 minutes, or until smooth and elastic. Form into a ball.

Lightly coat a very large bowl with a little oil. Add the dough and turn the ball to coat with the oil.

Cover the bowl and set aside in a warm place (80° to 85°), allowing the dough to rise for 1 hour, or until doubled in size. Lightly oil a baking sheet.

Punch down the dough and divide it into 10 pieces. Shape each piece into a roll and place on the prepared baking sheet. Cover and let rise in a warm place for 45 to 60 minutes, or until about doubled in size.

Preheat the oven to 375°. Bake the rolls for 20 to 30 minutes, or until lightly browned. Remove the rolls from the baking sheet and cool on a wire rack.

Per roll: 187 calories, 3.7 g. total fat (17% of calories), 1 g. monounsaturated fat, 0.4 g. polyunsaturated fat, 1.8 g. saturated fat, 6.6 g. protein, 34.4 g. carbohydrate, 4.6 g. dietary fiber, 28 mg. cholesterol, 231 mg. sodium

Makes 10

Whole-Wheat Monkey Bread

This bread is very special, not because of the ingredients but for the way the dough is shaped and the bread is eaten. The dough is torn into pieces, dipped in a small amount of butter or margarine and piled into a pan.

The baked bread is never cut but is torn from the bumpy-looking loaf. You can use any bread recipe, although this one is my favorite. There are pans made for baking monkey bread, but any small bundt or tube pan will do.

¼ cup honey
1 cup warm skim milk (110°–115°)
1 tablespoon active dry yeast
½ teaspoon salt
3 cups whole-wheat flour
1 tablespoon unsalted butter or margarine, melted

BAKING TIME: 30–40 MINUTES

In a large bowl, mix the honey and milk. Sprinkle the yeast on top. Set aside to proof for 5 to 10 minutes.

Stir in the salt and 1½ cups of the flour. Beat for 3 minutes with an electric mixer (or beat vigorously by hand).

Turn out onto a floured counter and knead in enough of the remaining flour to form a light, unsticky dough. Knead for 10 minutes, or until smooth and elastic. Form into a ball.

Lightly coat a very large bowl with a little oil. Add the dough and turn the ball to coat with the oil. Cover the bowl and set aside in a warm place (80° to 85°), allowing the dough to rise for 1 hour, or until doubled in size.

Lightly oil a 9″ × 5″ loaf pan.

Punch down the dough and break it into 12 roughly equal pieces. Dip one side of each piece in the butter or margarine and pile in the prepared pan. Cover and let rise for 30 minutes, or until doubled in size.

Preheat the oven to 375°. Bake for 30 to 40 minutes, or until the bread is lightly browned and sounds hollow when tapped on the bottom. Remove the bread from the pan and cool slightly on a wire rack. Serve hot. Pull the pieces from the loaf to eat.

(continued)

Per piece: 142 calories, 1.7 g. total fat (10% of calories), 0.8 g. monounsaturated fat, 0.3 g. polyunsaturated fat, 0.8 g. saturated fat, 5.2 g. protein, 28.9 g. carbohydrate, 3.8 g. dietary fiber, 3 mg. cholesterol, 101 mg. sodium

Makes 1 loaf; 12 pieces

Whole-Wheat and Honey Challah

Challah is a traditional egg bread baked for the Jewish Sabbath meal. It is both incredibly delicious and quite beautiful—a long braid with a deep brown glaze and often a sprinkling of poppy or sesame seeds.

My recipe uses whole-wheat flour and honey. It makes a very large loaf, but you can cut the ingredients in half to make a small one. I do, however, suggest making the large version. I know my own family eats this bread faster than any other I've ever baked, and leftovers are perfect for making cinnamon whole-grain French toast on the weekend.

The whole eggs give this bread its unique quality, and as you can see in the nutritional analysis, it still fits into a low-fat diet.

BAKING TIME: 40–45 MINUTES

2	cups warm water (110°–115°)
2	tablespoons honey
2	tablespoons active dry yeast
½	teaspoon salt
8–9	cups whole-wheat flour
4	tablespoons unsalted butter or margarine, melted
3	eggs
2	tablespoons water
2	tablespoons poppy seeds or sesame seeds

In a large bowl, mix the warm water and honey. Sprinkle the yeast on top.

Set aside to proof for 5 to 10 minutes.

Stir in the salt, then stir in 2 cups of the flour. Beat well for 3 minutes with an electric mixer (or beat vigorously by hand).

Add the butter or margarine and 2 of the eggs. Separate the remaining egg; add the white to the batter and reserve the yolk (cover and refrigerate) for a glaze.

Beat the mixture for another 2 minutes.

Turn out onto a floured counter and knead in enough of the remaining flour to form a workable dough. Knead for 10 minutes, adding enough flour to form an unsticky and slightly firm dough. Form into a ball.

Lightly coat a very large bowl (this dough rises very high) with a little oil.

Add the dough and turn the ball to coat with the oil. Cover the bowl and set aside in a warm place (80° to 85°), allowing the dough to rise for 1 hour, or until about doubled in size.

Lightly oil a baking sheet.

Punch down the dough and divide it into 4 equal pieces. Set 1 piece aside.

Roll the other 3 pieces into long strands and braid them together.

Pinch the ends together and tuck them under the loaf.

Place the braid on the prepared baking sheet.

Divide the remaining piece of dough into 3 more strands and braid to make a small loaf.

Center the small loaf on top of the larger one.

Cover and let rise in a warm place for about 30 to 45 minutes, or until almost doubled in size.

Preheat the oven to 350°.

Mix the reserved egg yolk with the 2 tablespoons water.

Brush the loaf with the egg wash and sprinkle with the poppy seeds or sesame seeds.

Bake for 40 to 45 minutes, or until the crust is browned and the bread sounds hollow when tapped on the bottom.

Remove the bread from the baking sheet and cool slightly on a wire rack.

Per slice: 175 calories, 3.8 g. total fat (18% of calories), 1 g. monounsaturated fat, 0.7 g. polyunsaturated fat, 1.6 g. saturated fat, 6.8 g. protein, 31.1 g. carbohydrate, 5.1 g. dietary fiber, 32 mg. cholesterol, 55 mg. sodium

Makes 1 very large loaf; 24 slices

Homemade Yeast Breads

Spanish Country Bread

This is a true European country bread: simple basic ingredients, a crispy flour-dusted crust and a wonderful, hearty, whole-grain flavor.

**BAKING TIME:
30–40
MINUTES**

1½	cups warm water (110°–115°)
1	tablespoon warm skim milk (110°–115°)
1	tablespoon active dry yeast
1½	teaspoons salt
3½	cups whole-wheat flour

In a large bowl, mix the water and milk. Sprinkle the yeast on top. Set aside to proof for 5 to 10 minutes.

Stir in the salt and 1½ cups of the flour. Beat well for 3 minutes with an electric mixer (or beat vigorously by hand).

Turn out onto a floured counter and knead in enough of the remaining flour to form a soft, unsticky dough. Knead for 10 minutes, or until smooth and elastic. Form into a ball.

Lightly coat a large bowl with a little oil. Add the dough and turn the ball to coat with the oil.

Cover the bowl and set aside in a warm place (80° to 85°), allowing the dough to rise for 45 minutes, or until doubled in size.

Lightly oil a baking sheet and sprinkle it with flour.

Punch down the dough and knead for a few minutes more. Shape into a round loaf and place on the prepared baking sheet.

Cover lightly and let rise in a warm place for 30 minutes, or until doubled in size.

Preheat the oven to 450°. Dust the top of the loaf with flour. Bake for 30 to 40 minutes.

Remove the bread from the baking sheet and cool on a wire rack.

Per slice: 122 calories, 0.7 g. total fat (5% of calories), 0.1 g. monounsaturated fat, 0.3 g. polyunsaturated fat, 0.1 g. saturated fat, 5.2 g. protein, 25.8 g. carbohydrate, 4.4 g. dietary fiber, 0 mg. cholesterol, 269 mg. sodium

Makes 1 loaf; 12 slices

Whole-Wheat French Bread

Whole-wheat flour produces a heavier, denser bread than white flour. The bread also has more flavor. For a lighter loaf, you can use half whole-wheat and half un-bleached flour.

The brick ovens that are traditionally used to make French bread account for its tender insides and crispy crust. To create a crispy crust at home, I improvise by spraying the loaves with water while they bake. If you have French-bread pans, use them instead of a baking sheet.

2½   cups warm water (110°–115°)
2   tablespoons active dry yeast
1   tablespoon salt
6–8   cups whole-wheat flour

**BAKING TIME:
25 MINUTES**

Pour the water into a large bowl and sprinkle the yeast on top. Set aside to proof for 5 to 10 minutes.

Add the salt, then stir in 2½ cups of the flour. Beat well for 3 minutes with an electric mixer (or beat vigorously by hand).

Turn out onto a floured counter and knead in enough of the remaining flour to form a soft, unsticky dough. Knead for 10 minutes, or until smooth and elastic. Form into a ball.

Lightly coat a very large bowl with a little oil. Add the dough and turn the ball to coat with the oil. Cover the bowl and set aside in a warm place (80° to 85°), allowing the dough to rise for 1 hour, or until doubled in size.

Lightly coat a baking sheet with no-stick spray and sprinkle with cornmeal.

Punch down the dough and divide it into 2 pieces. Shape into long, rounded loaves and place on the prepared baking sheet. Cover lightly and let rise in a warm place for 20 to 40 minutes, or until doubled in size.

Preheat the oven to 450°. Bake the loaves for 25 minutes; every 5 minutes during baking, open the oven door and use a clean plant sprayer to lightly mist the oven bottom and walls and the bread with water. Remove the bread from the pans and cool on a wire rack.

(continued)

Per slice: 105 calories, 0.6 g. total fat (5% of calories), 0.1 g. monounsaturated fat, 0.2 g. polyunsaturated fat, 0.1 g. saturated fat, 4.5 g. protein, 22.2 g. carbohydrate, 3.8 g. dietary fiber, 0 mg. cholesterol, 268 mg. sodium

Makes 2 loaves; 24 slices

Sprouted Wheat-Berry Bread

This bread has a sweet, nutty flavor and a nice chewy texture, thanks to the use of wheat berries (whole kernels of wheat). It's also a great sandwich bread. You'll have to plan ahead when making this bread because the wheat berries need 2 to 3 days to sprout.

BAKING TIME: 45–50 MINUTES

⅓	cup wheat berries
3	cups warm water (110°–115°)
2	tablespoons honey
1	tablespoon active dry yeast
1	tablespoon salt
6–7	cups whole-wheat flour

Approximately 2 to 3 days before you want to make this bread, place the wheat berries in a jar and cover generously with cold water. Let soak overnight. In the morning, drain off the water, rinse the berries, then drain well again. Place a piece of cheesecloth or mesh over the top of the jar, secure it with a rubber band and set the jar on a counter. Rinse and drain the berries each morning and evening. In a few days, when little white sprouts appear, the berries are ready to be used.

In a large bowl, mix the water and honey. Sprinkle the yeast on top. Set aside to proof for 5 to 10 minutes.

Stir in the salt and 2 cups of the flour. Beat well for 3 minutes with an electric mixer (or beat vigorously by hand).

Stir in the sprouted wheat berries. Turn out onto a floured counter and knead in enough of the remaining flour to form a workable dough. Knead for 10 minutes, or until smooth and elastic. Form into a ball.

Lightly coat a very large bowl with a little oil. Add the dough and turn the ball to coat it with the oil. Cover the bowl and set aside in a warm place (80° to 85°), allowing the dough to rise for 30 to 60 minutes, or until doubled in size.

Lightly oil two 9″ × 5″ loaf pans.

Punch down the dough and divide it in half. Shape the dough into 2 loaves and place in the prepared pans. Cover and let rise in a warm place for 30 minutes, or until doubled in size.

Preheat the oven to 500°. Place the loaves in the oven and immediately reduce the heat to 375°. Bake for 45 to 50 minutes, or until the loaves sound hollow when tapped on the bottom. Remove the bread from the pans and let cool on a wire rack.

Per slice: 116 calories, 0.6 g. total fat (4% of calories), 0.1 g. monounsaturated fat, 0.2 g. polyunsaturated fat, 0.1 g. saturated fat, 4.5 g. protein, 25 g. carbohydrate, 4.1 g. dietary fiber, 0 mg. cholesterol, 268 mg. sodium

Makes 2 loaves; 24 slices

Jewish Rye Bread

I created this bread using my childhood memories of the rye bread served in New York delis. It's great with sliced turkey or Swiss cheese and mustard. I love it toasted for breakfast with a little nonfat cream cheese, too. You can top the bread with kosher salt and extra caraway seeds if desired.

2	cups warm water (110°–115°)
2	tablespoons sugar
2	tablespoons active dry yeast
2	cups rye flour
1	tablespoon salt
2	tablespoons caraway seeds, lightly crushed
3	cups unbleached flour
1	egg
1	tablespoon water
1	tablespoon caraway seeds (optional)
1	tablespoon kosher salt (optional)

BAKING TIME: 30 MINUTES

Homemade Yeast Breads

In a large bowl, mix the warm water and sugar. Sprinkle the yeast on top. Set aside to proof for 5 to 10 minutes.

Add the rye flour. Beat well for 3 minutes with an electric mixer (or beat vigorously by hand).

Stir in the salt and crushed caraway seeds.

Turn out onto a floured counter and knead in enough of the unbleached flour to form a workable dough. Knead for 10 minutes, or until smooth and elastic. Form into a ball.

Lightly coat a large bowl with a little oil. Add the dough and turn the ball to coat with the oil.

Cover the bowl and set aside in a warm place (80° to 85°), allowing the dough to rise for 1 hour, or until doubled in size.

Lightly coat a baking sheet with no-stick spray.

Punch down the dough and divide it in half. Shape the dough into 2 round loaves and place on the prepared baking sheet.

Cover and let rise in a warm place for 45 minutes, or until doubled in size.

Fill a large baking dish with water and place on the bottom rack of the oven. Preheat the oven to 400°.

In a cup, lightly beat the egg and 1 tablespoon water with a fork. Brush the egg mixture over the loaves.

Sprinkle with 1 tablespoon caraway seeds and kosher salt (if using). Use a sharp knife to cut a few ½"-deep slits in the tops of the loaves.

Bake for 30 minutes, or until the loaves sound hollow when tapped on the bottom. Remove the bread from the pans and let cool on a wire rack.

Per slice: 99 calories, 0.6 g. total fat (6% of calories), 0.2 g. monounsaturated fat, 0.2 g. polyunsaturated fat, 0.1 g. saturated fat, 3.2 g. protein, 20.2 g. carbohydrate, 1.5 g. dietary fiber, 9 mg. cholesterol, 270 mg. sodium

Makes 2 loaves; 24 slices

Corn and Rye Bread

This bread has a nice flavor and good whole-grain texture. It is easy to slice and is terrific for sandwiches.

BAKING TIME:
45 MINUTES

2½ cups warm water (110°–115°)
1½ tablespoons molasses
1 tablespoon honey
1 tablespoon active dry yeast
4½–6 cups whole-wheat flour
¾ cup cornmeal
¾ cup rye flour
¼ cup poppy seeds
2 tablespoons caraway seeds
1½ tablespoons olive oil
½ teaspoon salt

Mix the water, molasses and honey in a large bowl. Sprinkle the yeast on top. Set aside to proof for 5 to 10 minutes.

Add 2½ cups of the whole-wheat flour.

Beat well for 3 minutes with an electric mixer (or beat vigorously by hand). Add the cornmeal, rye flour, poppy seeds, caraway seeds, oil and salt. Beat well.

Turn out onto a floured counter and knead in enough of the remaining whole-wheat flour to form a firm dough. Knead for 10 minutes, or until smooth and elastic. Form into a ball.

Lightly coat a large bowl with a little oil. Add the dough and turn the ball to coat with the oil.

Cover the bowl and set aside in a warm place (80° to 85°), allowing the dough to rise for approximately 1 hour, or until doubled in size.

Lightly oil two 9″ × 5″ loaf pans.

Punch down the dough and divide it in half. Knead for a few minutes and shape into loaves. Place the loaves in the prepared pans. Cover and let rise in a warm place for 45 minutes, or until doubled in size.

Preheat the oven to 350°. Bake for 45 minutes, or until the loaves sound hollow when tapped on the bottom. Remove the bread from the pans and cool on a wire rack.

Per slice: 125 calories, 2.2 g. total fat (15% of calories), 0.8 g. monounsaturated fat, 0.8 g. polyunsaturated fat, 0.3 g. saturated fat, 4.2 g. protein, 23.9 g. carbohydrate, 3.8 g. dietary fiber, 0 mg. cholesterol, 48 mg. sodium

Makes 2 loaves; 24 slices

Homemade Yeast Breads

Quick Onion-Pumpernickel Bread

This is an unusual yeast bread that doesn't require kneading. Quick Onion-Pumpernickel Bread has a mildly sweet flavor and a texture somewhere between that of a yeast bread and that of a quick bread. The hint of carob is an intriguing touch; you can replace the carob with cocoa powder if desired.

BAKING TIME: 30–35 MINUTES

1	cup warm water (110°–115°)
½	cup warm skim milk (110°–115°)
¼	cup molasses
2	tablespoons active dry yeast
3	tablespoons unsalted butter or margarine
4	tablespoons carob powder
2¼	cups whole-wheat flour
1	small onion, finely chopped
1	cup rye flour
1	teaspoon salt
1	teaspoon skim milk
2	teaspoons caraway seeds

In a large bowl, mix the water, warm milk and molasses. Sprinkle the yeast on top. Set aside to proof for 5 to 10 minutes.

In a small saucepan, melt the butter or margarine. Stir in the carob powder. Let cool.

Add the whole-wheat flour to the yeast mixture.

Beat well for 3 minutes with an electric mixer (or beat vigorously by hand). Add the onions, rye flour, salt and carob mixture. Beat for 3 minutes more.

Lightly oil a 9″ × 5″ loaf pan.

Pour the dough into the pan. Set aside in a warm place (80° to 85°) to rise for 30 minutes, or until doubled in size.

Preheat the oven to 375°.

Brush the top of the dough with the 1 teaspoon milk and sprinkle with the caraway seeds.

Bake for 30 to 35 minutes, or until the loaf sounds hollow when tapped on the bottom.

Remove the bread from the pan and cool on a wire rack.

Per slice: 164 calories, 3.8 g. total fat (20% of calories), 1 g. monounsaturated fat, 0.4 g. polyunsaturated fat, 2 g. saturated fat, 5.2 g. protein, 30.1 g. carbohydrate, 4.2 g. dietary fiber, 8 mg. cholesterol, 192 mg. sodium

Makes 1 loaf; 12 slices

Multigrain Black Bread

This hearty bread has a combination of whole grains that contribute to its dark color and fragrant aroma. This dough will be a bit sticky because of the large amount of nonwheat whole grains.

2½ cups warm water (110°–115°)
¼ cup molasses
2 tablespoons honey
2 tablespoons active dry yeast
3 cups whole-wheat flour
¾ cup cornmeal
¾ cup rolled oats
¾ cup oat bran or wheat bran
½ cup rye flour
⅓ cup carob powder or cocoa powder
3 tablespoons olive oil
2 teaspoons salt

BAKING TIME: 50–60 MINUTES

In a large bowl, mix the water, molasses and honey. Sprinkle the yeast on top. Set aside to proof for 5 to 10 minutes.

Add the whole-wheat flour. Beat well for 3 to 5 minutes with an electric mixer (or beat vigorously by hand). Cover and set aside in a warm place (80° to 85°) to rise for 30 minutes.

Stir in the cornmeal, oats, bran, rye flour, carob powder or cocoa, oil and salt. Turn out the dough onto a heavily floured counter and knead for 10 minutes, adding more whole-wheat flour as needed to form a moist but not too sticky dough. (Don't add too much flour, or the bread will be very heavy.) Form into a ball.

Coat a large bowl with a little oil. Add the dough and turn the ball to coat with the oil. Cover the bowl and set aside in a warm place (80° to 85°), allowing the dough to rise for 1 hour, or until doubled in size.

Punch down the dough.

Knead a few times and return it to the bowl.

Cover and let rise for 30 to 45 minutes, or until doubled in size.

Lightly oil a baking sheet and sprinkle with cornmeal.

Punch down the dough again and divide it in half.

Shape into 2 round loaves and place the loaves on the prepared baking sheet.

Cover and let rise in a warm place for 15 to 30 minutes.

Preheat the oven to 350°.

Bake for 50 to 60 minutes, or until the loaves sound hollow when tapped on the bottom.

Remove the bread from the baking sheet and let cool on a wire rack.

Per slice: 122 calories, 2.6 g. total fat (17% of calories), 1.5 g. monounsaturated fat, 0.5 g. polyunsaturated fat, 0.4 g. saturated fat, 3.9 g. protein, 23.7 g. carbohydrate, 3.5 g. dietary fiber, 0 mg. cholesterol, 184 mg. sodium

Makes 2 loaves; 24 slices

Minnesota Wild Rice Bread

Wild rice is not related to regular white or brown rice. It's actually an aquatic grass, although it is cooked and used like rice. I like wild rice that is cooked until it's chewy, not soggy. In this bread, the rice creates a slightly earthy flavor and texture that makes a hearty loaf of bread. You can cook wild rice ahead of time and refrigerate it until you're ready to use it.

BAKING TIME: 45 MINUTES

1½	cups water
¾	cup wild rice, rinsed
2½	cups warm water (110°–115°)
½	cup sugar or honey
2	tablespoons active dry yeast
5	cups whole-wheat flour

2   teaspoons salt
2–4   cups unbleached flour

In a medium saucepan, bring the 1½ cups water to a boil. Add the wild rice and return to a boil.

Reduce the heat to medium low and cook for 45 minutes, or until the water is absorbed.

Set aside to cool.

Pour the warm water into a large bowl. Stir in 1 tablespoon of the sugar or honey and sprinkle the yeast on top.

Set aside to proof for 5 to 10 minutes.

Stir in 2½ cups of the whole-wheat flour.

Beat well for 3 minutes with an electric mixer (or beat vigorously by hand). Add the salt, wild rice and remaining sugar or honey.

Turn out onto a floured counter and knead in the remaining 2½ cups whole-wheat flour and enough of the unbleached flour to form a workable dough. Knead for 10 minutes, or until smooth, elastic and only a little sticky.

Form into a ball.

Lightly coat a large bowl with a little oil. Add the dough and turn the ball to coat with the oil.

Cover the bowl and set aside in a warm place (80° to 85°), allowing the dough to rise for 1 hour, or until doubled in size.

Lightly oil two 9″ × 5″ loaf pans.

Punch down the dough and divide it in half.

Shape the dough into 2 loaves and place in the prepared pans.

Cover and let rise in a warm place for 30 to 45 minutes, or until doubled in size.

Preheat the oven to 350°.

Bake for 45 minutes, or until the loaves sound hollow when tapped on the bottom.

Remove the bread from the pans. Set aside to let cool on a wire rack.

> *Per slice: 160 calories, 0.7 g. total fat (4% of calories), 0.1 g. monounsaturated fat, 0.3 g. polyunsaturated fat, 0.1 g. saturated fat, 5.6 g. protein, 34.4 g. carbohydrate, 3.5 g. dietary fiber, 0 mg. cholesterol, 179 mg. sodium*

Makes 2 loaves; 24 slices

Olive Bread

Olives and whole-wheat flour pair up to create a whole-grain bread speckled with black flecks. You can add a little rosemary or sage for a flavor twist if desired.

BAKING TIME: 40 MINUTES

1	cup warm water (110°–115°)
1	tablespoon active dry yeast
3–3½	cups whole-wheat flour
1	teaspoon olive oil
1	onion, finely chopped
36	small black olives, pitted and chopped
1	teaspoon salt
½–1	teaspoon dried rosemary or sage (optional)

Pour the water into a large bowl and sprinkle the yeast on top. Set aside to proof for 5 to 10 minutes.

Add 1 cup of the flour. Beat well for 3 minutes with an electric mixer (or beat vigorously by hand).

Heat the oil in a small frying pan over medium heat.

Add the onions and cook for 5 minutes, or until soft.

Add to the dough.

Stir in the olives, salt and rosemary or sage (if using).

Turn out onto a floured counter and knead in enough of the remaining flour to form a soft, unsticky dough. Knead for 10 minutes, or until smooth and elastic. Form into a ball.

Lightly coat a large bowl with a little oil. Add the dough and turn the ball to coat with the oil.

Cover the bowl and set aside in a warm place (80° to 85°), allowing the dough to rise for 1 hour, or until doubled in size.

Lightly oil a baking sheet and sprinkle with flour.

Punch down the dough and knead for a few minutes more.

Shape into a round loaf and place on the prepared baking sheet.

Cover lightly and let rise in a warm place for 40 minutes, or until doubled in size.

Preheat the oven to 375°.

Dust the top of the loaf with flour.

Bake for 40 minutes. Remove the bread from the baking sheet and cool on a wire rack.

Per slice: 128 calories, 3 g. total fat (19% of calories), 1.6 g. monounsaturated fat, 0.4 g. polyunsaturated fat, 0.4 g. saturated fat, 4.9 g. protein, 23.6 g. carbohydrate, 4.3 g. dietary fiber, 0 mg. cholesterol, 237 mg. sodium

Makes 1 loaf; 12 slices

Sweet Potato and Honey Bread

For this loaf, I shred bright orange sweet potatoes (also known as yams) and incorporate them into a honey-sweetened dough. This is one of my favorite breads. It is soft and chewy warm from the oven, tastes excellent toasted for breakfast and is a great sandwich bread (my kids love it for lunch with natural peanut butter and fruit spread).

The recipe makes 3 large loaves. If you'd like, you can form some of the dough into dinner rolls. The bread and rolls freeze well, although they rarely make it to the freezer in our house.

3	cups warm water (110°–115°)
1½	cups honey
2	tablespoons active dry yeast
7½	cups whole-wheat flour
4	cups shredded sweet potatoes
2	teaspoons salt
6	cups unbleached flour

BAKING TIME: 45 MINUTES

In a large bowl, mix the water and 1 tablespoon of the honey. Sprinkle the yeast on top. Set aside to proof for 5 to 10 minutes.

Stir in 3 cups of the whole-wheat flour. Beat well for 3 minutes with an electric mixer (or beat vigorously by hand). Add the sweet potatoes, salt and remaining honey.

Turn out onto a floured counter and knead in the remaining 4½ cups whole-wheat flour and enough of the unbleached flour to form a workable dough. Knead for 10 minutes, or until smooth and elastic. Form into a ball.

(continued)

Lightly coat a large bowl with a little oil. Add the dough and turn the ball to coat with the oil. Cover the bowl and set aside in a warm place (80° to 85°), allowing the dough to rise for 1 hour, or until doubled in size.

Lightly oil three 9″ × 5″ loaf pans.

Punch down the dough and divide it into 3 pieces.

Shape into 3 loaves and place in the prepared pans.

Cover and let rise in a warm place for 30 to 45 minutes, or until doubled in size.

Preheat the oven to 350°.

Bake for 45 minutes, or until the loaves are brown on top and sound hollow when tapped on the bottom.

Remove the bread from the pans and let cool on a wire rack.

Per slice: 224 calories, 0.7 g. total fat (3% of calories), 0.1 g. monounsaturated fat, 0.3 g. polyunsaturated fat, 0.1 g. saturated fat, 6.1 g. protein, 49.8 g. carbohydrate, 3.7 g. dietary fiber, 0 mg. cholesterol, 123 mg. sodium

Makes 3 large loaves; 36 slices

Apple-Walnut Bread

This bread is filled with soft chunks of apple and crunchy bits of walnuts. Along with a hint of cinnamon, they create an incredible aroma while the bread is baking. This loaf is especially good for snacks and breakfast.

**BAKING TIME:
45 MINUTES**

2	cups warm water (110°–115°)
¾	cup honey
2	tablespoons active dry yeast
6–6½	cups whole-wheat flour
2	tart apples, peeled, cored and chopped
1	cup chopped walnuts
1	tablespoon ground cinnamon
2	teaspoons salt
2	cups unbleached flour

In a large bowl, mix the water and 1 tablespoon honey. Sprinkle the yeast on top. Set aside to proof for 5 to 10 minutes.

Stir in 2 cups of the whole-wheat flour. Beat well for 3 minutes with an electric mixer (or beat vigorously by hand).

Stir in the apples, walnuts, cinnamon, salt and remaining honey.

Stir in the unbleached flour.

Turn out onto a floured counter and knead in enough of the remaining whole-wheat flour to form a workable dough. Knead for 10 minutes, or until smooth, elastic and only a bit sticky.

Form into a ball.

Lightly coat a large bowl with a little oil.

Add the dough and turn the ball to coat with the oil.

Cover the bowl and set aside in a warm place (80° to 85°), allowing the dough to rise for 1 hour, or until doubled in size.

Lightly oil two 9" × 5" loaf pans.

Punch down the dough and divide it in half.

Shape the dough into 2 loaves and place in the prepared pans.

Cover and let rise in a warm place for 45 minutes.

Preheat the oven to 375°.

Bake for 45 minutes, or until the loaves sound hollow when tapped on the bottom.

Remove the bread from the pans and let cool on a wire rack.

Per slice: 213 calories, 3.7 g. total fat (15% of calories), 0.8 g. monounsaturated fat, 2.2 g. polyunsaturated fat, 0.3 g. saturated fat, 6.8 g. protein, 41 g. carbohydrate, 4.4 g. dietary fiber, 0 mg. cholesterol, 180 mg. sodium

Makes 2 loaves; 24 slices

Cinnamon-Raisin Swirl Bread

Raisins, cinnamon, honey and sugar are rolled inside this yeast bread. As you can imagine, it smells fabulous when baking.

When sliced, Cinnamon-Raisin Swirl Bread looks as good as it smells. Try it toasted.

This makes an excellent snack. In fact, it's a favorite in our house, so I double the recipe and make 4 loaves at a time. I freeze 2 loaves, put the third in the refrigerator and notice that the fourth is gone by the time it has cooled.

Dough

1   cup warm skim milk (110°–115°)
1   cup warm water (110°–115°)
¼   cup honey or maple syrup
1   tablespoon active dry yeast
½   teaspoon salt
4½–5½ cups whole-wheat flour
2   tablespoons unsalted butter or margarine, melted
1   tablespoon vanilla
½   teaspoon lemon extract or grated lemon rind
½   teaspoon ground cinnamon
¼   teaspoon ground nutmeg

Filling

¼   cup sugar or brown sugar
1   tablespoon ground cinnamon
½   teaspoon ground nutmeg
2   tablespoons honey
2   tablespoons unsalted butter or margarine, melted
¾   cup raisins

To make the dough: In a large bowl, mix the milk, water and honey or maple syrup. Sprinkle the yeast on top. Set aside to proof for 5 to 10 minutes.

Stir in the salt and 2 cups of the flour. Beat well for 3 minutes with an electric mixer (or beat vigorously by hand).

Stir in the butter or margarine, vanilla, lemon extract or lemon rind, cinnamon and nutmeg.

Turn out onto a floured surface and knead in enough of the remaining flour to form a workable dough. Knead for 10 minutes, or until smooth and elastic. Form into a ball.

Lightly coat a large bowl with a little oil. Add the dough and turn the ball to coat with the oil. Cover and set aside in a warm place (80° to 85°), allowing the dough to rise for 1 hour, or until doubled in size.

Lightly oil two 9″ × 5″ loaf pans.

Punch down the dough, knead it a few times and divide in half. Roll each piece into a rectangle (about 9″ × 12″).

To make the filling: In a cup, combine the sugar or brown sugar, cinnamon and nutmeg.

In another cup, mix the honey and butter or margarine.

Brush each piece of dough with the honey mixture. Sprinkle the sugar mixture and raisins on top.

Roll the dough lengthwise, pinch the edges closed and place in the prepared pans.

Cover and let rise in a warm place for 30 minutes, or until doubled in size.

Preheat the oven to 350°. Bake for 35 to 50 minutes, or until the tops are lightly browned.

Remove the bread from the pans and cool on a wire rack.

Per slice: 140 calories, 2.5 g. total fat (15% of calories), 0.7 g. monounsaturated fat, 0.3 g. polyunsaturated fat, 1.4 g. saturated fat, 3.8 g. protein, 27.5 g. carbohydrate, 3.1 g. dietary fiber, 6 mg. cholesterol, 52 mg. sodium

Makes 2 loaves; 24 slices

Muesli Bread

This is great for breakfast or snacks with jam or nonfat cream cheese. It's loaded with fruit, nuts, seeds and other ingredients that give it a hearty texture. If you like a really dense bread, substitute whole-wheat flour for the unbleached. This is one of Robert's favorite snack breads.

BAKING TIME: 45 MINUTES

2	cups warm water (110°–115°)
2	tablespoons honey
2	tablespoons active dry yeast
4–4½	cups unbleached flour
1	cup rolled oats
1	cup whole-grain flour (such as rye, corn, brown rice, oat or millet)
½	cup chopped dried apricots
½	cup raisins or other dried fruit
1	apple, peeled, cored and chopped
¼	cup chopped walnuts
¼	cup sunflower seeds
¼	cup pumpkin seeds

(continued)

Homemade Yeast Breads

¼   cup sesame seeds
¼   cup oat bran or wheat bran
1   tablespoon salt

In a large bowl, mix the water and honey. Sprinkle the yeast on top. Set aside to proof for 5 to 10 minutes.

Stir in 2 cups of the unbleached flour. Beat well for 3 minutes with an electric mixer (or beat vigorously by hand).

Add the oats, whole-grain flour, apricots, raisins or other dried fruit, apples, walnuts, sunflower seeds, pumpkin seeds, sesame seeds, bran and salt.

Turn out onto a floured counter and knead in enough of the remaining unbleached flour to form a workable dough that is slightly sticky. Knead for 10 minutes, or until smooth and elastic. Form into a ball.

Lightly coat a large bowl with a little oil. Add the dough and turn the ball to coat with the oil. Cover the bowl and set aside in a warm place (80° to 85°), allowing the dough to rise for 1 hour, or until doubled in size.

Lightly oil a baking sheet.

Punch down the dough and divide it in half. Shape into 2 round loaves and place on the prepared baking sheet. Cover and let rise in a warm place for 30 to 45 minutes, or until doubled in size.

Preheat the oven to 350°. Bake for 45 minutes, or until the loaves sound hollow when tapped on the bottom. Remove the bread from the baking sheet and let cool on a wire rack.

Per slice: 165 calories, 3.5 g. total fat (19% of calories), 0.9 g. monounsaturated fat, 1.8 g. polyunsaturated fat, 0.4 g. saturated fat, 5.2 g. protein, 29.6 g. carbohydrate, 2.4 g. dietary fiber, 0 mg. cholesterol, 269 mg. sodium

Makes 2 loaves; 24 slices

Whole-Wheat Cinnamon Rolls

Traditional cinnamon rolls are made with white flour and a sticky high-fat syrup. My version is low in fat and made with whole-grain flour. These very large rolls make a delicious and filling breakfast or snack.

⅓ cup warm water (110°–115°)
1 teaspoon + ½ cup honey
2 tablespoons active dry yeast
2 cups warm skim milk (110°–115°)
2 eggs
1 teaspoon salt
2 cups unbleached flour
5–6 cups whole-wheat flour
4 tablespoons unsalted butter or margarine, melted
1¾ cups brown sugar
3 tablespoons ground cinnamon
2 cups raisins (optional)

In a large bowl, mix the water and 1 teaspoon of the honey. Sprinkle the yeast on top. Set aside to proof for 5 to 10 minutes.

Stir in the milk, eggs, salt and remaining ½ cup honey. Add the unbleached flour and 2 cups of the whole-wheat flour. Beat well for 3 minutes with an electric mixer (or beat vigorously by hand).

Turn out onto a floured counter and knead in enough of the remaining whole-wheat flour to form a workable dough. Knead for 10 minutes, or until the dough is smooth and elastic. Form into a ball.

Coat a large bowl with a little oil. Add the dough and turn the ball to coat with the oil. Cover the bowl. Set aside in a warm place (80° to 85°), allowing the dough to rise for 1 hour, or until doubled in size.

Lightly oil a 12″ × 16″ baking pan, then brush with a little of the butter or margarine. Sprinkle with ¼ cup of the brown sugar and 1 tablespoon of the cinnamon.

Punch down the dough and turn out onto a lightly floured counter. Roll the dough into a large rectangle (approximately 18″ × 24″).

Brush the dough with the remaining butter or margarine. Sprinkle with the raisins (if using), the remaining 1½ cups brown sugar and the remaining 2 tablespoons cinnamon.

Beginning on the long side, roll up the dough and pinch the edges and ends closed. Using a sharp knife, slice the dough into 12 equal pieces.

Arrange the pieces, cut side up, in the pan (leaving about 1″

Homemade Yeast Breads

between pieces). Let rise in a warm place for 45 minutes, or until doubled in size.

Preheat the oven to 350°. Bake for 20 to 25 minutes, or until the rolls are browned on top. Remove the rolls from the oven and let cool in the pan.

Per roll: 557 calories, 6.4 g. total fat (10% of calories), 1.7 g. monounsaturated fat, 0.8 g. polyunsaturated fat, 3.1 g. saturated fat, 13.1 g. protein, 118.7 g. carbohydrate, 8 g. dietary fiber, 47 mg. cholesterol, 229 mg. sodium

Makes 12

French Breadstick Twists

These breadsticks are shaped into long twists. They are very moist and loaded with poppy seeds and sesame seeds.

BAKING TIME: 20–30 MINUTES

1¼	cups warm water (110°–115°)
2	tablespoons honey
1	tablespoon active dry yeast
½	teaspoon salt
1½	cups whole-wheat flour
1½	cups unbleached flour
1	egg white
1	tablespoon canola or olive oil
3	tablespoons poppy seeds
1	tablespoon sesame seeds
1	teaspoon garlic powder

In a large bowl, mix the water and honey. Sprinkle the yeast on top. Set aside to proof for 5 to 10 minutes.

Add the salt and 1 cup of the whole-wheat flour. Beat well for 3 minutes using an electric mixer (or beat vigorously by hand).

Turn out onto a floured counter and knead in the remaining ½ cup whole-wheat flour and enough of the unbleached flour to form a workable dough. Knead for 10 minutes, or until smooth and elastic. Form into a ball.

Lightly coat a large bowl with a little oil. Add the dough and turn the ball to coat with the oil. Cover the bowl and set aside in a warm place (80° to 85°), allowing the dough to rise for 1 hour, or until doubled in size.

Lightly oil a baking sheet.

Punch down the dough and divide it into 12 pieces. Roll each piece into a long strand and twist the ends several times to create spirals of dough.

Place the breadsticks on the prepared baking sheet, leaving room for them to expand. (Since the dough will tend to untwist a little, press down on the ends to hold them in place.)

Cover lightly and let rise in a warm place for 20 to 30 minutes, or until doubled in size.

In a cup, mix the egg white and oil. In another cup, mix the poppy seeds, sesame seeds and garlic powder.

Preheat the oven to 375°. Brush the breadsticks with the egg mixture and sprinkle with the seed mixture. Bake for 20 to 30 minutes, or until lightly browned. Cool slightly before serving.

Per breadstick: 149 calories, 2.9 g. total fat (17% of calories), 1 g. monounsaturated fat, 1.3 g. polyunsaturated fat, 0.3 g. saturated fat, 4.9 g. protein, 26.8 g. carbohydrate, 2.4 g. dietary fiber, 0 mg. cholesterol, 95 mg. sodium

Makes 12

Whole-Grain Bagels

If you're lucky enough to have a bagel shop in your area, look for bagels made with whole-wheat or multigrain flour. But if good ones aren't available in your area, it's easy to make your own. These whole-grain bagels freeze well and taste great as is or toasted.

Adding baking soda and cream of tartar to the water the bagels are boiled in prevents them from shrinking as they cook.

3   cups warm water (110°–115°)
3   tablespoons honey
2   tablespoons active dry yeast
1   teaspoon salt

BAKING TIME: 15–20 MINUTES

(continued)

Homemade Yeast Breads

8 cups whole-wheat flour
2 tablespoons baking soda
1 tablespoon cream of tartar

In a very large bowl, mix the water and honey. Sprinkle the yeast on top. Set aside to proof for 5 to 10 minutes.

Add the salt and 3 cups of the flour. Beat well for 3 minutes using an electric mixer (or beat vigorously by hand).

Turn out onto a floured counter and knead in enough of the remaining flour to form a workable but soft dough. Knead for 10 minutes, or until smooth and elastic. Form into a ball.

Lightly coat a very large bowl with a little oil. Add the dough and turn the ball to coat with the oil. Cover the bowl and set aside in a warm place (80° to 85°), allowing the dough to rise for 1 hour, or until doubled in size.

Bring a very large pot of water to a boil. Add the baking soda and cream of tartar.

Punch down the dough and divide into 16 pieces. Roll each piece into a rope 7" to 8" long. Put a drop of water at each end and pinch the ends together gently to form a circle.

Gently drop a few bagels into the boiling water (they expand, so don't crowd them). Boil for 2 minutes. Using a slotted spoon, turn the bagels over and boil for another 2 minutes.

Remove the bagels from the water and place on a wire rack to drain. Boil the remaining bagels in the same manner.

Lightly oil a baking sheet and place the bagels on it.

Preheat the oven to 400°. Bake for 15 to 20 minutes, or until crisp and lightly browned.

Per bagel: 220 calories, 1.2 g. total fat (5% of calories), 0.2 g. monounsaturated fat, 0.5 g. polyunsaturated fat, 0.2 g. saturated fat, 8.8 g. protein, 47.3 g. carbohydrate, 7.6 g. dietary fiber, 0 mg. cholesterol, 136 mg. sodium

Makes 16

Variations

Poppy seed: Lightly beat 1 egg white and brush some on top of each bagel before baking. Sprinkle with poppy seeds. (You could also use sesame seeds, minced onions or minced garlic in place of the poppy seeds.)

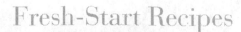
Fresh-Start Recipes

Per bagel: 225 calories, 1.5 g. total fat (6% of calories), 0.2 g. monounsaturated fat, 0.7 g. polyunsaturated fat, 0.2 g. saturated fat, 9.1 g. protein, 47.5 g. carbohydrate, 7.6 g. dietary fiber, 0 mg. cholesterol, 140 mg. sodium

Cinnamon-raisin: Increase the honey to ½ cup. Add ¾ cup raisins and 1 tablespoon ground cinnamon to the dough after beating it well but before incorporating more flour.

Per bagel: 262 calories, 1.2 g. total fat (4% of calories), 0.2 g. monounsaturated fat, 0.5 g. polyunsaturated fat, 0.2 g. saturated fat, 9 g. protein, 58.4 g. carbohydrate, 7.9 g. dietary fiber, 0 mg. cholesterol, 138 mg. sodium

Apple-cinnamon: Increase the honey to ½ cup. Add 2 cups peeled and chopped apples and 1 tablespoon ground cinnamon to the dough after beating it well but before incorporating more flour.

Per bagel: 251 calories, 1.3 g. total fat (4% of calories), 0.2 g. monounsaturated fat, 0.5 g. polyunsaturated fat, 0.2 g. saturated fat, 8.8 g. protein, 47.3 g. carbohydrate, 7.8 g. dietary fiber, 0 mg. cholesterol, 137 mg. sodium

Pumpernickel: Add 1 cup rye flour, 1 tablespoon molasses and 2 teaspoons caraway seeds to the dough after beating it well but before incorporating more flour.

Per bagel: 246 calories, 1.3 g. total fat (5% of calories), 0.2 g. monounsaturated fat, 0.5 g. polyunsaturated fat, 0.2 g. saturated fat, 9.4 g. protein, 53.1 g. carbohydrate, 8.4 g. dietary fiber, 0 mg. cholesterol, 138 mg. sodium

Stuffed Breads

It's easy to create stuffed breads. Just roll dough into a large rectangle and spread it with any number of ingredients. Then roll it up as you would a jelly roll before baking. When sliced, the bread will have filling swirled through it.

The savory stuffed breads that follow are excellent for

lunch or a light dinner. Serve them with a salad or soup to make a whole meal. They also make a flavorful snack.

Stuffed breads freeze well. They're delicious reheated, although they're good cold, too. Use my recipes as a starting point for your own creations. Here are some of my family's favorite fillings.

■ Smoked turkey breast, reduced-fat provolone cheese, Dijon mustard and roasted peppers

■ Sun-dried tomatoes, fresh basil, Parmesan and plum tomatoes

■ Black beans, part-skim sharp Cheddar cheese, jalapeño peppers, cilantro and nonfat sour cream

■ Ratatouille (page 281) and part-skim mozzarella cheese

■ Sautéed ground turkey breast, onions, mushrooms, carrots, thyme, basil, Dijon mustard and part-skim cheese

Stuffed Spinach and Feta Bread

If you prefer, you can replace the dough below with store-bought frozen dough. Just thaw it before proceeding with the recipe.

You can double the filling ingredients if you like, but I think the flavors are strong enough that it's not really necessary. For a heartier loaf, use all whole-wheat flour.

BAKING TIME: 45 MINUTES

Dough

2	cups warm water (110°–115°)
1	tablespoon sugar or honey
2	tablespoons active dry yeast
2	cups whole-wheat flour
1½	teaspoons salt
3–3½	cups unbleached flour

Filling

2	teaspoons olive oil
½	cup chopped red onions
10	cloves garlic, thinly sliced
10	ounces spinach, coarsely chopped
2	teaspoons sugar

Salt
Freshly ground black pepper
1   cup shredded part-skim Swiss cheese
4   ounces feta cheese, crumbled
1   egg, lightly beaten
2   tablespoons sesame seeds or poppy seeds

To make the dough: In a large bowl, mix the water and sugar or honey. Sprinkle the yeast on top. Set aside to proof for 5 to 10 minutes.

Add the whole-wheat flour and salt. Beat well for 3 minutes with an electric mixer (or beat vigorously by hand).

Turn out onto a floured counter and knead in enough of the unbleached flour to form a workable dough. Knead for 10 minutes, or until smooth and elastic. Form into a ball.

Lightly coat a large bowl with a little oil. Add the dough and turn the ball to coat with the oil. Cover the bowl and set aside in a warm place (80° to 85°), allowing the dough to rise for 1 hour, or until doubled in size.

To make the filling: Warm the oil in a large no-stick frying pan over medium heat.

Add the onions and garlic. Sauté for 3 minutes. Add the spinach, sugar and salt and pepper to taste.

Cook, stirring frequently, for 10 minutes, or until most of the liquid has evaporated. Set aside.

Lightly oil a baking sheet.

Punch down the dough and divide in half. Turn out onto a lightly floured counter and roll each piece into a 10″ × 15″ rectangle.

Sprinkle the Swiss, feta and spinach mixture evenly over the rectangles.

Beginning with the short side, roll up each rectangle and pinch the edges and ends closed.

Place the loaves, seam side down, on the prepared baking sheet, leaving room between them to allow for rising as they bake.

With a sharp knife, cut three 1″-deep slits on the top of each loaf. Brush the tops lightly with some of the egg and sprinkle with the sesame seeds or poppy seeds.

Preheat the oven to 350°. Bake for 45 minutes, or until the filling has burst out of the sides and the tops are nicely browned. Remove from the oven and let cool on the baking sheet for about 30 minutes before slicing and serving.

Per slice: 163 calories, 3.3 g. total fat (18% of calories), 0.8 g. monounsaturated fat, 0.4 g. polyunsaturated fat, 1.5 g. saturated fat, 7 g. protein, 26.6 g. carbohydrate, 2.6 g. dietary fiber, 13 mg. cholesterol, 307 mg. sodium

Makes 2 loaves; 20 slices

Vegetable Stuffed Bread

For variety, use vegetables other than the ones I suggest below. Asparagus, artichoke hearts, sun-dried tomatoes, peppers and broccoli all work well.

BAKING TIME: 45 MINUTES

Dough

2	cups warm water (110°–115°)
1	tablespoon sugar or honey
2	tablespoons active dry yeast
2	cups whole-wheat flour
1½	teaspoons salt
3–3½	cups unbleached flour

Filling

2	teaspoons olive oil
1	cup thinly sliced red onions
12	cloves garlic, thinly sliced
2	zucchini, quartered and thinly sliced
8	ounces mushrooms, sliced
¾	cup sliced roasted red peppers
½	cup chopped fresh parsley
3	tablespoons chopped fresh basil
	Salt
	Freshly ground black pepper
2	cups shredded part-skim mozzarella cheese
½	cup grated Parmesan cheese
1	egg, lightly beaten
2	tablespoons poppy seeds or sesame seeds

To make the dough: In a large bowl, mix the water and sugar or honey. Sprinkle the yeast on top. Set aside to proof for 5 to 10 minutes.

Add the whole-wheat flour and salt. Beat well for 3 minutes with an electric mixer (or beat vigorously by hand).

Turn out onto a floured counter and knead in enough of the unbleached flour to form a workable dough. Knead for 10 minutes, or until smooth and elastic. Form into a ball.

Lightly coat a large bowl with a little oil. Add the dough and turn the ball to coat with the oil. Cover the bowl and set aside in a warm place (80° to 85°), allowing the dough to rise for 1 hour, or until doubled in size.

To make the filling: Warm the oil in a large no-stick frying pan over medium heat. Add the onions and garlic; cook for 3 minutes. Add the zucchini, mushrooms, red peppers, parsley, basil and salt and black pepper to taste. Cook and stir for 15 minutes, or until most of the liquid has evaporated. Set aside.

Lightly oil a baking sheet. Punch down the dough and divide in half. Turn out onto a lightly floured counter and roll each piece of dough into a 10″ × 15″ rectangle.

Sprinkle the mozzarella, Parmesan and sautéed vegetables evenly over the rectangles. Beginning with the short side, roll up each rectangle and pinch the edges and ends closed. Place the loaves, seam side down, on the prepared baking sheet, leaving room between the loaves to allow for rising as they bake. With a sharp knife, cut three 1″-deep slits on the top of each loaf. Brush the tops lightly with the egg and sprinkle with the sesame seeds or poppy seeds.

Preheat the oven to 350°. Bake for 45 minutes, or until the filling has burst out of the sides and the tops are nicely browned. Remove from the oven and let cool on the baking sheet for about 30 minutes before slicing and serving.

Per slice: 180 calories, 4.1 g. total fat (20% of calories), 1.2 g. monounsaturated fat, 0.6 g. polyunsaturated fat, 1.8 g. saturated fat, 8.9 g. protein, 27.8 g. carbohydrate, 2.6 g. dietary fiber, 14 mg. cholesterol, 263 mg. sodium

Makes 2 loaves; 20 slices

Specialty Breads

You can make a wide variety of flavored breads using a basic dough recipe and whatever other ingredients you want. This is a dough that I especially like.

**BAKING TIME:
30–45
MINUTES**

1½	cups warm water (110°–115°)
4	tablespoons honey or sugar
1	tablespoon active dry yeast
2½	cups whole-wheat flour
1½	teaspoons salt
	Specialty ingredients (see below)
1–2	cups unbleached flour

In a large bowl, mix the water and 1 tablespoon of the honey or sugar. Sprinkle the yeast on top. Set aside to proof for 5 to 10 minutes.

Add 1½ cups of the whole-wheat flour and the remaining 3 tablespoons honey or sugar.

Beat well for 3 minutes with an electric mixer (or beat vigorously by hand).

Stir in the salt and your choice of specialty ingredients.

Turn out onto a floured counter and knead in enough of the remaining 1 cup whole-wheat flour and enough of the unbleached flour to form a workable dough. Knead for 10 minutes, or until smooth and elastic. Form into a ball.

Lightly coat a large bowl with a little oil. Add the dough and turn the ball to coat with the oil.

Cover the bowl and set aside in a warm place (80° to 85°), allowing the dough to rise for 1 hour, or until doubled in size.

Lightly oil a baking sheet.

Punch down the dough. Shape into a round loaf and place on the prepared baking sheet.

Cover and let rise in a warm place for 45 minutes, or until doubled in size.

Preheat the oven to 350°. Bake for 30 to 45 minutes, or until the loaf sounds hollow when tapped on the bottom. Remove the bread from the baking sheet and let cool on a wire rack.

Per slice (without specialty ingredients): 147 calories, 0.6 g. total fat (4% of calories), 0.1 g. monounsaturated fat, 0.2 g. polyunsaturated fat, 0.1 g. saturated fat, 4.9 g. protein, 32.1 g. carbohydrate, 3.4 g. dietary fiber, 0 mg. cholesterol, 268 mg. sodium

Makes 1 loaf; 12 slices

Specialty Ingredients

Sun-dried tomatoes and basil: Soak 1 to 2 ounces sun-dried tomatoes in boiling water for 5 minutes. Drain the tomatoes and slice or chop them. Add the tomatoes, ¼ cup grated Parmesan cheese and 3 tablespoons chopped fresh basil to the basic dough where indicated.

Per slice: 163 calories, 1.3 g. total fat (7% of calories), 0.3 g. monounsaturated fat, 0.3 g. polyunsaturated fat, 0.5 g. saturated fat, 6 g. protein, 33.8 g. carbohydrate, 3.6 g. dietary fiber, 2 mg. cholesterol, 310 mg. sodium

Cranberries and oranges: Add 1 cup dried cranberries, ½ cup honey and 1 tablespoon grated orange rind to the basic dough where indicated.

Per slice: 200 calories, 0.6 g. total fat (3% of calories), 0.1 g. monounsaturated fat, 0.2 g. polyunsaturated fat, 0.1 g. saturated fat, 4.9 g. protein, 45.9 g. carbohydrate, 4.3 g. dietary fiber, 0 mg. cholesterol, 269 mg. sodium

Jalapeño peppers and Cheddar: Add 4 ounces shredded part-skim sharp Cheddar cheese. You can also add the desired amount of canned chopped jalapeño peppers to the basic dough where indicated.

Per slice: 171 calories, 2 g. total fat (10% of calories), 0.1 g. monounsaturated fat, 0.2 g. polyunsaturated fat, 0.8 g. saturated fat, 6.9 g. protein, 32.8 g. carbohydrate, 3.5 g. dietary fiber, 5 mg. cholesterol, 402 mg. sodium

Saffron and toasted pine nuts: Soak ¼ teaspoon saffron threads in 2 tablespoons hot water for 15 minutes.

Toast ¼ cup pine nuts in a dry frying pan (or on a baking sheet in a 350° oven) just until they begin to brown (watch carefully; they burn easily).

Add the saffron and soaking water, pine nuts and ¼ cup honey to the basic dough where indicated.

Per slice: 186 calories, 2.3 g. total fat (11% of calories), 0.1 g. monounsaturated fat, 0.2 g. polyunsaturated fat, 0.1 g. saturated fat, 5.7 g. protein, 38.3 g. carbohydrate, 3.5 g. dietary fiber, 0 mg. cholesterol, 269 mg. sodium

Fennel seeds and anise seeds: Slightly crush ½ teaspoon fennel seeds and ½ teaspoon anise seeds.

Add the seeds, ½ cup honey and ¼ teaspoon almond extract to the basic dough where indicated.

Per slice: 191 calories, 0.6 g. total fat (3% of calories), 0.1 g. monounsaturated fat, 0.2 g. polyunsaturated fat, 0.1 g. saturated fat, 4.9 g. protein, 43.6 g. carbohydrate, 3.5 g. dietary fiber, 0 mg. cholesterol, 269 mg. sodium

Vegetables: In a food processor, combine ¼ cup coarsely chopped onions, 1 carrot, ½ green or sweet red pepper and 1 clove garlic. Finely chop using on/off turns. Add the vegetable mixture, ½ cup grated Parmesan cheese, 1 teaspoon dried basil and 1 teaspoon dried oregano to the basic dough where indicated.

Per slice: 172 calories, 1.9 g. total fat (10% of calories), 0.5 g. monounsaturated fat, 0.3 g. polyunsaturated fat, 0.9 g. saturated fat, 6.8 g. protein, 33.6 g. carbohydrate, 3.7 g. dietary fiber, 3 mg. cholesterol, 348 mg. sodium

References

Chapter 1

Page 5 "... immediate and lasting results." Prochaska, J. O., Norcross, J. C., and DiClemente, C. C. *Changing for Good* (New York: William Morrow, 1994).

Page 6 "... right steps at the right times." Ibid.: 57.

"... take charge of the steps required." J. J. Weaver et al. "A Review of Potential Moderating Factors in the Stress-Performance Relationship." U.S. Naval Training Systems Center Technical Reports v92-012 (1992): 84.

"... set themselves up for failure." Prochaska, Norcross and DiClemente. *Changing for Good*: 61.

Page 7 "... who watch their diets are physically inactive." Patterson, R. E., Haines, P. S., and Popkin, B. M. "Healthy Lifestyle Patterns of U.S. Adults." *Preventive Medicine* 23 (1994): 453–460.

Chapter 2

Page 11 "Your mood lifts." Weidner et al. "Improvements in Hostility and Depression in Relation to Dietary Change and Cholesterol Lowering: The Family Heart Study." *Annals of Internal Medicine* 117 (1992)(1): 820–823.

"Your grocery bills shrink." "Cutting Fat Makes Cents." *Prevention* (June 1994): 32.

"You're more alert and energetic." Wurtman, J. J., quoted in "Peak Performance Brain Food." *Omni* 2 (6)(April 1988): 67; Barnard, N. *Food for Life* (New York: Harmony Books, 1993): 129.

Page 12 "Less joint pain." Felson. "The Course of Osteoarthritis and Factors That Affect It." *Osteoarthritis* 19 (3)(Aug. 1993): 607–615.

"Lower blood pressure ..." Stein and Black. "The Role of Diet in the Genesis and Treatment of Hypertension." *Medical Clinics of North America* 77 (4)(July 1993): 831–847.

"... and cholesterol" "The Surprise Rewards of Weight Loss." *Prevention* (July 1994): 16.

"... developing gout, varicose veins ..." Ibid.

"... like carpal tunnel syndrome" Werner et al. "The Relationship between Body Mass Index and the Diagnosis of Carpal Tunnel Syndrome." *Muscle and Nerve* 17 (6)(June 1994): 632–636.

"... causes of death in the United States" M. Wootan et al. *Prescription: Good Nutrition*. (Washington: D.C.: Center for Science in the Public Interest, June 1994).

"... lead to fewer backaches ..." Kauppila et al. "Lumbar Disc Degeneration and Atherosclerosis of the Abdominal Aorta." *Spine* 19 (8)(1994): 923–929.

"... and recover from injury." Stallone. "The Influence of Obesity and Its Treatment on the Immune System." *Nutrition Reviews* 52 (2)(1994): 37–50. Jacobson, T. M. "Obesity and the Surgical Patient: Nursing Alert." *Ostomy Wound Management* 40 (2)(March 1994): 56–58, 60–63.

"... for the rest of their lives." Shattuck et al. "How Women's Adopted Low-Fat Diets Affect Their Husbands." *American Journal of Public Health* 82 (9)(Sept. 1992): 1244–1250.

"... their calories from fat." Miller et al. "Diet Composition, Energy Intake, and Exercise in Relation to Body Fat in Men and Women." *American Journal of Clinical Nutrition* 52 (1990): 426–430. Strain et al. "Food Intake of Very Obese Persons: Quantitative and Qualitative Aspects." *Journal of the American Dietetic Association* (1992): 199–204.

Page 13 "...cutting back on total calories." Kendall et al. "Weight Loss on a Low-Fat Diet: Consequences of the Imprecision of the Control of Food Intake in Humans." *American Journal of Clinical Nutrition* 53 (1991): 1124–1129.

Page 15 "...with their food than the calorie-cutters." Shah et al. "Comparison of a Low-Fat, Ad Libitum Complex-Carbohydrate Diet with a Low-Energy Diet in Moderately Obese Women." *American Journal of Clinical Nutrition* 59 (May 1994): 980–984.

"...as much weight as the calorie-cutters." Ibid.

"...reach a weight and stay there." Rodin et al. "Weight Cycling and Fat Distribution." *International Journal of Obesity* 14 (April 1990): 303–310.

Page 16 "...heart disease and cancer." "Childhood Origins of Lifestyle-Related Risk Factors for Coronary Heart Disease in Adulthood." *Nutrition and Health* 9 (2)(1993): 107–115.

"...isn't as significant a factor." Moerman et al. "Regional Fat Distribution as Risk Factor for Clinically Diagnosed Gallstones in Middle-Aged Men: A 25-Year Follow-Up Study." *International Journal of Obesity* 18 (1994): 435–439.

"...connected with infertility in women." Zaadstra. "Fat and Female Fecundity: Prospective Study of Effect of Body Fat Distribution on Conception Rates." *British Medical Journal* 306 (1993): 484–487.

"...lose your taste for fat." Miller et al. "Diet Composition, Energy Intake, and Exercise": 426–430. Urban et al. "Correlates of Maintenance of a Low-Fat Diet among Women in the Women's Health Trial." *Preventive Medicine* 21 (1992): 279–291.

"...after eating high-fat foods." Ibid.

"...weakening your immune system..." Kelley et al. "Concentration of Dietary N-6 Polyunsaturated Fatty Acids and the Human Immune System." *Clinical Immunology and Immunopathology* 62 (2)(1992): 240–244.

"...health problems, from impotence..." Butler et al. "Love and Sex after 60: How to Evaluate and Treat the Impotent Older Man." *Geriatrics* 49 (Oct. 1994): 27–32.

"...and gallstones..." Stone et al. "Gallbladder Emptying Stimuli in Obese and Normal-Weight Subjects." *Hepatology* 15 (1992): 758–795.

"...to heart disease..." Cunnane. "Childhood Origins of Lifestyle-Related Risk Factors." 30. Brace et al. "Factor VII Coagulant Activity and Cholesterol Changes in Premenopausal Women Consuming a Long-Term Cholesterol-Lowering Diet." *Arteriosclerosis and Thrombosis* 14 (8)(Aug. 1994): 1284–1289.

"...and cancer." Giovanucci et al. "A Prospective Study of Dietary Fat and Risk of Prostate Cancer." *Journal of the National Cancer Institute* 85 (19)(Oct. 1993): 1571–1579. Hankin, J. "Role of Nutrition in Women's Health: Diet and Breast Cancer." *Journal of the American Dietetic Association* 93 (9)(1993): 994–999. Black et al. "Effect of a Low-Fat Diet on the Incidence of Actinic Keratosis." *New England Journal of Medicine* 330 (18)(1994): 1272–1275. Alavanja et al. "Saturated Fat Intake and Lung Cancer Risk among Nonsmoking Women in Missouri." *Journal of the National Cancer Institute* 85 (23)(1993): 1906–1915.

"...defense against infection." Kelley et al. "Concentration of Dietary N-6 Polyunsaturated Fatty Acids."

"...to certain types of cancer." Giovanucci et al. "A Prospective Study of Dietary Fat." Hankin. "Role of Nutrition in Women's Health." Black et al. "Effect of a Low-Fat Diet." Alavanja et al. "Saturated Fat Intake and Lung Cancer Risk."

Page 17 "...organ located below the liver." W. W. LaMorte et al. "Increased Dietary Fat Content Accelerates Cholesterol Gallstone Formation in the Cholesterol-Fed Prairie Dog." *Hepatology* 18 (6)(Dec. 1993): 1498–1503.

"...condition that often requires surgery." Miller, B. F., and Keane, C. B. *Encyclopedia and Dictionary of Medicine, Nursing and Allied Health*, 5th ed. (Philadelphia: W. B. Saunders, 1993): 592–593.

References

" . . . than those who eat fat." Wyshak. "Dietary Animal Fat Intake, Calcium Intake, and Bone Fractures in Women 50 Years and Older." *Journal of Women's Health* 2 (4)(1993): 329–334.

" . . . complications associated with multiple sclerosis." Swank. "Multiple Sclerosis: Fat-Oil Relationship." *Nutrition* 7 (5): 368–376.

" . . . develop over many years." Cunnane. "Childhood Origins of Lifestyle-Related Risk Factors."

" . . . what we call a heart attack." Ibid.

" . . . slow the process or even reverse it." Willett, W. C. "Diet and Health: What Should We Eat?" *Science* 264 (April 22, 1994): 532–537.

Page 18 " . . . excess pounds of body fat." Linden and Chambers. "Clinical Effectiveness of Non-Drug Treatment for Hypertension: A Meta-Analysis." *Annals of Behavioral Medicine* 16 (1)(1994): 35–45.

" . . . with or without weight loss." Stein and Black. "The Role of Diet."

" . . . more complex carbohydrates than Americans do." Haffner et al. "Prevalence of Hypertension in Mexico City and San Antonio, Texas." *Circulation* 90 (3)(1994): 1542–1549.

" . . . gunked up with plaque." Butler et al. "Love and Sex after 60."

Page 19 " . . . is associated with lower back pain." Kauppila et al. "Lumbar Disc Degeneration and Atherosclerosis."

" . . . extra-cheese-please, high-fat diet." Giovanucci et al. "A Prospective Study of Dietary Fat."

" . . . skin cancer and lung cancer." Black et al. "Effect of a Low-Fat Diet." Alavanja et al. "Saturated Fat Intake and Lung Cancer Risk."

" . . . who ate a high-fat diet." Black et al. "Effect of a Low-Fat Diet."

" . . . their risk of developing lung cancer." Alavanja et al. "Saturated Fat Intake and Lung Cancer Risk."

Page 20 " . . . almost as many as lung cancer." Ensminger et al. *Foods and Nutrition Encyclopedia*, 2nd ed. (Clovis, Calif.: Pegus Press, 1994).

" . . . vegetables and whole grains." Willet et al. "Relation of Meat, Fat, and Fiber Intake to the Risk of Colon Cancer in a Prospective Study among Women." *New England Journal of Medicine* 323 (24)(1990): 1664–1672. Giovanucci et al. "Relationship of Diet to Risk of Colorectal Adenoma": 91–98.

" . . . oral, esophageal and pancreatic cancers." "Consumption of Meat and Fruit in Relation to Oral and Esophageal Cancer: A Cross-National Study." *Nutrition and Cancer* 19 (2)(1993): 169–179. "Effects of High-Fat Diet and Cholecystokinin Receptor Blockade on Pancreatic Growth and Tumor Initiation." *Carcinogenesis* 14 (4)(May 1993): 1021–1026.

" . . . more than 175,000 a year." Ensminger et al. *Foods and Nutrition Encyclopedia*.

" . . . the risk of breast cancer" Hankin. "Role of Nutrition in Women's Health."

" . . . contains a lot of fat." Ibid.

" . . . die of the disease." Jain et al. "Premorbid Diet and the Prognosis of Women with Breast Cancer." *Journal of the National Cancer Institute* 86 (18)(1994): 1390–1397.

Page 21 " . . . women who eat a fatty diet." Nordevang et al. "Dietary Habits and Mammographic Patterns in Patients with Breast Cancer." *Breast Cancer Research and Treatment* 26 (3)(1993): 207–215.

" . . . than people of normal weight." Stallone. "The Influence of Obesity and Its Treatment."

" . . . person of average weight." S. O. Norris et al. "Physiology of Wound Healing and Risk Factors That Impede the Healing Process." *Clinical Issues of Critical Care Nursing* 1 (1990): 545–562.

Page 22 " . . . affects over 13 million Americans." Tinker et al. "Diabetes Mellitus—A Priority Health Care Issue for Women." *Journal of the American Dietetic Association* 94 (9)(Sept. 1994): 976–985.

" . . . to convert food to energy." *American Medical Association Family Medical Guide*, 3rd ed., 1994: 558.

"...kidney failure and blindness." Ibid.: 559.

"...your risk is only about 1 in 20." Ibid.

"...diabetes runs in your family." Ibid.: 530.

"...have impaired glucose tolerance" Marshall. "Dietary Fat Predicts Conversion from Impaired Glucose Tolerance to NIDDM." *Diabetes Care* 17 (1)(1994): 50–56.

"...trouble metabolizing carbohydrates." Miller and Keane. *Encyclopedia and Dictionary of Medicine*: 618.

"...your risk of developing diabetes." Marshall. "Dietary Fat Predicts Conversion."

"...Type II diabetes increases threefold." Ibid.

Page 23 "...eliminate their need for insulin." *American Medical Association Family Medical Guide*.

"...protecting their hearts and blood vessels." Vessby et al. "Dietary Carbohydrates in Diabetes." *American Journal of Clinical Nutrition* 59 (suppl)(1994): 742S–746S.

"...childhood obesity increased 54 percent" Wolfe et al. "Overweight Schoolchildren in New York State: Prevalence and Characteristics." *American Journal of Public Health* 84 (5)(1994): 807–813.

"...one in four American children is overweight." Johnson and Birch. "Parents' and Children's Adiposity and Eating Style." *Pediatrics* 94 (5)(1994): 653–661.

"...and more emotional stress" Kern et al. "The Postingestive Consequences of Fat Condition Preferences for Flavors Associated with High Dietary Fat." *Physiology and Behavior* 54 (1994): 71–76.

"...those who plump up later in life." Wolfe et al. "Overweight Schoolchildren in New York State."

"...than their normal-weight peers." J. D. Sargent et al. "Obesity and Stature in Adolescence and Earnings in Young Adulthood: Analysis of a British Birth Cohort." *Archives of Pediatric Adolescent Medicine* 148 (7)(July 1994): 681–687.

"...who were killed in action." Strong et al. "Natural History of Aortic and Coronary Atherosclerotic Lesions in Youth." *Arteriosclerosis and Thrombosis* 13 (9)(1993): 1291–1298.

Page 24 "...fatty streaks in their coronary arteries." Strong et al. "Natural History."

"...fast foods and other fatty fare." Signiorelli and Lears. "Television and Children's Conceptions of Nutrition: Unhealthy Messages." *Health Communication* 4 (4)(1992): 245–257.

"...have sugary cereals for breakfast." Ibid.

"...high in artery-clogging fat." Whitaker et al. "School Lunch: A Comparison of the Fat and Cholesterol Content with Dietary Guidelines." *Journal of Pediatrics* 123 (1993): 857–862.

"...the way their parents eat." Johnson and Birch. "Parents' and Children's Adiposity."

"...eating habits to their children." Ibid.

Page 25 "...kids who eat fatty food." Shea et al. "Is There a Relationship Between Dietary Fat and Stature or Growth in Children Three to Five Years of Age?" *Pediatrics* 92 (4)(1993): 579–586.

"...what they like and what they don't." Kern et al. "The Postingestive Consequences of Fat Condition Preferences."

"...a traditional high-fat diet." Weidner et al. "Improvements in Hostility and Depression in Relation to Dietary Change and Cholesterol Lowering: The Family Heart Study." *Annals of Internal Medicine* 117 (1)(1992): 820–823.

Page 26 "...lower than the control group's." Shattuck et al. "How Women's Adopted Low-Fat Diets Affect Their Husbands."

"...a person in the high-fat group." "Cutting Fat Makes Cents."

"...smaller) clothes for everyone in the family!" Study at the Lipid

Research Clinic of George Washington University. *Muscle and Fitness* (Dec. 1992).

Chapter 3

Page 28 "...body fat may be, to some extent, inherited." A. J. Stunkard et al. "An Adoption Study of Human Obesity." *New England Journal of Medicine* 314 (4)(1986): 193–198; Greenwood, M., and Turkenkopf, I. *Genetic and Metabolic Aspects of Obesity* (New York: Churchill Livingstone, 1983): 193–205.

Page 30 "...convert 100 calories of fat into new body fat." Danforth. "Diet and Obesity." *Proceedings of the National Academy of Sciences U.S.A.* 82 (1985): 4866.

Page 31 "...turn the food into body fat." "Is Fat More Fattening?" *Tufts University Diet and Nutrition Letter* 4 (12)(Feb. 1987): 1–2; *Metabolism* 31 (1982): 1234–1242.

"...lose body fat and keep it off." L. H. Storlin et al. *American Journal of Physiology* 251 (1986): E576–E583.

"...difficult for your body to burn fat." Eckel, R. "Insulin Resistance: An Adaptation for Weight Maintenance." *Lancet* 340 (1990): 1452; Mc-Dougall, J. A. *The McDougall Program for Weight Loss* (New York: Dutton, 1994): 54.

"...in the hours that follow." A. Trembley et al. "Impact of Dietary Fat Content and Fat Oxidation on Energy Intake in Humans." *American Journal of Clinical Nutrition* 49 (1989): 799–805.

Page 32 "...60 percent of your calories from fat with every single bite." Mandelbaum-Schmid, J. "Are You Addicted to Fat?" *Health* (Jan./Feb. 1994): 28–29.

"...stored as body fat." Leibowitz, S. F., quoted in Marano, H. E. "Chemistry and Craving." *Psychology Today* (Jan./Feb. 1993): 30–36, 74.

"...even more fat-eating." Leibowitz, S. F. *Health* (Jan./Feb. 1994): 29; Leibowitz, S. F., quoted in Marano, H. E. "Chemistry and Craving."

" 'The mechanisms that enhance...' the research team." Leibowitz, S. F., quoted in *Health*.

Page 33 " '...signals to eat fat,' observes Dr. Bailey." Bailey, S., quoted in *Health* (Jan./Feb. 1994): 29.

"...storing more and using less." C. N. Sadur et al. "Fat Feeding Decreases Insulin Responsiveness of Adipose Tissue Lipoprotein Lipase." *Metabolism* 33 (1984): 1043–1047; Stamford, B. A., and Shimer, P. *Fitness without Exercise* (New York: Warner, 1990): 186–187; N. Torbay et al. "Insulin Increases Body Fat despite Control of Food Intake and Physical Activity." *American Journal of Physiology* 248 (1985): R120–R124.

"...high in both fat and sugar" Miller, W. C. *The Non-Diet Diet* (Englewood, Colo.: Taylor, 1993): 77.

"...right in the open door." Drewnowski, A. *Environmental Nutrition* 16 (10)(Oct. 1993): 6; L. B. Oscai et al. "Effects of Dietary Sugar and of Dietary Fat on Food Intake and Body Fat Content in Rats." *Growth* 5 (1987): 64–73; Oscai, L. B., and Miller, W. C. "Dietary-Induced Severe Obesity: Exercise Implications." *Medicine and Science in Sports and Exercise* 18 (1)(1985): 6–9; L. B. Oscai et al. "Effect of Dietary Fat on Food Intake, Growth, and Body Composition in Rats." *Growth* 48 (1984): 415–424.

"...the waist and stomach areas." Bouchard, C. "The Response to Long-Term Overfeeding in Identical Twins." *New England Journal of Medicine* 322 (1990): 1477–1482.

"...mental and physical fatigue." Wurtman, J. J. *Managing Your Mind and Mood through Food* (New York: HarperCollins, 1987).

Page 34 " 'This may be a contributor...' says Dr. Barnard." Barnard, N. *Food for Life* (New York: Harmony Books, 1993): 129.

Page 35 "...heart disease, for instance." Ornish, D. *Dr. Dean Ornish's Pro-*

gram for Reversing Heart Disease (New York: Random House, 1990): 25.

" . . . diets that were 40 percent fat." W. C. Willet et al. "Dietary Fat and Fiber in Relation to Risk of Breast Cancer: An 8-Year Follow-Up." *Journal of the American Medical Association* 268 (1992): 2037–2044.

" . . . the impact of low-fat eating." *Prevention's Stop Dieting and Lose Weight Cookbook* (Emmaus, Pa.: Rodale Press, 1994): x.

Page 36 " . . . 4 to 6 percent of daily calories as fat." Ornish, D. *Eat More, Weigh Less* (New York: HarperCollins, 1993): 20.

" . . . more fat from blood sugar and increase appetite." Astrup, A., and Raben, A. *European Journal of Clinical Nutrition* 32 (1992): 611–620; D. H. Ekwyn et al. *American Journal of Clinical Nutrition* 46 (1979): 1597–1611. Blundell, J. E., and Burley, V. J., in *Progress in Obesity Research*, Y. Oomura et al., eds. (London: John Libbey, 1990): 453–457.

" . . . and the balance monounsaturates." "Are You Eating Right? What 68 Nutrition Experts Really Think about Diet and Health." *Consumer Reports* (Oct. 1992): 644–653; J. Hallfrisch et al. "Modification of the United States' Diet to Effect Changes in Blood Lipids and Lipoprotein Distribution." *Atherosclerosis* 57 (2–3)(Nov. 1985): 179–188; Connor, S. L., and Connor, W. E. *The New American Diet* (New York: Simon & Schuster, 1986); Alabaster, O. *The Power of Prevention* (New York: Fireside, 1985): 87–88, 107.

" . . . important for many people." Willett, W. C. "Diet and Health: What Should We Eat?" *Science* 264 (April 22, 1994): 532–537.

Page 37 " . . . the 'bad' cholesterol) and promoting disease." Willett, W. C. "Diet and Health: What Should We Eat?"

Page 38 " . . . indicator of your ideal weight." Ratto, T. "The New Science of Weight Control." *Medical Self-Care* (March/April 1987): 29.

" . . . allow 'desirable' weights to creep up." J. E. Manson et al. "Body Weight and Longevity." *Journal of the American Medical Association* 257 (3)(Jan. 1987): 353–358.

Page 41 " . . . your body's Fat-Maker Switches." "Fat-Free Foods: Studies Show Calories Do Count." *Environmental Nutrition* 18 (4)(April 1995): 1–6.

" . . . people who restricted fat intake alone." Ibid.: 6.

" 'We're eating fat-free foods' . . . *Pounds*." Horbiah, J. *50 Ways to Lose Ten Pounds* (Lincolnwood, Ill.: Publications International, 1994).

Page 42 " . . . white rice and white flour." Gullo, S., quoted in O'Neill, M. *New York Times* (Feb. 8, 1995): C6.

" . . . compensate by eating more." Rolls, B., quoted in "Fat-Free Foods": 6.

Page 43 " . . . development of breast cancer." Story, J. *Federation Proceedings* 41 (Sept. 1982): 2797. A. Elias et al. *General Pharmacology* 15 (6)(1984): 535; E. Offenbacher, et al. *Diabetes* 29 (11)(Nov. 1980): 919.

Page 44 " . . . linked to gaining body fat." Miller. *Non-Diet Diet*: 75–77.

" 'People simply do not stop' . . . in New York City." Aronne, L., quoted in O'Neill. *New York Times*.

Page 45 " . . . by about 10 percent." J. W. Anderson et al. "Health Benefits and Practical Aspects of High-Fiber Diets." *American Journal of Clinical Nutrition* 59 (Suppl)(1994): 1242S–1247S; W. C. Miller et al. "Dietary Fat, Sugar and Fiber Predict Body Fat Content." *Journal of the American Dietetic Association* 94 (6)(June 1994): 612–615; Miles, C. W., "The Metabolizable Energy of Diets Differing in Dietary Fat and Fiber Measuring in Humans." *Journal of Nutrition* 122 (1992): 306–311.

Page 46 " . . . total fiber per day." Connor and Connor. *New American Diet*: 38; Alabaster. *Power of Prevention*: 127.

" . . . studied insulin for more than 30 years." Reaven, G., quoted in O'Neill. *New York Times*.

Page 47 " . . . insulin resistance and chronic disease." Simopoulos, A. P., quoted in O'Neill. *New York Times*.

" . . . craving fat or refined sugars." Barnard, N. *Food for Life*; Rodin, J. "Comparative Effects of Fructose, Aspartame, Glucose, and Water Preloads on

Calorie and Macronutrient Intake." *American Journal of Clinical Nutrition* 51 (1990): 428–435.

"Here's one more point to remember . . . California." Kenney, J., quoted in "Natural Weight Loss." *Prevention* (Sept. 1992): 52.

Page 48   ". . . as effectively as high-fiber, low-fat foods." J. Blundell et al. "Dietary Fat and the Control of Energy Intake: Evaluating the Effects of Fat on Meal Size and Post-Meal Satiety." *American Journal of Clinical Nutrition* 57 (suppl)(1993): 772S–778S.

Page 49   ". . . even when you sleep." Bailey, C. *Fit or Fat* (Boston: Houghton Mifflin, 1976).

Page 50   "New evidence shows . . . *Association*." Fiatarone et al. "High-Intensity Strength Training in Nonagenarians: Effect on Skeletal Muscle." *Journal of the American Medical Association* 263 (1990): 3029–3034; see also Evans, W., and Rosenberg, I. H. *Biomarkers: The 10 Determinants of Aging You Can Control* (New York: Simon & Schuster, 1991).

". . . on average, 350 extra calories." Mayo Clinic study, in press. "Natural Weight Control." *Prevention* (April 1993): 68.

Page 51   ". . . burn fat by about one-third." Suter, P. M., Schutz, Y., and Jequier, E. "The Effect of Ethanol on Fat Storage in Healthy Subjects." *New England Journal of Medicine* 326 (15)(1992): 983–987.

". . . increase the gain of body fat." J. V. Selby et al. *American Journal of Epidemiology* 1259 (1987): 979–988; Fowman, D. T. *Annals of Clinical Laboratory Science* 18 (1988): 181–189; M. J. Gerald et al. *Diabetes* 26 (1977): 780–785.

". . . come directly from alcohol—but many do." "Natural Weight Control."

Page 52   "But this is not the case, . . . Center." *Nutrition Review* 50 (9)(1994): 267–270; Flatt, J. P., quoted in Berg, F. M. "Alcohol Promotes Fat Storage." *Obesity and Health* 7 (6)(Nov./Dec. 1993): 107–108.

". . . two 48-hour sessions." Flatt, J. P., quoted in Berg. "Alcohol Promotes Fat Storage."

Page 53   ". . . contributes to abdominal fat gain." Suter, P., Schutz, Y., and Jequier, E. "The Effect of Ethanol on Fat Storage."

". . . as did the nondrinkers." *New England Journal of Medicine* 326 (1992): 983–987; *Nutrition Reviews* 50 (9)(1993): 267–270; *Obesity and Health* (Nov./Dec. 1993): 107–108, (Sept./Oct. 1993): 87–89, (Dec. 1989): 89, (June 1989): 41; *American Journal of Public Health* (Nov. 1990).

Page 54   ". . . keep their weight under control." Klesges, R. C., and Schumaker, S. "Understanding the Relations between Smoking and Body Weight and Their Importance to Smoking Cessation and Relapse." *Health Psychology* 11 (suppl)(1992): 1–3; Klesges, R. C. "How Cigarette Smoking and Weight Are Related." *Weight Control Digest* 4 (5)(Sept./Oct. 1994): 361–366.

" ' . . . a large minority of smokers do.' " Klesges. "How Cigarette Smoking and Weight Are Related": 363–366.

". . . increases the formation of body fat." *Lancet* (Oct. 30, 1965).

". . . twice as many smokers as nonsmokers have potbellies." *American Journal of Public Health* (Nov. 1990).

". . . the population's overindulgence in alcohol." *American Journal of Public Health* (Nov. 1990).

Page 55   ". . . to die prematurely of cancer." M. Criqui, et al. *Lancet* (Dec. 1994).

". . . to develop breast cancer." Boffetta, P., and Garfinkel, L. "Alcohol Drinking and Mortality among Men Enrolled in an American Cancer Society Study." *Epidemiology* 1 (5)(1990): 342–348.

". . . the risk for nondrinkers." W. C. Willet et al. "Moderate Alcohol Consumption and the Risk of Breast Cancer." *New England Journal of Medicine* 316 (1987): 1174–1180.

". . . risk of colon or rectal cancer by 78 percent." G. R. Howe et al. "Dietary Factors and Risk of Breast Cancer: Combined Analysis of 12 Case-Controlled Studies." *Journal of the National Cancer Institute* 82 (1990): 561–569.

Page 56 "... your basal (baseline) metabolic rate." *Journal of the National Cancer Institute* 85 (1993): 875.

"... in the evening than during the day." Callaway, C. W., cited in Rodin, J. *Body Traps* (New York: Morrow, 1992): 193.

" ' The truth is, if you eat' ... Association." Harper, P., quoted in "Burn Fat Faster." *Men's Health* (Nov. 1994): 26.

" 'The vast majority of overweight people' ... Center." Kenney, J., quoted in "Natural Weight Control." *Prevention* (July 1994): 133.

Page 57 "... significant benefits in just two weeks." J. A. Jenkins et al. "Nibbling versus Gorging: Metabolic Advantages of Increased Meal Frequency." *New England Journal of Medicine* 321 (14)(1989): 929–934.

"... deposits them in your body's fat cells." P. D. Kern et al. "The Effects of Weight Loss on the Activity and Expression of Adipose-Tissue Lipoprotein Lipase in Very Obese Humans." *New England Journal of Medicine* 322 (15)(1990): 1053–1059.

Page 58 "Water is a medium ... *Fat, Water Retention and You.*" Lindner, P. *Fat, Water Retention and You.* Cited in *Prevention's Lose Weight Guidebook 1992* (Emmaus, Pa.: Rodale Press, 1992): 16.

"... cause fat deposits to increase." Heus, M., Heus, G., and Heus, J. *Low-Fat for Life* (Barneveld, Wis.: Micamar, 1994): 87.

" 'The fatigue, simple headaches,' ... University of California, Davis." Applegate, L. *Power Foods* (Emmaus, Pa.: Rodale Press, 1991): 2.

Page 59 "... eliminate accumulated wastes as well." McArdle, W. D., Katch, F. I., and Katch, V. L. *Exercise Physiology: Energy, Nutrition, and Human Performance* (Philadelphia: Lea & Febiger, 1986): 451; Swarth, J. *Stress and Nutrition* (San Diego: Health Media of America, 1986): 23; Brooks, G. A., and Fahey, T. D. *Exercise Physiology: Human Bioenergetics and Its Applications* (New York: Macmillan, 1985): 462.

Page 60 "... more overweight they are." *International Journal of Obesity* 17 (2)(1993): 69–76.

Page 61 "The unhealthy relationship ... Friedman, M.D." Tucker, Larry, A., and Friedman, Glenn M., cited in *Prevention's Lose Weight Guidebook 1993* (Emmaus, Pa.: Rodale Press, 1993): 151–152.

Page 62 "... twice as likely to be obese." Tucker, Larry, A., and Bagwell, Marilyn, cited in *Prevention's Lose Weight Guidebook 1993* (Emmaus, Pa.: Rodale Press, 1993): 152.

"... extra snacking into account." *Prevention's Lose Weight Guidebook 1993* (Emmaus, Pa.: Rodale Press, 1993): 153.

"... to prop yourself up." Barnard, N. *Food for Life.*

Page 63 "... deprived of good-quality sleep." "Overeating? Get Some Sleep?" *Tufts University Diet and Nutrition Letter* 12 (9)(Nov. 1994): 1–2.

"... poorer-quality sleep—than ever before." Bliwise, D., quoted in "Overeating?"

"Research has shown ... University of Chicago." Rechtschaffen, A., quoted in "Overeating?"

Page 64 "... increased body fat, researchers have found." Ghinassi, F. "Coping with Stress and Eating." *Weight Control Digest* 4 (2)(March/April 1994): 335–338.

"... foods high in fat and refined sugar" Rookus, M. A. "Changes in Body Mass Index in Young Adults in Relation to Number of Life Events Experienced." *International Journal of Obesity* 12 (1988): 29–39.

"... a great deal of added body fat." Sternberg, B. "Relapse in Weight Control: Definitions, Processes, and Prevention Strategies." In Marlatt, G. A., and Gordon, J. R., eds. *Relapse Prevention: Maintenance Strategies in the Treatment of Addictive Behaviors* (New York: Guilford Press, 1985): 521–545. B. Linde et al. *American Journal of Physiology* 256 (1989): E12–E18.

"... storing more body fat." Mirkin, G. *Getting Thin* (Boston: Little, Brown, 1983): 62–63, 84–85.

"... your sense of calmness and control." See for example: Hendler, S. S. *The*

Oxygen Breakthrough (New York: Pocket Books, 1991); Nathan, R. G., Staats, T. E., and Rosch, P. J. *The Doctors' Book of Instant Stress Relief* (New York: Ballantine, 1989); and Fried, R. *The Breath Connection* (New York: Plenum, 1991).

Chapter 4

Page 70   "...fat-burning metabolism and energy." Hager, D. L. "Why Breakfast Is Important." *Weight Control Digest* 3 (1)(Jan./Feb. 1993): 225–226.

"...when you turn it on." Stamford, B. A., and Shimer, P. *Fitness without Exercise* (New York: Warner, 1990); Zak, V., Carlin, C., and Vash, P. D. *The Fat-to-Muscle Diet* (New York: Berkley, 1988): 30; Natow, A. B., and Heslin, J. *The Fat Attack Plan* (New York: Pocket Books, 1990): 42, 165.

"...fat-storing processes instead." Zak, Carlin, and Vash. *Fat-to-Muscle Diet.*

"...biological rhythms into higher revs." Ibid.

Page 71   " 'It's calorie-burning'...Center." Zak, Carlin, and Vash. *Fat-to-Muscle Diet.*

"...from 7,000 to 12,000 lux." C. H. Czeisler et al. "Bright Light Induction of Strong (Type O) Resetting of the Human Circadian Pacemaker." *Science* 244 (June 16, 1989): 1328–1333; C. H. Czeisler et al. "Human Sleep: Its Duration and Organization Depend on Its Circadian Phase." *Science* 210 (Dec. 12, 1980); Kronauer, R., and Czeisler, C. H., quoted in "Jet Lag Breakthrough." *Condé Nast's Traveler* (Sept. 1989): 35–36.

Page 72   "...more energy and higher metabolism." Lamberg, L. *Bodyrhythms: Chronobiology and Peak Performance* (New York: Morrow, 1994): 42.

"...increase your morning metabolism." Zak, Carlin, and Vash. *Fat-to-Muscle Diet*; Stamford and Shimer. *Fitness without Exercise*: 41, 44.

"...the exercise habit one year later." *Prevention's Lose Weight Guidebook 1992* (Emmaus, Pa.: Rodale Press, 1992): 142.

Page 73   "...more likely to be fat than glycogen." Sheats, C. *Lean Bodies* (Dallas: Summit Group, 1992): 25.

"...the calories they burn come from fat." Wilcox, A., cited in "Fat Burns as Sun Rises." *Prevention* (Oct. 1986): 67.

Page 74   "Enjoy a Great-Tasting, Low-Fat Breakfast" D. G. Schlundt et al. "The Role of Breakfast in the Treatment of Obesity." *American Journal of Clinical Nutrition* 55 (1992): 645–651; *Obesity and Health* 6 (12)(Nov./Dec. 1992): 103.

" 'Most times you lose control.' " Stone, K. *Snack Attack* (New York: Warner, 1991): 33, 87.

Page 75   " 'When you wake up'...the researchers say." Zak, Carlin, and Vash. *Fat-to-Muscle Diet.*

"In addition, 'you will be hungry'...Minnesota." Callaway, C. W. *The Callaway Diet* (New York: Bantam, 1991): 192.

Page 76   "...that prime you for an active day." Lamberg, L. *Bodyrhythms*; *Prevention's Lose Weight Guidebook 1993* (Emmaus, Pa.: Rodale Press, 1993): 148.

"...the fat-burning rate for the whole day." D. A. Jenkins et al. *American Journal of Clinical Nutrition* 35 (1982): 1339–1346.

Page 78   "...double what they are after lunch." J. E. Nester et al. *Diabetes Care* 11 (1988): 755–760.

Chapter 5

Page 79   "...overeat, especially at night." Lamb, L. E. *The Weighting Game: The Truth about Weight Control* (New York: Lyle Stuart, 1988). "There are millions of people in the United States who are suffering from undernutrition—a simple lack of calories because they have been on unwise diets...," says Dr. Lamb, cardiologist and medical consultant to the President's Council on Physical Fitness and Sports. "As metabolism slows, there is less demand for oxygen. [And] fatigue is the single most commonly experienced symptom by individuals on a diet overly restricted in calories."

"So instead of stuffing . . . *Nutrition*." D. A. Jenkins et al. "Nibbling versus Gorging: Metabolic Advantages of Increased Meal Frequency." *New England Journal of Medicine* 321 (4)(Oct. 5, 1989): 929–934. Jones, P. J., Leitch, C. A., and Pederson, R. A. "Meal-Frequency Effects on Plasma Hormone Concentrations and Cholesterol Synthesis in Humans." *American Journal of Clinical Nutrition* 57 (6)(1993): 868–874; S. L. Edelstein et al. "Increased Meal Frequency Associated with Decreased Cholesterol Concentrations." *American Journal of Clinical Nutrition* 55 (1992): 664–669.

Page 80 " . . . more food during the day." Edelstein et al. "Increased Meal Frequency."

" . . . conversion of sugar to body fat." Mirkin, G. *Getting Thin* (Boston: Little, Brown, 1983): 62–65, 195; Darden, E. *A Day-by-Day 10-Step Program* (Dallas: Taylor, 1992): 26.

" . . . smaller, healthier insulin response." Miller, W. C. *The Non-Diet Diet* (Englewood, Colo.: Morton, 1991): 88.

Page 81 "Adults make an average . . . Boston." Blackburn, G. L., cited in *Environmental Nutrition* 16 (2)(Feb. 1993): 1.

Page 82 " ' . . . by the time you eat dinner.' " Podell, R. N. *The G-Index Diet* (New York: Warner, 1993): 262.

" . . . high-fat, high-sugar foods." Leibowitz, S. F. quoted in Marano, H. E. "Chemistry and Craving." *Psychology Today* (Jan./Feb. 1993): 30–36, 74.

" . . . more fat late at night." Marano. "Chemistry and Craving."

"And 'it's when you make changes' . . . California." Hanson, D., quoted in "Natural Weight Loss." *Prevention* (Jan. 1994): 121.

Page 83 " . . . a Fat-Maker Switch by mistake." *Obesity and Health* 3 (2)(Feb. 1989): 4; Brandon, J. E. *Health Values* (May/June 1987).

Page 84 " . . . the body responds in a similar way." Blundell, J. E., and Hill, A. J. "Paradoxical Effects of an Intense Sweetener (Aspartame) on Appetite." *Lancet* (May 10, 1986): 1092–1093; Brala, P. M., and Hagen, R. L. "Effects of Sweetness Perception and Caloric Value of a Preload on Short-Term Intake." *Physiology and Behavior* 30 (1983): 1–9; Porikos, K. P., and Friedman, M. I. "Drinking Saccharin Increases Food Intake and Preference." *Appetite* 12 (1989): 1–10.

" . . . turn the ingested fuel into fat." D. G. Bruce et al. "Cephalic Phase Metabolic Responses in Normal Weight Adults." *Metabolism* 36 (1987): 721–725; Geiselman, P. J. "Sugar-Induced Hyperphagia: Is Hyperinsulinemia, Hypoglycemia, or Any Other Factor a 'Necessary' Condition?" *Appetite* 11 (Suppl)(1988): 26–34; Rodin, J. "Insulin Levels, Hunger, and Food Intake: An Example of Feedback Loops in Body Weight Control." *Health Psychology* 4 (1985): 1–24; J. Rodin et al. "Effect of Insulin and Glucose on Feeding Behavior." *Metabolism* 34 (1985): 826–831; C. Simon et al. "Cephalic Phase Insulin Secretion in Relation to Food Presentation in Normal and Overweight Subjects." *Physiology and Behavior* 36 (1986): 465–469; Porikos and Friedman. "Drinking Saccharin"; VanderWeele, D. A. "Hyperinsulinism and Feeding: Not All Sequences Lead to the Same Behavioral Outcome or Conclusions." *Appetite* 6 (1985): 47–52; Vasselli, J. R. "Carbohydrate Ingestion, Hypoglycemia, and Obesity." *Appetite* 6 (1985): 53–59.

" ' . . . for fats in some people.' " Callaway, C. W. *The Callaway Diet* (New York: Bantam, 1991): 194.

" . . . need to be weighed, too." Blundell, J. E., and Hill, A. J. "Paradoxical Effects"; Blundell, J. E., and Hill, A. J. "Artificial Sweeteners and the Control of Appetite." In D. Worden et al., eds. *The Future of Predictive Evaluation* vol. 2 (Lancaster: MTP Press, 1987): 263–282; Brala, P. M., and Hagen, R. L. "Effects of Sweetness Perception"; Rolls, B. J., Hetherington, M. and Laster, L. J. "Comparison of the Effects of Aspartame and Sucrose on Appetite and Food Intake." *Appetite* 11 (1988): 62–67; Porikos, K. P., Booth, G., and Van Itallie,

T. B. "Effect of a Covert Nutritive Dilution on the Spontaneous Food Intake of Obese Individuals." *American Journal of Clinical Nutrition* 30 (1977): 1638–1644; T. B. Van Itallie et al. "Use of Aspartame to Test the 'Body Weight Set Point' Hypothesis." *Appetite* 11 (1988): 68–72.

" '...no miracle cure from artificial sweeteners.' " Barnard. *Food for Life*: 109.

"...fat-forming processes into overdrive." Hallfrisch, J. "Metabolic Effects of Dietary Fructose." *Federation of American Societies for Experimental Biology Journal* 4 (1990): 2652; Roongpisuthpong, C. *Diabetes Research and Clinical Practice* 14 (1991): 123.

Page 85 " 'Guard against generation of'... Center." Vash, P. D. "Outsmarting the Fat Cell." *Shape* (March 1987): 72–74.

" '...stuffs these fats into fat cells.' " McDougall, J. A. *The McDougall Program for Maximum Weight Loss* (New York: Dutton, 1994): 64.

"...reinforce your taste for sweet foods." Ornish, D. *Eat More, Weigh Less* (New York: HarperCollins, 1993): 43.

" 'Artificial sweeteners may impede'... Dr. McDougall." McDougall. *The McDougall Program*: 73.

Page 86 " '...help you break the habit.' " Barnard, N. *Food for Life* (New York: Harmony Books, 1993): 107–108.

"Eating smaller, nutritious meals... Rossi, Ph.D." Rossi, E. L., with Nimmons, D. *The 20-Minute Break* (Los Angeles: Jeremy Tarcher, 1991): 122–123.

Page 90 " '   energy reserves are restored.' " Ibid.

Chapter 6

Page 92 "...exercise or hard physical labor." McArdle, W. D., Katch, F. I., and Katch, V. L. *Exercise Physiology: Energy, Nutrition, and Human Performance* (Philadelphia: Lea & Febiger, 1986): 451.

Page 93 " 'Drinking generous amounts of water'... Boston." Blackburn, G. L., quoted in *Prevention* (Sept. 1992): 50.

"...successful, lasting weight loss." Miller, W. C. *The Non-Diet Diet* (Englewood, Colo.: Morton, 1993): 83–84.

" '...to warm it to core body temperature," Darden, E. *A Day-by-Day 10-Step Program* (Dallas: Taylor, 1992): 43.

Page 94 " '...metabolizing stored fat into usable energy—is minimized.' " Ibid.: 11.

" 'Because a deficiency of water'... *Brain Power*." Mark, V. H. *Brain Power: A Neurosurgeon's Complete Program to Maintain and Enhance Brain Fitness throughout Your Life* (New York: Houghton Mifflin, 1989).

"...helping to decrease fatigue." McArdle, Katch, and Katch. *Exercise Physiology*; Hanson, P. G. *The Joy of Stress* (Kansas City: Andrews, McMeel & Parker, 1987): 27.

Page 95 "...withdraw from the caffeine on Saturday and Sunday." R. Griffiths et al. *New England Journal of Medicine* (Oct. 15, 1992).

"...caffeine may increase metabolism." A. G. Dulloo et al. "Normal Caffeine Consumption: Influence on Thermogenesis and Daily Energy Expenditure in Lean and Postobese Human Volunteers." *American Journal of Clinical Nutrition* 49 (1)(1989): 44–50.

" '...whatever food they eat.' " Rodin, J. *Body Traps* (New York: Morrow, 1992): 194.

Page 96 "...which is table sugar)." Miller. *The Non-Diet Diet*: 75–77.

"...can contribute to obesity." Ibid.: 92.

Chapter 7

Page 100 " 'Any activity that increases'... Dr. Blair." Blair, S. N. *Living with Exercise* (Dallas: LEARN Education Center, 1991): 18.

References

Page 102 " . . . neutralize natural cravings for high-fat foods." Grilo, C. M., Wilfley, D. E., and Brownell, K. D. "Physical Activity and Weight Control: Why Is the Link So Strong?" *Weight Control Digest* 2 (3)(May/June 1992): 153–160; Grilo, C. M., Brownell, K. D., and Stunkard, A. J. "The Metabolic and Psychological Importance of Exercise in Weight Control." In Stunkard, A. J., and Walden, T. A., eds. *Obesity: Theory and Therapy* (New York: Raven Press, 1992); Piscatella, J. C. *Controlling Your Fat Tooth* (New York: Workman, 1991): 100–104. Various studies cited in Piscatella. *Controlling Your Fat Tooth*: 101.

" 'Research is even showing' . . . California." Hanson, D., quoted in "Natural Weight Control." *Prevention* (Jan. 1994): 114.

" ' . . . we feel depressed and anxious.' " Johnsgard, K., quoted in *Prevention's Lose Weight Guidebook 1994* (Emmaus, Pa.: Rodale Press, 1994): 19–20.

Page 103 " 'A staggering quarter of a million deaths' . . . Sports Medicine." "Just Do It, Even If It's Just a Little." *Tufts University Diet and Nutrition Letter* 11 (8)(Oct. 1993): 1.

" . . . maintaining weight-loss success." Grilo, Wifley, and Brownell. "Physical Activity and Weight Control." K. N. Pavlou et al. "Exercise as an Adjunct to Weight Loss and Maintenance in Moderately Obese Subjects." *American Journal of Clinical Nutrition* 49 (1989): 1115–1123; S. Kayman. "Maintenance and Relapse after Weight Loss in Women: Behavioral Aspects." *American Journal of Clinical Nutrition* 52 (1990); 800–807.

" . . . higher, undesired weights after dieting." Kayman et al. "Maintenance and Relapse after Weight Loss in Women."

" . . . cravings for high-fat food." Piscatella. *Controlling Your Fat Tooth*.

" . . . helps reduce excess body fat." *International Journal of Obesity* 13 (1989): 4.

" . . . tend to outlive inactive people." "Just Do It."

" . . . little progress is being made." *Obesity and Health* 8 (1)(Jan./Feb. 1994): 7–9.

" . . . quit during the first year." *Physician and Sports Medicine* 14 (11)(1986): 24. Miller, W. C. "Exercise: Americans Don't Think It's Worth It!" *Obesity and Health* 8 (2)(March/April 1994): 29, 38.

" . . . becomes less active with each passing year." Piscopo, J. *Fitness and Aging* (New York: Wiley, 1985).

" . . . after every set of active minutes." *Weight Control Digest* 3 (4)(July/Aug. 1993): 276.

Page 104 "Middle-age Americans . . . Boston." Blackburn, G. L., quoted in Helmich, N. *USA Today* (March 30, 1992).

" . . . to handle everday stress." Dienstbier, R. "Arousal and Physiological Toughness: Implications for Mental and Physical Health." *Psychological Bulletin* 96 (10)(1989): 84–100; "The Toughness Response." *Advances* 7 (1)(1990): 6–7.

" . . . stressful situations and daily hassles." Bartlett, S. J. "Exercise, Stress Reduction, and Overweight." *Weight Control Digest* 4 (3)(May/June 1994): 353–355.

" . . . increase your energy and alertness." Moore-Ede, M. *The Twenty-Four-Hour Society* (Reading, Mass.: Addison-Wesley, 1993): 55–56.

Page 105 "You can lose a pound . . . Blacksburg." Walberg-Rankin, J., quoted in *Men's Health* (Jan./Feb. 1994): 83.

" . . . helps you fight fat." Blair, S., quoted in "Natural Weight Control." *Prevention* (Jan. 1993): 38.

Page 106 " ' . . . little measurable cardiovascular improvement.' " Duncan, J., quoted in *Prevention's Lose Weight Guidebook 1994* (Emmaus, Pa.: Rodale Press, 1994): 3.

"When both parents are active, . . . and Obesity." National Institutes of Health Conference on Physical Activity and Obesity, (Dec. 1992). Reported in *Obesity and Health* 8 (1)(Jan./Feb. 1994): 10.

References

Page 107 " 'These little motions' . . . Michigan.' " Kuntzleman, C., quoted in "Natural Weight Loss." *Prevention* (March 1994): 73.

Page 108 " . . . body fat for storage." Marano, H. E. "Chemistry and Craving." *Psychology Today* (Jan./Feb. 1993): 30–36, 74.

" . . . do it with the TV on." Myers, D. G. *The Pursuit of Happiness* (New York, Morrow, 1992): 76, 77–79, 206–207.

Page 109 " . . . digestive processes are still going on." Stamford, B. "Meals and the Timing of Exercise." *Physician and Sports Medicine* 17 (11)(Nov. 1989): 151. Stamford, B. A., and Shimer, P. *Fitness without Exercise* (New York: Warner, 1990): 44, 128; Stamford, B. "Meals and the Timing of Exercise." J. M. Davis et al. "Weight Control and Calorie Expenditure: Thermogenic Effects of Pre-Prandial and Post-Prandial Exercise." *Addictive Behavior* 14 (3)(1989): 347–351; Poehlman, E. T., and Horton, E. S. "The Impact of Food Intake and Exercise on Energy Expenditure." *Nutrition Reviews* 47 (5)(May 1989): 129–137.

"By 'pulling oxygen into the body' . . . Kentucky." Stamford and Shimer. *Fitness without Exercise*: 44.

" . . . raising energy levels and lowering tension." Thayer, R. E. "Energy, Tiredness, and Tension Effects of a Sugar Snack versus Moderate Exercise." *Journal of Personality and Social Psychology* 52 (1987): 119–125.

Page 110 " . . . gained more productive hours in a day." "Natural Weight Control." *Prevention* (June 1993): 50.

" . . . a conditioned person's heart." McArdle, W. D., Katch, F. I., and Katch, V. I. *Exercise Physiology: Energy, Nutrition, and Human Performance* (Philadelphia: Lea & Febiger, 1986).

Page 111 " . . . assessed over a 20-year period." Cooper, K. H. Personal communications (Aug. 21, 1986; May 15, 1988; January 25, 1994).

Page 113 " . . . increase aerobic activities." Cooper, K. H. *The Aerobics Way* (New York: Bantam, 1977): 44.

" . . . risk of developing atherosclerosis." Cooper, K. H. *The Aerobics Program for Total Well-Being* (New York: Bantam, 1988): 113.

" . . . hungry long after the meal is over." Grilo, C. M., Wilfley, D. E., and Brownell, K. D. "Physical Activity and Weight Control: Why Is the Link So Strong?" *Weight Control Digest* 2 (3)(May/June 1992): 153–160; Grilo, C. M., Brownell, K. D., and Stunkard, A. J. "The Metabolic and Psychological Importance of Exercise in Weight Control." In Stunkard, A. J., and Walden, T. A., eds. *Obesity: Theory and Therapy* (New York: Raven Press, 1992); Piscatella *Controlling Your Fat Tooth*: 100–104. Stephens, T. "Physical Activity and Mental Health in the United States and Canada: Evidence from Four Population Surveys." *Preventive Medicine* 17 (1988): 35–47; Hogan, J. "Personality Correlates of Physical Fitness." *Journal of Personality and Social Psychology* 56 (1989): 284–288; Tucker, L. A. "Physical Fitness and Psychological Disorders." *International Journal of Sport Psychology* 21 (1990): 185–201.

Page 114 " . . . for more than ten hours." J. M. Davis et al. "Weight Control and Calorie Expenditure"; Gleeson, M. "Effects of Physical Exercise on Metabolic Rate and Dietary Induced Thermogenesis." *British Journal of Nutrition* 47 (1982): 173; R. Bielinski et al. "Energy Metabolism during the Postexercise Recovery in Man." *American Journal of Clinical Nutrition* 42 (1985): 69–82.

Page 115 " . . . a moderate exercise routine." U.S. Department of Health and Human Services, Public Health Service. *Exercise and Your Heart*. Pub. No. 83–1677 (Washington, D.C.: National Institutes of Health, 1981).

" ' . . . wish to seek medical advice.' " Hage, P. "Exercise Guidelines: Which to Believe?" *Physician and Sports Medicine* 10 (1982): 23.

" ' . . . unusual signs or symptoms,' the ACSM advises." American College of Sports Medicine. *Guidelines for Graded Exercise Testing Prescription*, 4th ed. (Philadelphia: Lea & Febiger, 1991).

" . . . cause injuries to your joints." Yessis, M. *Secrets of Soviet Sports Fitness and Training* (New York: M. Evans, 1987): 71–78; Lawrence, R. M., and Rosenzweig, S. *Going the Distance* (Los Angeles: Jeremy Tarcher, 1987):

26–27; Shellock, F. G. "Physiological Benefits of Warm-Up." *Physician and Sports Medicine* 11 (10)(Oct. 1983): 134–139; Shyne, K. "To Stretch or Not to Stretch?" *Physician and Sports Medicine* 10 (9)(Sept. 1982): 137–140.

"...such as the thighs." Sharkey, B. J. *New Dimensions in Aerobic Fitness* (Champaign, Ill.: Human Kinetics, 1991): 25–26.

Page 116 "...the lower end of this range." Bailey, C., and Bishop, L. *The Fit or Fat Woman* (Boston: Houghton Mifflin, 1989): 44–45.

Page 118 " '...take pressure off yourself,' he concluded." France, K. "Competitive versus Non-Competitive Thinking during Exercise: Effects on Norepinephrine Levels." Paper presented at the annual meeting of the American Psychology Association, Toronto, Canada (Aug. 1984).

" 'One of the jobs of adrenaline'...Dr. Stamford." Stamford, B., quoted in "Natural Weight Loss." *Prevention* (May 1992): 35.

" '...stores of fat in the abdominal area.' " Ibid.

Chapter 8

Page 121 "Studies point to the conclusion...work productivity." Grandjean, E. *Fitting the Task*, rev. ed. (New York: Taylor & Francis, 1988).

Page 122 " '...away from the brain.' " Wurtman, J. J., quoted in "Peak Performance Brain Food." *Omni* 2 (6)(April 1988): 67.

"...the pro-fat hormone estrogen." E. K. Hamalainen et al. *Journal of Steroid Biochemistry* 20 (1984): 459–464; Goldin, B. R., and Gorbach, S. L. *American Journal of Clinical Nutrition* 48 (1988): 787–790.

Page 123 "To an astonishing extent, ...Ontario." Weingarten, H., quoted in Goldberg, J. "The Taste of Desire." *American Health* (Oct. 1990): 52.

" 'That isn't the choice at all.' " Ornish, D., quoted in *Newsweek* (May 27, 1991): 53.

Page 124 "...aggressiveness in normal, healthy people." Spring. "Carbohydrates: Methodological Review."

"...with either protein-rich or carbohydrate-rich foods." Wurtman, J. J. *Managing Your Mind and Mood through Food* (New York: HarperCollins, 1987): 27.

Page 125 " '...the arrow is pointing toward storage,' says Dr. Stamford." Stamford, B., quoted in "Natural Weight Loss." *Prevention* (May 1992): 105.

Page 127 "It accounts for almost 10 percent...Service." "Nutrition Flash!" *Self* (Sept. 1992): 76.

Page 128 "These spices may help...studies." Schiffman, S. "The Use of Flavor to Enhance the Efficacy of Reducing Diets." *Hospital Practice* 21 (7)(1986): 44H–44R; Quebec studies cited in *Prevention's Lose Weight Guidebook 1992* (Emmaus, Pa.: Rodale Press, 1992): 64; Henry, C. J. K., and Emergy, B. "Effect of Spiced Food on Metabolic Rate." *Human Nutrition: Clinical Nutrition* 40C (1986): 165–168.

Chapter 9

Page 132 "...metabolize fats more slowly than others." Elias, M. "Hostility, Anxiety May Hold Key to Heart Attack." *USA Today* (April 15, 1994).

" '...high anger levels just doesn't work,' she notes." Stoney, C., quoted in Elias. "Hostility, Anxiety May Hold Key to Heart Attack."

" '...whatever situation you're in.' " Williams, R., quoted in "Natural Weight Control." *Prevention* (July 1994): 134.

Page 133 "These chemicals in turn...Maryland." Leathwood, P., and Pollet, P. "Diet-Induced Mood Changes in Normal Populations." *Journal of Psychiatric Research* 17 (1983): 147–15; H. Lieberman, et al. "The Behavioral Effects of Food Constituents: Strategies Used in Studies of Amino Acids, Protein, Carbohydrates and Caffeine." *Nutrition Reviews* (Suppl)(May 1986): 61–69; H. Lieberman et al. "Mood, Performance and Sensitivity: Changes Induced by Food Constituents." *Journal of Psychiatric Research* 17 (1984): 135–145;

Spring, B. "Effects of Foods and Nutrients on the Behavior of Normal Individuals." In Wurtman, J. J., and Wurtman, R. J., eds. *Nutrition and the Brain*, Vol. 7 (New York: Raven Press, 1986): 1–47; Christensen, L. "Impact of Dietary Change on Emotional Distress." *Journal of Abnormal Psychology* 94 (1985): 565–579; Wurtman and Wurtman. *Nutrition and the Brain*.

" . . . more cortisol than those with less fat there." Rebuffe-Scrive, M., quoted in *Prevention* (July 1994): 136.

" . . . than their nonstressed counterparts." *International Journal of Obesity* 17 (1993): 597–604.

" . . . plays a role in abdominal fat distribution." Berg, F. S. "Risks Focus on Visceral Obesity, May Be Stress Linked." *Obesity and Health* 7 (5)(Sept./Oct. 1993): 87–89.

Page 134 " . . . wandering off to your abdomen for storage." *Obesity Research* 1 (3)(1993): 206–222.

" . . . including slower fat-burning." B. Linde et al. *American Journal of Physiology* 256 (1989): E12–E18.

" . . . keep cortisol levels down." *Prevention* (July 1994).

" . . . lead to major, lasting changes." Prochaska, J. O., Norcross, J. C., and DiClemente, C. C. *Changing for Good* (New York: Morrow, 1994).

" ' . . . accumulating and overwhelming you.' " Nathan, R. G., Staats, T. E., and Rosch, P. J., *The Doctors' Guide to Instant Stress Relief* (New York: Ballantine, 1989): xxiii, 4.

" 'Whether it's meditation' . . . Boston." Benson, H., quoted in *Prevention* (July 1994): 136.

Page 135 " . . . successful, lasting weight loss and good lifelong health." Council on Scientific Affairs, American Medical Association. "Treatment of Obesity in Adults." *Journal of the American Medical Association* 260 (17)(1988): 2547–2551. Rock, C. L., and Coulston, A. M. "Weight Control Approaches: A Review by the California Dietetic Association." *Journal of the American Dietetic Association* 88 (1988): 44–48. R. R. Weinsier et al. "Recommended Therapeutic Guidelines for Professional Weight Control Programs." *American Journal of Clinical Nutrition* 40 (1984): 865–872.

" . . . a general loss of control." "Breathing Linked to Personality." *Psychology Today* (July 1983): 109; Teich, M., and Dodelcs, G. "Mind Control: How to Get It, How to Use It, How to Keep It." *Omni* (Oct. 1987): 53–60.

Page 136 " ' . . . can do to improve your life.' " Hendler, S. S. *The Oxygen Breakthrough* (New York: Simon & Schuster, 1989): 7, 8, 94.

" . . . with optimal levels of oxygen." Winter, A., and Winter, R. *Build Your Brain Power* (New York: St. Martin's Press, 1986): 70.

" . . . lost elasticity of lung tissue." Kannel, W. B., quoted in Maleskey, G. "What It Means When You're Short of Breath." *Prevention* (Dec. 1985): 75.

" . . . 4 liters of oxygen per minute." Winter and Winter. *Build Your Brain Power*: 65.

Page 137 " . . . energy production in the body." Hendler. *Oxygen Breakthrough*.

" . . . one quart a minute." Funk, E. "Avoiding Altitude Sickness." *Summit County Journal* (Breckenridge, Colo.: 1978): 7.

" . . . accomplish the same work." Asimov, I. *Isaac Asimov on the Human Body and the Human Brain* (New York: Bonanza Books, 1984): 236.

Page 139 " . . . power of the word becomes stronger." Nathan, Staats, and Rosch, P. J., *The Doctors' Guide*: 56–58.

" . . . to whatever situation arises." Mark, V. H., and Mark, J. P. *Brain Power: A Neurosurgeon's Complete Program to Maintain and Enhance Brain Fitness throughout Your Life* (Boston: Houghton Mifflin, 1989); Mark, V. H., and Mark, J. P. *Reversing Memory Loss* (Boston: Houghton Mifflin, 1991).

" . . . and around your eyes." Stroebel, C. H. *QR: The Quieting Reflex* (New York: Berkley Books, 1987).

Page 140 " 'Changing your thoughts' . . . Harvard Medical School." Ghinassi, F. "Coping with Stress and Eating." *Weight Control Digest* 4 (2)(March/April 1994): 335–338.

Page 141 "...you handle everyday stress." Bartlett, S. J. "Exercise, Stress Reduction and Overweight." *Weight Control Digest* 4 (3)(May/June 1994). 353–355.

"...boost of mental and physical energy." Emery, G. *Rapid Relief from Emotional Distress* (New York: Ballantine, 1988); Moore-Ede, M. *The Twenty-Four-Hour Society* (Reading, Mass.: Addison-Wesley, 1993); Lamberg, L. *Bodyrhythms: Chronobiology and Peak Performance* (New York: Morrow, 1994).

" 'Exercise has a powerful impact'...New York." Motta, R., quoted in *Prevention's Lose Weight Guidebook 1994* (Emmaus, Pa.: Rodale Press, 1994): 9.

"...and improves stress control." Daniel, M. "Opiate Receptor Blockade by Naltrexone and Mood State after Physical Activity." *British Journal of Sports Medicine* 26 (1992): 111; Raglin, J. "Exercise and Mental Health." *Sports Medicine* 9 (1990): 323.

"...over a one-year period." King, A. C., Taylor, C. B., and Haskell, W. L. "Effects of Differing Intensities and Formats of 12 Months of Exercise Training on Psychological Outcomes in Older Adults." *Health Psychology* 12 (1993): 292–300.

Page 142 " '...to produce higher levels of cortisol.' " Dienstbier, R. "Arousal and Physiological Toughness: Implications for Mental and Physical Health." *Psychological Bulletin* 96 (10)(1989): 84–100; "The Toughness Response." *Advances* 7 (1)(1990): 6–7.

" '...and marital happiness,' they observe." Notarius, C., and Markman, H. *We Can Work It Out: Making Sense Out of Marital Conflict* (New York: Putnam, 1993): 29.

Page 143 "For a variation,...Pennsylvania." Seligman, M. E. P. *What You Can Change and What You Can't* (New York: Knopf, 1993): 132.

Page 144 " '...gained 15 pounds of fat' " Westcott, W., quoted in "Natural Weight Control." *Prevention* (June 1994): 60.

Page 145 "...muscle, fat, bone and related tissues." National Institutes of Health report. Cited in Hellmich, N. "Most Battle the Bulge without a Strategy." *USA Today* (March 30, 1992).

"...or even every week." "Swear Off the Scales for Good and Still Lose." *Environmental Nutrition* 16 (11)(Nov. 1993): 3.

" 'The focus should be on healthy'...*Living without Dieting*." Foreyt, J., quoted in Fletcher, A. M. *Thin for Life* (Shelburne, Vt.: Chapters, 1994): 56.

Page 146 "...late-night standby—milk and cookies." Simonson, M., quoted in "Natural Weight Loss." *Prevention* (Sept. 1992): 58.

" '...or because I'm upset?' " :41. Ibid.

"Watching television for long periods...Maryland." *Prevention's Lose Weight Guidebook 1993* (Emmaus, Pa.: Rodale Press, 1993): 155.

"...16 percent below resting levels." "Television Trance Slows Metabolism." *Environmental Nutrition* 15 (6)(June 1992): 1; Klesges, R. C. Report to the Society of Behavioral Medicine.

Page 147 " '...it is absolutely critical.' " Foreyt, J., quoted in "Natural Weight Loss." *Prevention* (Jan. 1994): 117.

Page 149 "...teachers to students is 18 to 1." Crum, T. F. *The Magic of Conflict* (New York: Simon & Schuster, 1987): 120.

"...to as much as 8 to 1." Ray, M., and Myers, R. *Creativity in Business* (New York: Doubleday, 1986): 48–49.

"...self-sabotaging behavior patterns." King, G. A., Polivy, J., and Herman, P. C. "Cognitive Aspects of Dietary Restraint: Effects on Personal Memory." *International Journal of Eating Disorders* 10 (3)(May 1991): 313–321.

" '...enmesh you in painful emotions.' " Nash, J. D. *Maximize Your Body Potential* (Palo Alto, Calif.: Bull, 1986): 206.

"A sense of failure...Massachusetts." Hutchinson, M. G. *Transforming Body Image* (Trumansburg, N.Y.: Crossing Press, 1985): 35. Heatherton, T. F., Polivy, J., and Herman, C. P. "Dietary Restraint: Some Current Findings and Speculations." *Psychology of Addictive Behaviors* 4 (2)(1990): 100–106; Heatherton, T. F., Polivy, J., and Herman, C. P. "Effects of Distress on Eating:

The Importance of Ego-Involvement." *Journal of Personality and Social Psychology* 62 (5)(May 1992): 801–803.

Page 151 "... back from stressful situations." Ljungdahl, L. "Laugh If This Is a Joke." *New England Journal of Medicne* 261 (1989): 558; K. M. Dillon et al. "Positive Emotional States and Enhancement of the Immune System." *International Journal of Psychiatry in Medicine* 15 (1)(1985–1986): 13–18; P. Eckman et al. "Autonomic Nervous System Activity Distinguishes among Emotions." *Science* 221 (1983): 1208–1210; A. L. S. Berk et al. *Clinical Research* 36 (1988): 121, 435A; A. L. S. Berk et al. *The Federation of American Societies for Experimental Biology Journal* 2 (1988): A1570.

"... and to avoid exercise." Grilo, C. M., and Schiffman, S. "Longitudinal Investigation of the Abstinence Violation Effect in Binge Eaters." *Journal of Consulting and Clinical Psychology* 62 (1994): 611–619. C. M. Grilo et al. "The Social Self, Body Dissatisfaction, and Binge Eating in Obese Females." *Obesity Research* 2 (1994): 24–27.

Page 152 "Ask yourself 'Is it' ... *From Stress to Strength*." Eliot, R. S. *From Stress to Strength* (New York: Bantam, 1994).

"... also shortening your life." Williams, R., and Williams, V. *Anger Kills* (New York: Times Books, 1993).

"... unexpected fatal heart attack." Williams and Williams. *Anger Kills*; Eliot. *From Stress to Strength*; Eliot, R. S., and Breo, D. *Is It Worth Dying For?* (New York: Bantam, 1989); Tavris, C. *Anger: The Misunderstood Emotion* (New York: Simon & Schuster, 1982).

"... certain forms of cancer." M. Watsom et al. *Psychological Medicine* 21 (1991): 51–57; Seligman, M. E. P. *Learned Optimism* (New York: Knopf, 1991): 167–178.

"... can eventually destroy relationships." Williams and Williams. *Anger Kills*.

" 'Besides, laughing burns calories.' " Therrien, M., quoted in *Prevention's Lose Weight Guidebook 1992* (Emmaus, Pa.: Rodale Press, 1992): 125.

"... leaving us feeling more relaxed." Lefcourt, H. M., and Martin, R. A. *Humor and Life Stress* (New York: Springer-Verlag, 1986); A. M. Nezu et al. "Sense of Humor as a Moderator of the Relation between Stressful Events and Psychological Distress: A Prospective Analysis." *Journal of Personality and Social Psychology* 54 (1988): 520–525.

"... and strengthened immune response." Chapman, A., and Foot, H. *Handbook of Humor and Laughter: Theory, Research and Applications* (New York: John Wiley, 1982); K. M. Dillon et al. "Positive Emotional States and Enhancement of the Immune System." *International Journal of Psychiatry in Medicine* 15 (1)(1985–1986): 13–18; "Laughing toward Longevity." *University of California, Berkeley, Wellness Letter* (June 1985): 1; "The Mind Fights Back" *Washington Post*; Brody. "Laughter." *New York Times*.

Chapter 10

Page 156 "... the muscles is reduced metabolism." Lamb, L. E. *The Weighting Game: The Truth about Weight Control* (New York: Lyle Stuart, 1988): 147–148.

"... providing a remarkable metabolic boost." Evans, W., and Rosenberg, I. H. *Biomarkers: The 10 Determinants of Aging You Can Control* (New York: Simon & Schuster, 1991): 44.

" 'To wage war effectively against body fat,' ... Kentucky." Stamford, B. A., and Shimer, P. *Fitness without Exercise* (New York: Warner, 1991): 71.

Page 157 "... even when you sleep." Bailey, C. *Fit or Fat*, rev. ed. (Boston: Houghton Mifflin, 1993).

"... even when you're resting." Evans, W., quoted in "Bodybuilding for the Nineties." *Nutrition Action Health Letter* (June 1992): 1–7.

"... weight machines or body-weight calisthenic exercises." American College of Sports Medicine. *Guidelines for Exercise Testing and Prescription*

4th ed. (Philadelphia: Lea & Febiger, 1991): 112–113.

"Muscle-making resistance exercise . . . University Park." Evans, W., cited in "Fat to Firm at 40-Plus." *Prevention* (Aug. 1994): 59–63, 136.

" . . . stubborn layers of excess body fat." Wilmore, J. H., in "Ask the Expert." *Weight Control Digest* 1 (5)(July/Aug. 1991); Westcott, W. L. "Exercise Sessions Can Make the Difference in Weight Loss." *Perspective* 13 (1987): 42–44; Westcott, W. L. *Strength Fitness*, 3rd ed. (Dubuque, Ia.: W. C. Brown, 1991): 3, 74–75; Westcott, W. L. "Strength Training: How Much Is Enough?" *IDEA Today* (Feb. 1991): 33–35; Westcott, W. L. "The Magic of 'Fast Fitness': They Enjoy It More and Do It Less." *Perspective: The Journal of Professional Directors of YMCAs* (Jan. 1992): 14–16; Wilmore, J. H. "Alterations to Strength, Body Composition and Anthropometric Measurements Consequent to 10-Week Weight Training Program." *Medicine and Science in Sports and Exercise* 6 (1974): 133–138; Westcott, W. L., Toomey, K., and Doherty, A. "Strength Training, Body Composition, and Spot Reducing." (1992).

" 'Our oldest exerciser is 100 years old.' " Evans. "Bodybuilding for the Nineties": 5.

Page 158 "To make a comparison of the two, . . . Sports Medicine." Westcott. "Exercise Sessions"; Westcott. *Strength Fitness*.

" . . . studies reported similar results." Westcott. "Strength Training"; Westcott. "The Magic of 'Fast Fitness'."

" ' . . . as part of a normal human body.' " Drinkwater, B., quoted in Hogan, C. "Strength." *American Health* (Nov. 1988): 55–59.

" . . . levels of 'bad' LDL cholesterol." T. W. Boyden et al. "Resistance Exercise Training Is Associated with Decreases in Serum Low-Density Lipoprotein Cholesterol Levels in Premenopausal Women." *Archives of Internal Medicine* 153 (1)(Jan. 11, 1993): 97–100.

Page 160 " . . . without injury or muscle strain." Evans and Rosenberg. *Biomarkers*: 119.

Page 161 " 'Without the eccentric component' . . . School." Fiatarone, M., quoted in *Prevention* (Feb. 1992): 55.

Page 162 " . . . angle of the pelvis." Cailliet, R. *Understand Your Backache* (Philadelphia: F. A. Davis, 1984): 118–121; Mensendieck, E. M. *Look Better, Feel Better* (New York: Harper & Row, 1954): 48.

" . . . difference in your waistline." F. I. Katch et al. "Effects of Sit-Up Exercise Training on Adipose Tissue Cell Size and Activity." *Research Quarterly for Exercise and Sport* 55 (1984): 242–247; Clark, N. "Sit-Ups Don't Melt Ab Flab." *Runner's World* (March 1985): 32.

" . . . which causes pelvic tilt." Sharkey, B. J. *Physiology of Exercise* (Champaign, Ill.: Human Kinetics, 1984): 336; Cailliet. *Understand Your Backache*: 122–124; Cailliet, R., and Gross, L. *The Rejuvenation Strategy* (Garden City, N.Y.: Doubleday, 1987).

Page 163 "Sometimes called voluntary contractions . . . *Weight Control.*" Lamb. *Weighting Game*: 201.

Page 164 " . . . toning your upper abdominal area." Pirie, L. *Getting Built* (New York: Warner Books, 1984): 146–148.

Page 167 " . . . fitness and good posture." Lagerwerff, E. B., and Perlroth, K. A. *Mensendieck Your Posture and Your Pains* (New York: Anchor/Doubleday, 1973): 148–150; Yessis, M. "Back in Shape." *Sports Fitness* (June 1986): 46, 76; Yessis, M. "The Midsection: Your Essential Link." *Sports Fitness* (April 1985): 91–93; Daniels and Worthingham. *Therapeutic Exercise*: 59.

Page 168 "As you gently lower your legs . . . Los Angeles." Cailliet. *Understand Your Backache*: 116.

" . . . and strengthen your back." Ibid.; Cailliet. *Rejuvenation Strategy*; White, A. A. *Your Aching Back* (New York: Bantam, 1984); Imrie, D., and Barbuto, L. *The Back Power Program* (New York: Wiley, 1990); Swezey, R. L., and Swezey, A. M. *Good News for Bad Backs* (New York: Knightsbridge, 1990).

Page 173 " . . . instead of lifting weights." Evans and Rosenberg. *Biomarkers*: 127.

"Sitting in a normal position, . . . Dr. Stamford." Stamford and Shimer. *Fitness without Exercise*: 88

Chapter 11

Page 183 " . . . the breaking point. " Rossi, L. *The 20-Minute Break* (Los Angeles: Jeremy Tarcher, 1992).

Page 184 " . . . more intense than your evening activities." Mackoff, B. *The Art of Self-Renewal* (Los Angeles: Lowell House, 1992).

Page 186 " . . . the slower rhythms of home." Miller, E. E. *Software for the Mind* (Berkeley, Calif.: Celestial Arts, 1988); Sheikh, A. A., ed. *Imagery: Current Theory, Research, and Application* (New York: Wiley Interscience, 1984); Marks, D. F., ed. *Theories of Image Formation* (New York: Brandon House, 1986); Suinn, R. M. *Seven Steps to Peak Performance* (Lewiston, N.Y.: Hans Huber, 1986).

Page 187 " . . . increased energy and better health." Kaplan, R. "The Role of Nature in the Context of the Workplace." *Landscape and Urban Planning* 26 (1993): 193–201; *Mental Medicine Update* 2 (2)(Fall 1993).

" . . . with extra energy and excitement." Imber-Black, E., and Roberts, J. *Rituals for Our Time* (New York: HarperCollins, 1992); O'Neil, J. R. *The Paradox of Success* (New York: Tarcher/Putnam, 1993).

" . . . when they are primed to fall." "Natural Weight Loss." Moore-Ede, M. *The Twenty-Four-Hour Society* (Reading, Mass.: Addison-Wesley, 1993); Wyman, J. W. *The Light Book* (Los Angeles: Jeremy Tarcher, 1990).

Page 188 " . . . to play a practical joke." deBono, E. *Serious Creativity* (New York: HarperCollins, 1993).

" . . . among 70 percent of them." Ziv, A., and Gadish, O. *Journal of Social Psychology* 129 (1990): 759–768.

Page 189 "Evidence shows that . . . *Last.*" Nagler, W. *The Dirty Half Dozen* (New York: Warner, 1991): 47–48.

" . . . tempt you to eat more." Stone, K. *Snack Attack* (New York: Warner, 1991): 156.

" . . . and total calorie intake." *Prevention* (Sept. 1992): 51.

Chapter 12

Page 191 " . . . other big-time problems." Liebman, B. "The Last Supper?" *Nutrition Action Health Letter* 21 (4)(May 1994): 6–7; American Heart Association's 20th Science Forum. January 17–20, 1993. *Environmental Nutrition* 16 (3)(March 1993): 1.

Page 192 " . . . with more physical activity." "Better to Eat the Main Meal Earlier?" *Tufts University Diet and Nutrition Letter* 11 (4)(June 1993): 1.

Page 193 "The late, heavy meal . . . *Anti-Fat Nutrients.*" Clouatre, D. *The Complete Guide to Anti-Fat Nutrients* (San Francisco: Pax, 1993): 106.

"If you eat a large evening meal . . . research has shown." Lipetz. *Good Calorie Diet* (New York: HarperCollins, 1992): 66; T. M. S. Wolever et al. *American Journal of Clinical Nutrition* 48 (1988): 1041–1047.

" . . . depending on when they ate." Proceedings of the Tenth International Congress on Nutrition.

Page 194 " . . . what we've eaten, according to Dr. Smith." Smith, A. F., cited in DeAngelis, T. "On a Diet? Don't Trust Your Memory." *Psychology Today* (Oct. 1989): 12.

" 'The first and perhaps most important' . . . Yale University." Brownell, K. D. *The LEARN Program for Weight Control* (Dallas: LEARN Education Center, 1991): 15.

" . . . records lost the most weight." K. J. Streit et al. "Food Records: A Predictor and Modifier of Weight Change in a Long-Term Weight Loss Program." *Journal of the American Dietetic Association* 91 (1991): 213–216.

Page 195 "...than bland, boring food." Schiffman, S. "The Use of Flavor to Enhance the Efficacy of Reducing Diets." *Hospital Practice* 21 (7)(1986): 44H–44R.

Page 196 "...digesting, absorbing and utilizing it." Ibid.; *Prevention's Lose Weight Guidebook 1992* (Emmaus, Pa.: Rodale Press, 1992): 64.

"...a fat-burning, metabolism-raising effect." Henry, C. J. K., and Emery, B. "Effect of Spiced Food on Metabolic Rate." *Human Nutrition: Clinical Nutrition* 40C (1986): 165–168.

"...mental and physical fatigue." Wurtman, J. J. *Managing Your Mind and Mood through Food* (New York: HarperCollins, 1987); Chafetz, M. *Smart for Life* (New York: Penguin, 1993); Lamberg, L. *Bodyrhythms: Chronobiology and Peak Performance* (New York: Morrow, 1994).

Page 197 "...sometimes borders on sleepiness." Wurtman. *Managing Your Mind and Mood*; Chafetz. *Smart for Life*; Lamberg. *Bodyrhythms*; Somer, E. *Food and Mood* (New York: Henry Holt, 1995).

"...known as catecholamines." Wurtman. *Managing Your Mind and Mood*; Chafetz. *Smart for Life* Lamberg. *Bodyrhythms*.

"In contrast, 'rock 'n' rollers'...Baltimore." Simonson, M., quoted in *Prevention's Lose Weight Guidebook 1992* (Emmaus, Pa.: Rodale Press, 1992): 133.

Page 198 "...you're likely to consume." *Tufts University Diet and Nutrition Letter* 9 (4)(June 1991): 1–2.

"...the high-decibel hangout." Ferber, C., and Cabanac, M. "Influence of Noise on Gustatory Affective Ratings and Preference for Sweet or Salt." *Appetite* 8 (1987): 229–235; McCarron, A., and Tierney, K. J. "The Effect of Auditory Stimulation on the Consumption of Soft Drinks." *Appetite* 13 (1989): 155–159; T. C. Roballey et al. "The Effect of Music on Eating Behavior." *Bulletin of the Psychonomic Society* 23 (1985): 221–222.

"...stored as body fat." *Prevention's Lose Weight Guidebook 1992* (Emmaus, Pa.: Rodale Press, 1992): 133.

"...continue eating when full." *Health Values* (May/June 1987); "What Is a Slender Eating Style?" *Obesity and Health* 3 (2)(Feb. 1989): 4.

"...slowly and lengthening the meal." Spiegel, T. A., Wadden, T. A., and Foster, G. D. "Objective Measurement of Eating Rate during Behavioral Treatment of Obesity." *Behavior Therapy* 22 (1991): 61–67.

"...enhance the enzyme activity." D. R. Morse et al. "Oral Digestion of a Complex-Carbohydrate Cereal: Effects of Stress and Relaxation on Physiological and Salivary Measures." *American Journal of Clinical Nutrition* 49 (1)(1989): 97–105.

Page 199 "...may be slow, sustained walking." *Prevention* (July 1994).

"...take less of a toll." *Prevention's Lose Weight Guidebook 1993* (Emmaus, Pa.: Rodale Press, 1993): 166.

"Plus, a walk...Minnesota." Hauri, P., and Linde, S. *No More Sleepless Nights* (New York: Wylie, 1992).

"While carbohydrates are the body's fuel...Institute." Duncan, J., quoted in *Prevention* (Aug. 1994): 63.

Page 200 "...exercised before their meal." J. M. Davis et al. "Weight Control and Calorie Expenditure: Thermogenic Effects of Pre-Prandial and Post-Prandial Exercise." *Addictive Behaviors* 14 (1989): 347–351.

"...as much as 50 percent." Clouatre, D. *The Complete Guide to Anti-Fat Nutrients* (San Francisco: Pax, 1993): 107; Davis et al. "Weight Control"; Gleeson, M. "Effects of Physical Exercise on Metabolic Rate and Dietary-Induced Thermogenesis." *British Journal of Nutrition* 47 (1982): Bielinski et al. "Energy Metabolism during the Postexercise Recovery in Man." *American Journal of Clinical Nutrition* 42 (1985); Darden, E. *A Day-by-Day 10-Step Program* (Dallas: Taylor, 1992): 75.

"'...just as it's winding down.'" Roffers, M. "Nutrition Myths."

"If you walk after a meal, you may burn 15 percent...magazine."

"Natural Weight Control." *Prevention* (April 1993): 67.

" '... so it burns more calories.' " Stamford, B., quoted in "Natural Weight Control." *Prevention* (April 1993): 67.

"Light evening exercise ... have shown." Stamford, B. "What Time Should You Exercise?" *The Physician and Sports Medicine* 14 (8)(Aug. 1986): 162.

"... had some low-intensity exercise." Stamford, B. "Meals and the Timing of Exercise." *The Physician and Sports Medicine* 17 (11)(Nov. 1989): 151. Roffers, M. "Nutrition Myths." *Medical Self-Care* (March/April 1986): 52.

Page 201 "... and sustained sexual attraction.)" Rossi, E. L. *The 20-Minute Break* (Los Angeles: Jeremy Tarcher, 1991).

" '... scheduled at consistent times.' " Hagerman, F. C. quoted in "Natural Weight Loss." *Prevention* (March 1994): 70.

Chapter 13

Page 204 " '... dependent on adequate deep rest.' " Darden, E. *A Day-by-Day 10-Step Program* (Dallas: Taylor, 1992): 77.

"... even while you sleep." Department of Nutrition and Dietetics at King's College, University of London. "Train Your Body to Trim Your Tummy." *Prevention* (May 1994): 51.

"... cover up with a single sheet." Darden. *Day-by-Day*: 81–82.

Page 205 "... the more your sleep improves." C. M. Shapiro et al. "Fitness Facilitates Sleep." *European Journal of Applied Physiology* 53 (1984): 1–4; Baekland, F., study cited in Mirkin, G., *Dr. Gabe Mirkin's Fitness Clinic* (Chicago: Contemporary Books, 1986); Shapiro, C., and Zloty, R. B., cited in Mirkin. *Fitness Clinic*.

"... the increased body temperature." Sewitch, D. "Slow Wave Sleep Deficiency Insomnia: A Problem in Thermo-Down Regulation at Sleep Onset." *Psychophysiology* 24 (1987): 200–215; Perl, J. *Sleep Right in Five Nights* (New York: Morrow, 1993): 232–233.

" '... with fewer awakenings,' they note." Hauri, P., and Linde, S. *No More Sleepless Nights* (New York: Wiley, 1990): 130–131.

"... within three hours of bedtime." J. A. Horne et al. *Sleep* 10 (1987): 383–392; Willensky, D. "Hints for Sound Sleep." *American Health* (May 1992): 50.

"... wave patterns in your brain." South African study on low-calorie diets and disrupted sleep, in *American Journal of Clinical Nutrition*. Reported in *Self* (Sept. 1994): 90.

Page 206 "... low-fat, low-protein snacks." Lamberg, L. *Bodyrhythms: Chronobiology and Peak Performance* (New York: Morrow, 1994): 46; Wurtman, J. J. *Managing Your Mind and Mood through Food* (New York: HarperCollins, 1987).

"... state of mind and calm emotions." Wurtman. *Managing Your Mind and Mood*; Chafetz, M. D., ed. *Nutrition and Neurotransmitters: The Nutrient Bases of Behavior* (New York: Prentice-Hall, 1990); Somer, E. *Food and Mood* (New York: Henry Holt, 1995).

" '... without time pressure,' says Dr. Hauri." Lamberg, L. "The Boy Who Ate His Bed ... And Other Mysteries of Sleep." *American Health* (Nov. 1990): 56.

Page 207 "... a learned association with sleeplessness." Perl. *Sleep Right*: 213.

"... known as free running." Ibid.: 205.

Page 208 "... asleep the next night." Broughton, R. "Performance and Evoked Potential Measures of Various States of Daytime Sleepiness." *Sleep* 5 (Suppl. 2)(1982); Dott: *Asleep in the Fast Lane*: 138; Hauri, P. "Behavioral Treatment of Insomnia." *Medical Times* 107 (6)(1986): 36–47; Regestein, Q. R. "Practical Ways to Manage Insomnia." *Medical Times* 107 (6)(1986): 19–23.

" . . . your body's biological rhythms." Hauri, P. "Behavioral Treatment of Insomnia"; Regestein. "Practical Ways to Manage Insomnia."
" . . . your sleep/wake rhythm." Perl. *Sleep Right*: 195, 209.

Chapter 14

Page 212 " . . . daily ritual of connection." Imber-Black, E., and Roberts, J. *Rituals for Our Times* (New York: HarperCollins, 1992).

Chapter 15

Page 226 " . . . used in limited quantities." Walford, R. L. *The 120-Year Diet* (New York: Simon & Schuster, 1986): 256; Grundy, S. M. "Comparison of Monounsaturated Fatty Acids and Carbohydrates for Lowering Plasma Cholesterol." *New England Journal of Medicine* 314 (12)(March 20, 1986): 745-748; S. M. Grundy et al. "Rationale of the Diet-Heart Statement of the American Heart Association, Report of the Nutrition Committee." *Circulation* 65 (4)(1982): 841A; Mensink, R. P., and Katahn, M. B. "Effect of Monounsaturated Fatty Acids versus Complex Carbohydrates on High-Density Lipoproteins in Healthy Men and Women." *Lancet* (Jan. 17, 1987): 122-124.

"Additionally, olive oil may help . . . University." "Will Olive Oil Lower Your Blood Pressure?" *Tufts University Diet and Nutrition Letter* 5 (7)(Sept. 1987): 1.

" . . . lead to stroke and heart attack." Grundy. "Comparison of Monounsaturated Fatty Acids"; Grundy et al. "Rationale of the Diet-Heart Statement"; Mensink and Katahn. "Effect of Monounsaturated Fatty Acids."

" . . . the way other oils can." *Journal of the National Cancer Institute* 72 (1984): 745; *Federation Proceedings* 43 (1984): 614; *Nutrition Action* (July/Aug. 1986): 5.

Page 230 " . . . low-fat or nonfat dairy products." Snowdon, D. A., and Phillips, R. L. "Does a Vegetarian Diet Reduce the Occurrence of Diabetes?" *American Journal of Public Health* 75 (5)(May 1985): 507–512; "Position of the American Dietetic Association: Vegetarian Diets." *Journal of the American Dietetic Association* 88 (3)(March 1988): 351; Ballentine, R. *Transition to Vegetarianism* (Honesdale, Pa.: Himalayan Institute, 1987); Liebman, B. "Are Vegetarians Healthier Than the Rest of Us?" *Nutrition Action* (June 1983): 8; Burr, M. L., and Sweetnam, P. M. "Vegetarianism, Dietary Fiber, and Mortality." *American Journal of Clinical Nutrition* 36 (5)(Nov. 1982): 873–877; Dwyer, J., quoted in *Environmental Nutrition* (May 1987).

" . . . an average of 9 percent." P. Maenpaa et al. "Effects of a Low-Fat Lactovegetarian Diet on Health Parameters of Adult Subjects." *Ecology of Food and Nutrition* 25 (3)(1991): 255–267.

" . . . exhibit fewer feelings of anger." "Better Eating Goes to Your Head." *Tufts University Diet and Nutrition Letter* 11 (1)(March 1993): 2.

" . . . the rest of the U.S. population." Burr and Sweetnam. "Vegetarianism, Dietary Fiber, and Mortality"; Liebman. "Are Vegetarians Healthier?"

Page 231 " . . . stronger immune system, studies show." Snowdon and Phillips. "Does a Vegetarian Diet Reduce the Occurrence of Diabetes?"; "Position of the American Dietetic Association"; *Australian and New Zealand Journal of Medicine* (Aug. 1984); Ballentine. *Transition*; Liebman. "Are Vegetarians Healthier?"; *British Medical Journal* 291 (July 6, 1985); *Journal of the Royal Society of Medicine* 79 (June 1986).

Page 232 " ' . . . contain a thousand times more.' " *Mutagen Research* 72 (1980): 511.

Chapter 16

Page 247 " . . . in America's 620,000 restaurants." This section was adapted from Cooper, R. K. *Health and Fitness Excellence* (Boston: Houghton Mifflin, 1989).

Subject

Index

Note: <u>Underscored</u> page references indicate boxed text. **Boldface** references indicate illustrations. *Italic* references indicate tables. For a listing of recipes and main ingredients, see the Recipe Index beginning on page 462.

A

Abdominal exercises, 161–68
abdominal roll-ups,
164–65, **164**
abdominal vacuum exercise,
<u>162</u>
exhalation roll-ups, 165–66,
165
reverse trunk rotations,
167–68, **167**
transpyramid breathing exercise, 163–64
twisting exhalation roll-ups,
166–67, **166**
Abdominal fat
from alcohol, 53
cancer risk from, 21–22
health risks from, 15–16
from smoking, <u>54</u>
stress and, 133–34
Abdominal roll-ups, for
abdominal toning,
164–65, **164**
Abdominal vacuum exercise,
for abdominal toning,
<u>162</u>
Adenosine triphosphate
(ATP), breathing and,
135–36
Adrenaline
release of, during exercise,
118
stress and, 132
Aerobic exercise, 110–11
resistance training and,
158
heart rate and, 109–10

Alcohol
  cutting back on, 53
  effects of, 50–55
American food, low-fat, 253
American Heart Association,
    248
American Spoon Foods, mail-
    order supplies from,
    262
Anger
  effect of, on life span, 152
  management of, 142–44
Antioxidants, in fruits and veg-
    etables, 230
Antipasto, quick recipe for,
    217–18
Appetizers
  low-fat, 188–89
  restaurant, 248–49
  Spanish, 252
Arm curls, for upper arm ton-
    ing, 173–74, **174**
Arm exercises. *See* Upper arm
    exercises
Artificial sweeteners
  in beverages, 96
  food cravings from, 84, 85
Atherosclerosis, causes of, 17

B

Back, muscle-toning exercises
    for, 168–73
Back-of-the-upper-arm
    extensions, for upper
    arm toning, 174–75,
    175
Back pain
  abdominal exercises and,
    161–62
  dietary fat and, 18–19
Beans. *See also* Legumes
  quick recipes for, 221
  refried, in pita, 217

Behavior modification, for
    stress management,
    134–35
Bircher-Benner Muesli, 77
Blood clots, dietary fat and, 18
Blood pressure. *See* High blood
    pressure
Blood sugar
  alcohol consumption and, 51
  from carbohydrates, 43
  converted to fat, 42
  function of, 43
  morning depletion of, 75–76
  smoking and, 54
  stress and, 65
  sugar consumption and, 43
Body temperature
  fat-burning and, 204
  insomnia and, 205–6
Breads
  as appetizer, 189
  freezing, 213
  homemade, 232
  quick, 239–41
  quick recipes for, 222
  stocking up on, 256
  whole-grain, in restaurants,
    250
Breakfast
  as metabolism booster,
    74–78
  skipping
    how to avoid, 76
    pitfalls of, 55, 56, 57, 122
Breast cancer
  alcohol and, 55
  dietary fat and, 20–21
Breathing
  diaphragmatic, 136–38, 138
  for stress management, 64,
    135–38
Burgers
  fat in, 129–30
  quick recipes for, 217

Butter, fat composition of, *36*

Buttock exercises
hip raises, 178, 180, **180**
modified knee bends, 175–76, **176**

C

Caffeine, effects of, 94–95
Cajun cuisine, low-fat, 253
Calf raises, for lower leg toning, 180–81, **181**
California cuisine, low-fat, 253
Calories, daily limit of, 38–40, *39*
Cancer. *See also specific types*
alcohol and, 55
anger and, <u>152</u>
dietary fat and, 16, 19–22
vegetarianism and, 231–32
Canned goods, stocking up on, 256–57
Canola oil, uses for, <u>226</u>
Carbohydrates, <u>43</u>
as alternative to high-fat foods, 30–31
complex
benefits of, <u>43</u>, 44
for breakfast, 76
calming effects of, <u>124</u>
for insulin resistance, 47
fat burning from, 13
sleepiness from, 197
Cereals
for breakfast, 76
whole-grain, 250
cooking, *236–37*, 238–39
Cheese, as appetizer, 189
Chef's Catalog, The, mail-order supplies from, 262

Chest and shoulder raises, for chest, shoulder and upper back toning, 171–72, **171**
Chest crosses, for chest, shoulder and upper back toning, 172–73, **172**
Chest exercises
chest and shoulder raises, 171–72, **171**
chest crosses, 172–73, **172**
modified push-ups, 170–71, **170**
Children, dietary fat and, 9, 23–25
Chili pepper, fat-burning effect of, 196
Chinese food, low-fat, 252–53
Chips, fat in, 126
Chocolate, low-fat, 90
Cholesterol
food label information on, <u>214</u>
lipoproteins and, <u>14</u>
vegetarianism and, 231
Clots, blood, dietary fat and, 18
Coconut oil, in snacks, <u>81</u>
Coffee, 97
Colorectal cancer
alcohol and, 55
dietary fat and, 20
Condiments, 233
low-fat substitutions for, *228*
stocking up on, 259–60
Cooking, low-fat
learning, 7–8
shopping for, 261–62
supplies for, 255–60
utensils for, 260–61
Cortisol, fat storage and, 132–33, 134, 142
Couscous, quick recipe for, 219

Crackers, as appetizer, 189
Cravings, for fat, 32–33
Cue words, for stress manage-
    ment, 138–39, *138*

D

Daily Calorie Limit, calculat-
    ing, 38–40, *39*
Daily Dietary Fat Budget,
    estimating, 40, *40*
Dairy products
    fat in, 128
    low-fat substitutions for,
        228
    stocking up on, 257
Dean and Deluca, mail-order
    supplies from, 262
Dehydration
    causes of, 91–92
    effects of, 94
    hidden, 58–60
Deli foods, low-fat, 253–54
Desserts
    delaying, after dinner,
        198–99
    during the evening, 201–2
    low-fat, 130, 201–2, *202*,
        229
    in restaurants, 250
Diabetes. *See also* Insulin
    dietary fat and, 22–23
    insulin resistance and,
        46–47
Diamond Organics, mail-order
    supplies from, 262
Diaphragmatic breathing,
    136–38, *137*
Diets. *See also* Weight loss
    low-calorie vs. low-fat, 15
Dining-out strategies,
    247–54
Dinner
    appetizers before, 188–89

changing habits concerning,
    191–202
delaying dessert after,
    198–99
exercise after, 108–9, 112,
    199–201, *200*
low-fat suggestions for, *195*
pace of, 197–98
protein for, 196–97
recommended calories in,
    193–94
timesaving ideas for, 194
timing of, 192–93
Dips, fat in, 126
Dressings, salad. *See* Salad
    dressings
Dry goods, stocking up on,
    257–58

E

Eating out, strategies for,
    247–54
Eating slowly, as fat-burner,
    42
Eggs, low-fat substitutions for,
    228
Eicosapentaenoic acid (EPA),
    health benefits of, *218*
Emotional state, low-fat
    lifestyle and, 25–26
Endometrial cancer, dietary
    fat and, 21
Energy
    from protein, 196–97
    regaining late-afternoon,
        183–89
Entrées, choosing, in restau-
    rants, 249
EPA, health benefits of, *218*
Estrogen
    cancer risk and high levels
        of, 21–22
    high-fat diet and, 122

Ethnic foods, low-fat, 250–54
Exercise
    aerobic (*see* Aerobic exer-
        cise)
    after dinner, 108–9,
        199–201, 200
    for afternoon energy,
        185–86
    benefits of, 113, 114
    effects of, on
        life span, 100–101,
            102–3
        stress levels, 103–4
        weight loss, 103
    fan use during, 118
    finding time for, 99–102,
        104–9, 110, 112–13
    guidelines for, 114–19
    morning, as metabolism
        booster, 72–74, 74
    muscle-toning, 49 (*see also*
        Muscle-toning exer-
        cises)
    standing as, 105
    for stress management,
        141–42
    to counteract inactivity, 61
    walking as (*see* Walking)
Exercise equipment, 108, 112
Exercise tolerance test, 115
Exhalation roll-ups, for ab-
        dominal toning,
        165–66, **165**

F

Fat, abdominal. *See* Abdomi-
        nal fat
Fat, body, from high-fat foods,
        30, 31
Fat, dietary
    children and, 9, 23–25
    cravings for, 32–33
    daily budget for, 40, *40*

    effect of, combined with
        sugar, 125
    food label information on,
        214
    monounsaturated, *36*, 37
    percentage of calories from,
        35–38
    polyunsaturated, 18, *36*, 37
    saturated, *36*, 37
    storage of, 12–13, 30, 31,
        33
    substitutions for, 31, 85–86,
        227, *228–29*
Fat burning, 4, 5, 6, 7
Fatigue
    from high-fat foods,
        33–34
    late afternoon, 183–89
Fiber, dietary
    food label information on,
        214
    insulin resistance and,
        46–47
    recommended daily intake
        of, 46
    satisfying appetite with,
        47–48
    types of, 45–46
Fish
    low-fat substitutions for,
        229
    omega-3 fatty acids in, 218
    quick recipes for, 219, 222
Flatulence, from beans, 242
Flavorings, 233
    low-fat substitutions for,
        228
Flour
    stocking up on, 258
    whole-grain
        cooking with, *236–37*
        for quick breads, 239,
            241
        refined vs., 235

Food costs, reduced, from low-
fat lifestyle, 26
Food journal, for tracking effects of food, 133
Food labels, understanding information from, 214
Food processor, 261
Food records, for weight loss,
194, 194
France, eating habits in,
192–93
Free radicals, fruits and vegetables and, 230
French food, low-fat, 251–52
French fries, fat in, 130
Fried foods
fat in, 130
in restaurants, 248
Fruits
anti-aging effects of, 230
fiber in, 47
pureed, 218–19
as snacks, 82
sugar in, 83–85

G

Galanin, fat cravings from,
32–33
Gallstones, dietary fat and,
16–17
Garlic, peeling, 219
Garlic press, 261
Gas, intestinal, from beans,
242
Glucose. *See* Blood sugar
Glucose tolerance
diabetes risk and, 22
insulin resistance and, 46
Glycogen
appetite and, 47
depletion of, in morning, 75
Grains
stocking up on, 258

whole
cooking, 235, *236–37*,
238
cooking time for, 223
importance of, 225–27,
234–35
Guilt, stress from, 150

H

Hamburgers
fat in, 129–30
quick recipes for, 217
HDL cholesterol, 14, 113,
218, 231
Heart attacks
anger and, 152
causes of, 17
among French, 192
Heart disease
in children, 23–24
dietary fat and, 17
wine and, 53–55
Heart rate monitor, for measuring pulse, 117
Herbs, stocking up on, 258–59
High blood pressure
from anger, 152
dietary fat and, 17–18
from insulin resistance, 46
High-density lipoprotein
(HDL), 14, 113, 218,
231
High-fat foods
body fat gained from, 30, 31
low-fat substitutions for,
228–29
Hip raises, for buttocks toning, 178, 180, **180**
Hoagies, fat in, 128–29
Humor, for stress manage-
ment, 151–53, 188
Hydrogenated oils, health
problems from, 34

Hypertension. *See* High blood pressure

I

Ice water, as fat-burner, 6, 42, 92, 93–94
Immune system
dietary fat and, 16
overweight and, 21
Impotence, dietary fat and, 18
Inactivity, weight gain from, 60–62
Indian food, low-fat, 252
Ingredients
mail-order sources of, 261–62
stocking up on, 255–60
Insomnia, body temperature and, 205–6
Insulin
alcohol consumption and, 51
blood sugar reduced by, 42, 43
for diabetes, 22, 23
fat storage and, 31, 33, 42, 42, 86, 125
Insulin resistance, from low-fiber eating, 46–47
Italian food, low-fat, 250–51

J

Japanese food, low-fat, 253

K

Kitchen
equipment, 261
stocking, 256–60
Knee bends
for afternoon energy, 186

modified, for thigh and buttocks toning, 175–76, **176**
Knee-to-chest lifts, for lower back toning, 169, **169**
Knives, kitchen, 261

L

Labels, food, understanding information from, 214
Laughter, for stress management, 151–53, 188
LDL cholesterol, 14, 158, 218
Leftovers, as snacks, 87
Leg exercises, 180–81, **181**. *See also* Thigh exercises
Legumes. *See also* Beans
buying, 241–42
cooking times for, *243*
importance of, 225–27
precooked, 213, 244–45
presoaking, 213, 242–43
quick-cook method for, 244
Lemon juicer, 261
Light
as energy booster, 187
as metabolism booster, 71–72, 72
Linoleic acid, sources of, 18
Lipoprotein lipase, fat storage and, 33
Lipoproteins, cholesterol and, 14. *See also* HDL cholesterol; LDL cholesterol
Low-density lipoprotein (LDL), 14, 158, 218
Lower back exercises
pelvic tilt movements, 170, **170**
seated lower back stretches, 169, **169**
single knee-to-chest lifts, 169, **169**

Lower leg exercises
  standing calf raises,
    180–81, **181**
Low-fat diets, vs. low-calorie
  diets, 15
Low-fat foods. *See also spe-*
  cific foods and meals
  mail-order sources of,
    261–62
  overeating, pitfalls of, 41,
    42, 44
  quick recipes for, <u>220–22</u>
  stocking up on, 255–60
  suggestions for, <u>195</u>
Low-Fat Living Program
  benefits of, 11–26
  cooking skills for, 7–8
  skillpower vs. willpower in,
    4, 6–7
  "Switchbreaks" in, 5–6
  weight loss from, 9
Low-Fat Living 3-plus-4 Eating Plan
  benefits of, 8, 80, <u>83</u>
  snacks for, <u>88–89</u>
Lunch
  energy from, <u>124</u>
  importance of, 121–22
  low-fat, 122–30
  skipping, 121–22
Lung cancer, dietary fat and,
  19–20

M

Mail-order food suppliers,
  261–62
Maximal graded exercise test
  (MaxGXT), <u>115</u>
Mayonnaise, fat in, 128
Meal planning, <u>31</u>
  quick recipes for,
    215–19
  shortcuts for, 219, 223

timesaving tips for, 211–13,
  215
to avoid meal skipping, <u>57</u>
Meals, size of, 79–80
Meal skipping, pitfalls of,
  55–57, 121–22
Meats
  low-fat substitutions for,
    229
  reducing consumption of,
    227, 231, 232–34
Metabolism
  carbohydrates and, 13
  effect of television on,
    146–47
  fat-storing, 33
  morning, increasing,
    69–78
Mexican food
  fat in, 129
  low-fat, 251
  quick recipes for, 217
Mixer, handheld electric, 261
Monounsaturated fat
  effects of, <u>37</u>
  in oils, *36*, <u>226</u>
Muesli, Bircher-Benner, <u>77</u>
Multiple sclerosis, dietary fat
  and, 17
Muscle loss, 156
Muscle tone, fat burning and,
  48–50
Muscle-toning exercises, <u>49</u>
  abdominal, 161–68
  buttocks, 175–76, 178, 180
  chest, 170–73
  from chores, 181–82
  fat-burning from, 156–58
  guidelines for, 158–61
  lower back, 168–70
  lower leg, 180–81
  sample schedule for, <u>179</u>
  shoulder, 170–73
  sleep and, 203–4

thigh, 175–78
upper arm, 173–75
upper back, 170–73
Mustard, fat-burning effect of,
196

N

Neck rotations, for afternoon
energy, 185
Negative thinking, stress from,
146–51, 148, 151
Neurotransmitters, food and,
133
Nonfat foods, pitfalls of
overeating, 41, 42, 44

O

Oatmeal, for breakfast, 75,
76, 77
Obesity
causes of, 12
childhood, 23
immune system and, 21
Oils
fat composition of, 36
hydrogenated, 34
low-fat substitutions for,
229
monounsaturated, 37, 226
pure vegetable, in snacks, 81
stocking up on, 259–60
types of fatty acids in, 37
Olive oil, uses for, 226
Omega-3 fatty acids, health
benefits of, 218
Oriental dishes, quick recipes
for, 216
Osteoporosis
calcium and, 125–26
dietary fat and, 17
Ovarian cancer, dietary fat
and, 21

Overeating
handling guilt over, 150
of low-fat and nonfat foods,
41, 42, 44
from sleep deprivation,
62–63
of snacks, 86
from stress, 146
Overweight. See Obesity

P

Palm-kernel oil, in snacks, 81
Palm oil, in snacks, 81
Pans, no-stick, 261
Pasta
quick recipes for, 220
sauces for, 128, 220, 250
stocking up on, 256
variations of, 216
Pelvic tilt movements, for
lower back toning,
170, **170**
Pilaf, quick recipe for, 216
Pita bread, for pizza, 215–16
Pizza
fat in, 129
low-fat substitutions for,
215–16
low-fat toppings for, 251
PMHR, for exercise, 116,
116
Polyunsaturated fat
effects of, 37
function of, 18
in oils, 36
Potbelly. See Abdominal fat
Poultry, quick recipes for, 217,
222
Predicted maximal heart rate
(PMHR), for exercise,
116, 116
Prostate cancer, dietary fat
and, 19

Protein
   for breakfast, 76
   for dinner, 196–97
   as energy source, 124
   fat burning from, 13
Push-ups, modified, for chest, shoulder and upper back toning, 170–71, **170**

Q

Quick breads, 239–41

R

Record-keeping, of food intake, 194, 194
Refried beans, in pita sandwich, 217
Relaxation. *See also* Stress, management of
   breathing for, 64, 135–38
Resistance training. *See also* Muscle-toning exercises
   aerobic exercise and, 158
   fat-burning from, 157–58
   guidelines for, 158–61
Restaurant dining, guidelines for, 247–54
Reverse trunk rotations, for abdominal toning, **167**, 167–68
Rice
   cooking time for, 223
   quick recipes for, 221
   white vs. brown, 235

S

Salad bars, 126–27, 249
Salad dressings
   fat in, 127
   low-fat, 233, 249
   quick recipes for, 220–21
Salads
   ingredients for, 233
   preparing greens for, 215
   quick recipes for, 220–21
Salad spinner, 261
Salt, substitutions for, 227
Sandwiches
   quick recipes for, 222
   submarine, 128–29
Sandwich spreads, fat in, 128
Saturated fat
   effects of, 37
   in oils, *36*
Sauces, low-fat substitutions for, *228*
Seafood. *See* Fish
Seasonings, stocking up on, 258–60
Seated leg extensions, for thigh toning, 176–77, **177**
Second wind, late afternoon, 183–89
Serotonin, sleep and, 197
Shopping, mail-order, for low-fat foods, 261–62
Shoulder exercises
   chest and shoulder raises, 171–72, **171**
   chest crosses, 172–73, **172**
   modified push-ups, 170–71, **170**
Shoulder shrugs, for afternoon energy, 185–86
Side dishes, low-fat substitutions for, *229*
Skin cancer, dietary fat and, 19
Sleep
   effect of exercise on, 114
   ensuring quality of, 63, 203–8

insomnia, body temperature and, 205–6
poor-quality, overeating from, 62–63
Smoking, weight and, 54
Snacks
    benefits of, 79–81, 86–87, 90
    calories in, 82–83
    during the evening, 201–2
    fat grams in, 82
    from leftovers, 87
    low-fat, 188–89, 229
    overeating, 86
    skipping, pitfalls of, 55, 57
    suggestions for, 88–89
    timing of, 81–82, 90
Sodium, food label information on, 214
Soups
    as appetizers, 189
    fat in, 126
    low-fat, 249
    quick recipes for, 221–22
Southwest Gourmet Gallery, mail-order supplies from, 262
Spanish food, low-fat, 252
Spices
    as fat-burners, 128, 196
    stocking up on, 258–59
Squash, quick cooking of, 223
Standing, as exercise, 105
Standing calf raises, for lower leg toning, 180–81, 181
Standing side leg raises, for thigh toning, 177–78, 178
Staples, stocking up on, 255–60
Starches, types of, 43
Stews, quick recipes for, 221–22

Strength training. See Muscle-toning exercises
Stress
    causes of
        guilt, 150
        negative thinking, 146–51, 148, 151
        TV watching, 146–47
    effect of, on
        fat-burning, 63–65, 131–34
        life span, 152
        overeating, 146
        sleep, 207, 208
    during exercise, 117
    management of, 134–53
        with breathing, 64, 135–38
        with exercise, 141–42
        with humor, 151–53
    vegetarianism and, 231
Stretches, seated, for lower back toning, 169, 169
Submarine sandwiches, fat in, 128–29
Sucrose. See Sugar
Sugar, effects of
    combined with fat, 125
    on health, 43
Sunlight, as metabolism booster, 72
Supplies
    mail-order, 261–62
    stocking up on, 255–60
Sweeteners
    artificial, food cravings from, 84, 85
    in beverages, 96
    health effects of, 43, 44
    low-fat substitutions for, 228
    stocking up on, 260

T

Tapas, 252
Target heart rate zone, for exercise, <u>116</u>, 116–17
Teas, 97
Television watching. See TV watching
Thermic effect of food, metabolism and, 13
Thigh exercises
  modified knee bends, 175–76, **176**
  seated leg extensions, 176–77, **177**
  standing side leg raises, 177–78, **178**
Torso turns, for afternoon energy, 186
Trans-fatty acids, health problems from, <u>34</u>
Transpyramid breathing exercise, for abdominal toning, 163–64, **163**
Travel, low-fat food for, 254
TV watching
  stress from, 146–47
  weight gain from, 61–62
Twisting exhalation roll-ups, for abdominal toning, 166–67, **166**

U

Upper arm exercises
  arm curls, 173–74, **174**
  back-of-the-upper-arm extensions, 174–75, **175**
Upper back exercises
  chest and shoulder raises, 171–72, **171**
  chest crosses, 172–73, **172**
  modified push-ups, 170–71, **170**

Utensils
  for low-fat cooking, 260–61
  mail-order sources of, 261–62

V

Vegetables
  anti-aging effects of, <u>230</u>
  as meat substitute, 233
  quick recipes for, <u>221</u>
  as snacks, <u>82</u>
Vegetarian dishes, low-fat, 254
Vegetarianism, health benefits of, 230–32
Very-low density lipoprotein (VLDL), <u>14</u>

W

Walking
  after eating, 108–9, 199–201, <u>200</u>
  as exercise, 106, 107, 108, 112, 199–201, <u>200</u>
Walnut Acres, mail-order supplies from, 262
Water
  consumption of, tracking, <u>96</u>
  as fat-burner, <u>6</u>, <u>42</u>, 92, 93–94
  importance of, 58–60, 91–97
  with lunch, 125–26
Water containers, <u>59</u>
Weigh-ins, disadvantages of, 144–45
Weight, determining ideal, 38–39
Weight control, smoking and, <u>54</u>
Weight cycling, disadvantages of, 15

Weight gain, from TV watching, 61–62
Weight loss
  benefits of, 11–12
  food records for, 194, _194_
  from low-fat diet, 15, 35
  and timing of meals, 193
Whole grains
  cooking, 235, _236–37_, 238
  cooking time for, 223
  importance of, 225–27, 234–35

Willpower, fallacy of, 6–7
Wine
  health benefits of, 53–55
  heart disease and, 192
Wrist circles, for afternoon energy, 186

Y

Yams, quick cooking of, 223

Recipe

Index

Note: <u>Underscored</u> page
references indicate boxed text.

A

Acorn squash
  Autumn's Acorn Cheddar
    Soup, 296
Active dry yeast, for bread,
  385
Almonds
  Almond and Hazelnut
    Biscotti, 358–59
  Broccoli Lemon Amandine,
    347
  Cinnamon, Raisin and Nut
    Spread, 380
Angel food cake
  Whole-Grain Cocoa Angel
    Food Cake, 366–67
Angel hair pasta
  Angel Hair Pasta with Fresh
    Tomato Sauce, 320
Appetizers
  Baba Ghanoush,
    380–81
  Black Olive and Pimento
    Spread, 379–80
  Cinnamon, Raisin and Nut
    Spread, 380
  Cucumber and Yogurt
    Spread, 381–82
  Lentil Spread in Pita
    Pockets, 305–6
  Sweet Pea Guacamole,
    289
Apples
  Apple Crisp, 375–76
  Apple Crumb Pie, 373–74
  Apple Spice Cake, 363–64
  Apple-Walnut Bread,
    410–11
Applesauce, as fat substitute,
  <u>298</u>

B

Bagels
  Whole-Grain Bagels,
    417–19
Baked goods. *See also spe-
    cific types*
  storing leftover, <u>271</u>

Baking soda
    Oatmeal Soda Bread, 273
Balsamic vinegar
    Balsamic Splash, 348
    Four-Bean Salad with Bal-
        samic Vinaigrette, 290
Bananas
    Banana Bread, 364–65
Bars
    Lemon Delicacy Bars,
        371–72
    Sweet Potato–Cherry
        Squares with Orange
        Icing, 370–71
Basil
    Mixed Green Salad with
        Creamy Fresh Basil
        Dressing, 321
Basmati rice
    Brown Basmati Rice with
        Lemon, 318–19
Beans, 290
    Four-Bean Salad with Bal-
        samic Vinaigrette, 290
    refried
        Tacos, 315–16
    Southwestern Black Beans,
        323–24
Beets
    European Mixed Vegetable
        Salad, 347–48
    Greens with Baby Beets,
        Toasted Walnuts and
        Maple-Raspberry
        Vinaigrette, 354
Biscotti
    Almond and Hazelnut
        Biscotti, 358–59
Biscuits
    Green Chili and Cheddar
        Buttermilk Biscuits, 270
Black beans
    Southwestern Black Beans,
        323–24

Black bread
    Multigrain Black Bread,
        405–6
Bread crumbs, homemade,
    280
Breads
    biscuits
        Green Chili and Cheddar
            Buttermilk Biscuits, 270
    freezing, 273
    muffins
        Gingerbread Muffins, 298
    quick
        Banana Bread, 364–65
        Cracked-Wheat Quick
            Bread, 280
        Oatmeal Soda Bread, 273
        Old-Fashioned Corn-
            bread, 304–5
        Pumpkin-Cranberry
            Bread, 362–63
        Zucchini Spice Bread,
            361–62
    scones
        Raspberry-Currant
            Scones, 360–61
    stuffed, 419–26
    yeast
        Apple-Walnut Bread,
            410–11
        basic ingredients of,
            385–86
        Cinnamon-Raisin Swirl
            Bread, 411–13
        Corn and Rye Bread,
            402–3
        Country Farmhouse
            Bread, 391–92
        French Breadstick Twists,
            416–17
        Honey Cracked-Wheat
            Bread, 392–93
        Honey Dinner Rolls, 394
        Jewish Rye Bread, 401–2

Breads *(continued)*
 yeast *(continued)*
  Minnesota Wild Rice
   Bread, 406–7
  Muesli Bread, 413–14
  Multigrain Black Bread,
   405–6
  Olive Bread, 408–9
  proofing yeast for, 386
  Quick Onion-Pumper-
   nickel Bread, 404–5
  Spanish Country Bread,
   398
  Specialty Breads, 424–26
  Sprouted Wheat-Berry
   Bread, 400–401
  steps in baking, 386–91
  Stuffed Spinach and Feta
   Bread, 420–22
  Sweet Potato and Honey
   Bread, 409–10
  Vegetable Stuffed Bread,
   422–23
  Whole-Grain Bagels,
   417–19
  Whole-Wheat and Honey
   Challah, 396–97
  Whole-Wheat Cinnamon
   Rolls, 414–16
  Whole-Wheat French
   Bread, 399–400
  Whole-Wheat Monkey
   Bread, 395–96
Breadsticks
 French Breadstick Twists,
  416–17
Broccoli
 Broccoli Lemon Amandine,
  347
 Linguine Frittata with
  Broccoli, 271–72
Brownies
 Dutch Cocoa Fudge Brown-
  ies, 372–73

Burgers
 Turkey Burgers, 329
Butter, getting more flavor
 from, 313

C

Caesar salad
 Caesar-Style Salad, 344
Cakes
 Apple Spice Cake,
  363–64
 Carrot-Pineapple Cake,
  365–66
 Chocolate Cream Cheese
  Delight, 367–68
 Sour Cream Coffee Cake,
  369
 Whole-Grain Cocoa Angel
  Food Cake, 366–67
Carrots
 Carrot-Pineapple Cake,
  365–66
 European Mixed Vegetable
  Salad, 347–48
 Honey-Glazed Baby Car-
  rots, 334
 Old-Fashioned Chicken and
  Vegetable Stew,
  352–53
Challah
 Whole-Wheat and Honey
  Challah, 396–97
Cheddar cheese
 Autumn's Acorn Cheddar
  Soup, 296
 Green Chili and Cheddar
  Buttermilk Biscuits,
  270
Cheese
 Autumn's Acorn Cheddar
  Soup, 296
 Chocolate Cream Cheese
  Delight, 367–68

Green Chili and Cheddar Buttermilk Biscuits, 270

Lemon Linguine Parmesan, 313

Mesclun Greens with Italian Parmesan Vinaigrette, 327–28

part-skim, 325

Ratatouille and Grilled Mozzarella Sandwiches, 281–82

Stuffed Spinach and Feta Bread, 420–22

Swiss Dijon Chicken Rolls, 345

Cheesecake
Chocolate Cream Cheese Delight, 367–68

Cherries
Cherry Pie, 374–75

Red-Leaf Lettuce with Pine Nuts, Cherries and Dried-Tomato Vinaigrette, 338–39

Sweet Potato–Cherry Squares with Orange Icing, 370–71

Chestnuts
Roasted Chestnut and Wild Rice Soup, 292–93

Chicken
Chicken and Wheat Berry Salad, 278–79

Chicken Baked with Sherry-Peach Sauce, 332–33

Chicken Cutlets with Raspberry Vinaigrette, 312–13

Chicken Salad with Peaches and Pecans, 277–78

ground, 329

Old-Fashioned Chicken and Vegetable Stew, 352–53

Santa Fe Chicken Fajitas, 322–23

Southwestern Chicken Chili, 303–4

Swiss Dijon Chicken Rolls, 345

Village Paella, 349–51

Chick-peas
Four-Bean Salad with Balsamic Vinaigrette, 290

Hummus in Pita Sandwiches, 275

Middle Eastern Baked Falafel, 283–85

Children under two, fat intake of, 264

Chili
Southwestern Chicken Chili, 303–4

Thick and Hearty Vegetable Chili, 302–3

Chili peppers
Green Chili and Cheddar Buttermilk Biscuits, 270

Chinese noodles
Oriental Noodles, 299–300

Chips
Pita Chips, 378–79

Wonton Chips, 300–301

Chocolate. See Cocoa

Cinnamon
Cinnamon, Raisin and Nut Spread, 380

Cinnamon-Raisin Swirl Bread, 411–13

Whole-Wheat Cinnamon Rolls, 414–16

Cocoa
Chocolate Cream Cheese Delight, 367–68

Dutch Cocoa Fudge Brownies, 372–73

Whole-Grain Cocoa Angel Food Cake, 366–67

Coffee cake
 Sour Cream Coffee Cake,
  369
Cookies
 Almond and Hazelnut Bis-
  cotti, 358–59
 Chewy Oatmeal-Raisin
  Cookies, 356
 Old-Fashioned Molasses
  Cookies, 357
 Whole-Grain Mandelbrot,
  359–60
Cooking sprays, 332
Corkscrew pasta
 Tex-Mex Pasta Salad,
  294–95
Corn
 Colorful Corn Relish, 297
Cornmeal
 Corn and Rye Bread, 402–3
 Old-Fashioned Cornbread,
  304–5
Coulis
 Raspberry Coulis, 378
Couscous
 Couscous Pilaf, 333
Cracked wheat
 Cracked-Wheat Quick
  Bread, 280
 Honey Cracked-Wheat
  Bread, 392–93
Cranberries
 Pumpkin-Cranberry Bread,
  362–63
Cream cheese
 Black Olive and Pimento
  Spread, 379–80
 Chocolate Cream Cheese
  Delight, 367–68
 Cinnamon, Raisin and Nut
  Spread, 380
Crisps
 Apple Crisp, 375–76
Croutons, homemade, 321

Cucumbers
 Cucumber and Red Grape
  Salad, 282–83
 Cucumber and Yogurt
  Spread, 381–82
 Dilled Cucumber Salad,
  285
 Israeli Salad, 276
Currants
 Raspberry-Currant Scones,
  360–61

D

Desserts
 Almond and Hazelnut
  Biscotti, 358–59
 Apple Crisp, 375–76
 Apple Crumb Pie, 373–74
 Apple Spice Cake,
  363–64
 Banana Bread, 364–65
 Carrot-Pineapple Cake,
  365–66
 Cherry Pie, 374–75
 Chewy Oatmeal-Raisin
  Cookies, 356
 Chocolate Cream Cheese
  Delight, 367–68
 Dutch Cocoa Fudge Brown-
  ies, 372–73
 Lemon Delicacy Bars,
  371–72
 Lemon Tapioca Pudding,
  376–77
 Old-Fashioned Molasses
  Cookies, 357
 Perfect Pumpkin Pudding,
  377–78
 Pumpkin-Cranberry Bread,
  362–63
 Raspberry Coulis, 378
 Sour Cream Coffee Cake,
  369

Recipe Index

Sweet Potato–Cherry
Squares with Orange
Icing, 370–71
Whole-Grain Cocoa Angel
Food Cake, 366–67
Whole-Grain Mandelbrot,
359–60
Zucchini Spice Bread,
361–62
Dijon mustard
Swiss Dijon Chicken Rolls,
345
Dips. *See* Spreads
Dressings, salad
Balsamic Splash, 348
Citrus-Season Salad with
Ginger-Horseradish
Dressing, 307
Creamy Garlic Dressing,
314–15
Four-Bean Salad with
Balsamic Vinaigrette,
290
Greens with Baby Beets,
Toasted Walnuts and
Maple-Raspberry
Vinaigrette, 354
Mesclun Greens with Italian
Parmesan Vinaigrette,
327–28
Mixed Green Salad with
Creamy Fresh Basil
Dressing, 321
Mixed Greens with Peach
and Pecan Dressing,
274
Red- and Green-Leaf
Lettuce with Maple-
Walnut Dressing,
351
Red-Leaf Lettuce with Pine
Nuts, Cherries and
Dried-Tomato Vinai-
grette, 338–39

Spinach Salad with Pears,
Walnuts and Warm
Mustard Vinaigrette,
334–35

E
Eggplant
Baba Ghanoush, 380–81
Ratatouille and Grilled
Mozzarella Sand-
wiches, 281–82
Eggs
Linguine Frittata with
Broccoli, 271–72
Egg whites, as substitute for
whole eggs, 272
Evaporated skim milk
as low-fat alternative, 349
for mock whipped cream,
315

F
Fajitas
Santa Fe Chicken Fajitas,
322–23
Falafel
Middle Eastern Baked
Falafel, 283–85
Fats, in yeast breads, 386
Feta cheese
Stuffed Spinach and Feta
Bread, 420–22
Fettuccine
Fettuccine with Roasted
Red Pepper Sauce,
336–37
Greek Pasta Salad,
286–87
Fish
Picante Seafood Veracruz,
317
Village Paella, 349–51

Flour, for yeast breads, 384, 385, 391

French fries
Spicy French Potatoes, 330

French-style dishes
French Breadstick Twists, 416–17
Ratatouille and Grilled Mozzarella Sandwiches, 281–82
Whole-Wheat French Bread, 399–400

Frittatas
Linguine Frittata with Broccoli, 271–72

G

Garlic
Creamy Garlic Dressing, 314–15
Vegetable Stuffed Bread, 422–23

Gazpacho
Thick and Zesty Gazpacho, 268–69

Ginger
Citrus-Season Salad with Ginger-Horseradish Dressing, 307

Gingerbread
Gingerbread Muffins, 298

Gnocci
Pasta Rustica, 342–43

Grains
Brown Basmati Rice with Lemon, 318–19
Chicken and Wheat Berry Salad, 278–79
Couscous Pilaf, 333
Mexicali Rice, 324–25
Minnesota Wild Rice Bread, 406–7

Roasted Chestnut and Wild Rice Soup, 292–93
Sprouted Wheat-Berry Bread, 400–401
Village Paella, 349–51

Grapes
Cucumber and Red Grape Salad, 282–83

Great Northern Beans
Four-Bean Salad with Balsamic Vinaigrette, 290

Greek-style dishes
Cucumber and Yogurt Spread, 381–82
Greek Pasta Salad, 286–87

Green beans
Four-Bean Salad with Balsamic Vinaigrette, 290
Fresh Green Bean Salad, 330–31
Old-Fashioned Chicken and Vegetable Stew, 352–53
Specialty Green Beans, 337–38

Green-leaf lettuce
Greens with Baby Beets, Toasted Walnuts and Maple-Raspberry Vinaigrette, 354
Red- and Green-Leaf Lettuce with Maple-Walnut Dressing, 351

Greens
Greens with Baby Beets, Toasted Walnuts and Maple-Raspberry Vinaigrette, 354
Mesclun Greens with Italian Parmesan Vinaigrette, 327–28
Mixed Green Salad with Creamy Fresh Basil Dressing, 321

Mixed Greens with Peach and Pecan Dressing, 274

Red- and Green-Leaf Lettuce with Maple-Walnut Dressing, 351

Red-Leaf Lettuce with Pine Nuts, Cherries and Dried-Tomato Vinaigrette, 338–39

Salad Nouveau, 314

Guacamole
Sweet Pea Guacamole, 289

H

Halibut
Picante Seafood Veracruz, 317

Village Paella, 349–51

Hazelnut
Almond and Hazelnut Biscotti, 358–59

Herbs
dried vs. fresh, 268
freezing, 276

Honey
Honey Cracked-Wheat Bread, 392–93

Honey Dinner Rolls, 394

Honey-Glazed Baby Carrots, 334

Sweet Potato and Honey Bread, 409–10

Whole-Wheat and Honey Challah, 396–97

Horseradish
Citrus-Season Salad with Ginger-Horseradish Dressing, 307

Hummus
Hummus in Pita Sandwiches, 275

I

Italian-style dishes
Caesar-Style Salad, 344

Mesclun Greens with Italian Parmesan Vinaigrette, 327–28

Pasta Rustica, 342–43

White Pizza, 325–27

K

Kidney beans
Four-Bean Salad with Balsamic Vinaigrette, 290

L

Leftovers
baked goods, 271
for lunch, 342

Legumes
Four-Bean Salad with Balsamic Vinaigrette, 290

Hummus in Pita Sandwiches, 275

Lentil Spread in Pita Pockets, 305–6

Middle Eastern Baked Falafel, 283–85

Southwestern Black Beans, 323–24

Sweet Pea Guacamole, 289

Lemons
Broccoli Lemon Amandine, 347

Brown Basmati Rice with Lemon, 318–19

Lemon Delicacy Bars, 371–72

Lemon Linguine Parmesan, 313

Lemon Tapioca Pudding, 376–77

Lentils
Lentil Spread in Pita Pock-
ets, 305–6
Linguine
Lemon Linguine Parmesan,
313
Linguine Frittata with
Broccoli, 271–72
Liquid smoke, 322
Lunch
leftovers for, 342
menus for, 266–67

M

Main dishes
Angel Hair Pasta with Fresh
Tomato Sauce, 320
Chicken Baked with
Sherry-Peach
Sauce, 332–33
Chicken Cutlets with
Raspberry Vinaigrette,
312–13
Old-Fashioned Chicken and
Vegetable Stew,
352–53
Pasta Rustica, 342–43
Pepper-Seared Sea Scal-
lops, 336
Picante Seafood Veracruz,
317
Santa Fe Chicken Fajitas,
322–23
Swiss Dijon Chicken Rolls,
345
Tacos, 315–16
Thai Stir-Fry, 339–41
Turkey Burgers, 329
Village Paella, 349–51
White Pizza, 325–27
Mandelbrot
Whole-Grain Mandelbrot,
359–60

Maple syrup
Greens with Baby Beets,
Toasted Walnuts and
Maple-Raspberry
Vinaigrette, 354
Red- and Green-Leaf
Lettuce with Maple-
Walnut Dressing, 351
Menus
dinner, 310–11
lunch, 266–67
Mesclun greens
Mesclun Greens with Italian
Parmesan Vinaigrette,
327–28
Mexican-style dishes
Mexicali Rice, 324–25
Picante Seafood Veracruz,
317
Quesadillas, 288
Santa Fe Chicken Fajitas,
322–23
Southwestern Chicken
Chili, 303–4
Sweet Pea Guacamole,
289
Tacos, 315–16
Thick and Hearty Vegetable
Chili, 302–3
Middle Eastern–style dishes
Baba Ghanoush,
380–81
Hummus in Pita Sand-
wiches, 275
Israeli Salad, 276
Middle Eastern Baked
Falafel, 283–85
Milk, evaporated skim
as low-fat alternative, 349
for mock whipped cream,
315
Molasses
Old-Fashioned Molasses
Cookies, 357

Monkey bread
  Whole-Wheat Monkey
    Bread, 395–96
Moroccan-style dishes
  Couscous Pilaf, 333
Mozzarella
  Ratatouille and Grilled
    Mozzarella Sand-
    wiches, 281–82
Muesli
  Bircher-Benner Muesli, 77
  Muesli Bread, 413–14
Muffins
  Gingerbread Muffins, 298
Mushrooms
  Ratatouille and Grilled
    Mozzarella Sand-
    wiches, 281–82
  Vegetable Stuffed Bread,
    422–23
Mustard
  Spinach Salad with Pears,
    Walnuts and Warm
    Mustard Vinaigrette,
    334–35
  Swiss Dijon Chicken Rolls,
    345

N

Noodles
  Oriental Noodles, 299–300
Nutmeg
  Baked Yams with Nutmeg
    Cream, 318
Nuts
  Almond and Hazelnut
    Biscotti, 358–59
  Apple-Walnut Bread,
    410–11
  Broccoli Lemon Amandine,
    347
  Chicken Salad with Peaches
    and Pecans, 277–78

Cinnamon, Raisin and Nut
  Spread, 380
Greens with Baby Beets,
  Toasted Walnuts and
  Maple-Raspberry
  Vinaigrette, 354
Mixed Greens with Peach
  and Pecan Dressing,
  274
Red- and Green-Leaf
  Lettuce with Maple-
  Walnut Dressing, 351
Red-Leaf Lettuce with Pine
  Nuts, Cherries and
  Dried-Tomato Vinai-
  grette, 338–39
Roasted Chestnut and Wild
  Rice Soup, 292–93
Spinach Salad with Pears,
  Walnuts and Warm
  Mustard Vinaigrette,
  334–35
toasting, 338

O

Oats
  Bircher-Benner Muesli,
    77
  Chewy Oatmeal-Raisin
    Cookies, 356
  Muesli Bread, 413–14
  Oatmeal Soda Bread, 273
Oils, for greasing baking pans,
  386
Olives
  Black Olive and Pimento
    Spread, 379–80
  Olive Bread, 408–9
Onions
  Quick Onion-Pumpernickel
    Bread, 404–5
  Vegetable Stuffed Bread,
    422–23

Oranges
  Sweet Potato–Cherry
    Squares with Orange
    Icing, 370–71
Oriental-style dishes
  Hot-and-Sour Soup,
    341–42
  Oriental Noodles, 299–300
  Thai Stir-Fry, 339–41

P

Parmesan cheese
  Lemon Linguine Parmesan,
    313
  Mesclun Greens with Italian
    Parmesan Vinaigrette,
    327–28
Parsnips
  Old-Fashioned Chicken
    and Vegetable Stew,
    352–53
Pasta
  Angel Hair Pasta with Fresh
    Tomato Sauce, 320
  broth for tossing, 294
  choosing, 286
  Fettuccine with Roasted Red
    Pepper Sauce, 336–37
  Greek Pasta Salad, 286–87
  Lemon Linguine Parmesan,
    313
  Linguine Frittata with Broc-
    coli, 271–72
  Oriental Noodles,
    299–300
  Pasta Rustica, 342–43
  Tex-Mex Pasta Salad,
    294–95
Peaches
  Chicken Baked with Sherry-
    Peach Sauce, 332–33
  Chicken Salad with Peaches
    and Pecans, 277–78

Mixed Greens with Peach
  and Pecan Dressing,
  274
Pears
  Spinach Salad with Pears,
    Walnuts and Warm
    Mustard Vinaigrette,
    334–35
Peas
  Sweet Pea Guacamole, 289
Pecans
  Chicken Salad with Peaches
    and Pecans, 277–78
  Mixed Greens with Peach
    and Pecan Dressing,
    274
Pepper, black
  Pepper-Seared Sea Scallops,
    336
Peppers
  Fettuccine with Roasted Red
    Pepper Sauce, 336–37
  Green Chili and Cheddar
    Buttermilk Biscuits, 270
  Israeli Salad, 276
  Ratatouille and Grilled
    Mozzarella Sand-
    wiches, 281–82
  Vegetable Stuffed Bread,
    422–23
Picante sauce
  Picante Seafood Veracruz,
    317
Pies
  Apple Crumb Pie, 373–74
  Cherry Pie, 374–75
Pilaf
  Couscous Pilaf, 333
Pimentos
  Black Olive and Pimento
    Spread, 379–80
Pineapple
  Carrot-Pineapple Cake,
    365–66

Pine nuts
  Red-Leaf Lettuce with Pine
    Nuts, Cherries and
    Dried-Tomato Vinai-
    grette, 338–39
Pita bread
  Hummus in Pita Sand-
    wiches, 275
  Lentil Spread in Pita Pock-
    ets, 305–6
  Peasants' Salad Pita
    Pockets, 291–92
  Pita Chips, 378–79
Pizza
  White Pizza, 325–27
Potatoes
  Mashed Potatoes with a
    Difference, 346
  Old-Fashioned Chicken and
    Vegetable Stew, 352–53
  Spicy French Potatoes, 330
Poultry
  Chicken and Wheat Berry
    Salad, 278–79
  Chicken Baked with Sherry-
    Peach Sauce, 332–33
  Chicken Cutlets with Rasp-
    berry Vinaigrette,
    312–13
  Chicken Salad with Peaches
    and Pecans, 277–78
  fat in, 278
  ground, 329
  Old-Fashioned Chicken and
    Vegetable Stew,
    352–53
  Santa Fe Chicken Fajitas,
    322–23
  Southwestern Chicken
    Chili, 303–4
  Swiss Dijon Chicken Rolls,
    345
  Turkey Burgers, 329
  Village Paella, 349–51

Puddings
  Lemon Tapioca Pudding,
    376–77
  Perfect Pumpkin Pudding,
    377–78
Pumpernickel bread
  Quick Onion-Pumpernickel
    Bread, 404–5
Pumpkin
  Perfect Pumpkin Pudding,
    377–78
  Pumpkin-Cranberry Bread,
    362–63

Q

Quesadillas, 288
Quick breads. See Breads,
  quick

R

Raisins
  Chewy Oatmeal-Raisin
    Cookies, 356
  Cinnamon, Raisin and
    Nut Spread,
    380
  Cinnamon-Raisin Swirl
    Bread, 411–13
Raspberries
  Chicken Cutlets with
    Raspberry Vinaigrette,
    312–13
  Raspberry Coulis,
    378
Raspberry jam
  Raspberry-Currant Scones,
    360–61
Raspberry vinegar
  Greens with Baby Beets,
    Toasted Walnuts and
    Maple-Raspberry
    Vinaigrette, 354

Ratatouille
  Ratatouille and Grilled
    Mozzarella Sand-
    wiches, 281–82
Red-leaf lettuce
  Red- and Green-Leaf
    Lettuce with Maple-
    Walnut Dressing, 351
  Red-Leaf Lettuce with Pine
    Nuts, Cherries and
    Dried-Tomato Vinai-
    grette, 338–39
Refried beans
  Tacos, 315–16
Relishes
  Colorful Corn Relish, 297
Rice. *See also* Wild rice
  Brown Basmati Rice with
    Lemon, 318–19
  Mexicali Rice, 324–25
  Village Paella, 349–51
Rolls
  Honey Dinner Rolls, 394
  shaping, 390
  Whole-Wheat Cinnamon
    Rolls, 414–16
Rye flour
  Corn and Rye Bread, 402–3
  Jewish Rye Bread, 401–2

S

Salad dressings. *See* Dress-
    ings, salad
Salads
  Caesar-Style Salad, 344
  Chicken Salad with Peaches
    and Pecans, 277–78
  Citrus-Season Salad with
    Ginger-Horseradish
    Dressing, 307
  Colorful Corn Relish, 297
  Cucumber and Red Grape
    Salad, 282–83
  Dilled Cucumber Salad,
    285
  European Mixed Vegetable
    Salad, 347–48
  Fresh Green Bean Salad,
    330–31
  Greek Pasta Salad, 286–87
  Greens with Baby Beets,
    Toasted Walnuts and
    Maple-Raspberry
    Vinaigrette, 354
  Israeli Salad, 276
  Mesclun Greens with Italian
    Parmesan Vinaigrette,
    327–28
  Mixed Green Salad with
    Creamy Fresh Basil
    Dressing, 321
  Mixed Greens with Peach
    and Pecan Dressing,
    274
  Peasants' Salad Pita Pock-
    ets, 291–92
  Red- and Green-Leaf
    Lettuce with Maple-
    Walnut Dressing, 351
  Red-Leaf Lettuce with Pine
    Nuts, Cherries and
    Dried-Tomato Vinai-
    grette, 338–39
  Salad Nouveau, 314
  Spinach Salad with Pears,
    Walnuts and Warm
    Mustard Vinaigrette,
    334–35
  Tex-Mex Pasta Salad,
    294–95
Salmon
  Picante Seafood Veracruz,
    317
Salt, in yeast breads, 385–86
Sandwiches
  Hummus in Pita Sand-
    wiches, 275

Lentil Spread in Pita Pockets, 305–6
Peasants' Salad Pita Pockets, 291–92
Ratatouille and Grilled Mozzarella Sandwiches, 281–82
Sauces
low-fat ingredients for, 283
Raspberry Coulis, 378
Scallops
Pepper-Seared Sea Scallops, 336
Picante Seafood Veracruz, 317
Village Paella, 349–51
Scones
Raspberry-Currant Scones, 360–61
Seafood. See Fish; Shellfish
Seasonings
for low-fat dishes, 298
Shellfish
Pepper-Seared Sea Scallops, 336
Picante Seafood Veracruz, 317
Thai Stir Fry, 339–41
Village Paella, 349–51
Shells, pasta
Pasta Rustica, 342–43
Sherry
Chicken Baked with Sherry-Peach Sauce, 332–33
Shrimp
Thai Stir-Fry, 339–41
Village Paella, 349–51
Side dishes
Baked Yams with Nutmeg Cream, 318
Broccoli Lemon Amandine, 347
Brown Basmati Rice with Lemon, 318–19

Couscous Pilaf, 333
Fettuccine with Roasted Red Pepper Sauce, 336–37
Honey-Glazed Baby Carrots, 334
Lemon Linguine Parmesan, 313
Mashed Potatoes with a Difference, 346
Mexicali Rice, 324–25
Southwestern Black Beans, 323–24
Specialty Green Beans, 337–38
Spicy French Potatoes, 330
Snacks. See also Desserts
Baba Ghanoush, 380–81
Black Olive and Pimento Spread, 379–80
Cinnamon, Raisin and Nut Spread, 380
Cucumber and Yogurt Spread, 381–82
Pita Chips, 378–79
Snapper
Picante Seafood Veracruz, 317
Soups
Autumn's Acorn Cheddar Soup, 296
Hot-and-Sour Soup, 341–42
Roasted Chestnut and Wild Rice Soup, 292–93
Thick and Zesty Gazpacho, 268–69
Sour cream
Sour Cream Coffee Cake, 369
Southwestern-style dishes
Santa Fe Chicken Fajitas, 322–23
Southwestern Black Beans, 323–24

Southwestern-style dishes
    (continued)
    Southwestern Chicken
        Chili, 303–4
    Tex-Mex Pasta Salad,
        294–95
Spanish-style dishes
    Spanish Country Bread, 398
    Thick and Zesty Gazpacho,
        268–69
    Village Paella, 349–51
Spinach
    Spinach Salad with Pears,
        Walnuts and Warm
        Mustard Vinaigrette,
        334–35
    Stuffed Spinach and Feta
        Bread, 420–22
Spreads
    Baba Ghanoush, 380–81
    Black Olive and Pimento
        Spread, 379–80
    Cinnamon, Raisin and Nut
        Spread, 380
    Cucumber and Yogurt
        Spread, 381–82
    Lentil Spread in Pita
        Pockets, 305–6
    Sweet Pea Guacamole, 289
Squares
    Sweet Potato–Cherry
        Squares with Orange
        Icing, 370–71
Squash. *See also* Pumpkin;
        Zucchini
    acorn
        Autumn's Acorn Cheddar
        Soup, 296
Stews
    Old-Fashioned Chicken and
        Vegetable Stew,
        352–53
Stir-fries
    Thai Stir-Fry, 339–41

Sun-dried tomatoes
    Red-Leaf Lettuce with Pine
        Nuts, Cherries and
        Dried-Tomato Vinai-
        grette, 338–39
Sweeteners, in yeast breads,
        385
Sweet potatoes
    Mashed Potatoes with a Dif-
        ference, 346
    Old-Fashioned Chicken and
        Vegetable Stew,
        352–53
    Sweet Potato and Honey
        Bread, 409–10
    Sweet Potato–Cherry
        Squares with Orange
        Icing, 370–71
Swiss cheese
    Swiss Dijon Chicken Rolls,
        345
Swordfish
    Picante Seafood Veracruz,
        317

T

Tacos, 315–16
Tangerines
    Citrus-Season Salad with
        Ginger-Horseradish
        Dressing, 307
Tapioca
    Lemon Tapioca Pudding,
        376–77
Tex-Mex-style dishes. *See*
        Southwestern-style
        dishes
Thai-style dishes
    Thai Stir-Fry, 339–41
Tomatoes
    Angel Hair Pasta with Fresh
        Tomato Sauce, 320
    Israeli Salad, 276

Red-Leaf Lettuce
with Pine Nuts,
Cherries and Dried-
Tomato Vinaigrette,
338–39
Thick and Zesty Gazpacho,
268–69
Tortillas
Quesadillas, 288
Turkey
ground, <u>329</u>
Turkey Burgers, 329

V

Vegetables. *See also specific
vegetables*
Old-Fashioned Chicken and
Vegetable Stew, 352–53
Thick and Hearty Vegetable
Chili, 302–3
Vegetable Stuffed Bread,
422–23
Vinaigrette
Chicken Cutlets with Rasp-
berry Vinaigrette,
312–13
Four-Bean Salad with Bal-
samic Vinaigrette, 290
Greens with Baby Beets,
Toasted Walnuts and
Maple-Raspberry
Vinaigrette, 354
Mesclun Greens with Italian
Parmesan Vinaigrette,
327–28
Red-Leaf Lettuce with Pine
Nuts, Cherries and
Dried-Tomato Vinai-
grette, 338–39
Spinach Salad with Pears,
Walnuts and Warm
Mustard Vinaigrette,
334–35

Vinegar, balsamic
Balsamic Splash, 348
Four-Bean Salad with Bal-
samic Vinaigrette, 290

W

Walnuts
Apple-Walnut Bread,
410–11
Cinnamon, Raisin and Nut
Spread, 380
Greens with Baby Beets,
Toasted Walnuts and
Maple-Raspberry
Vinaigrette, 354
Red- and Green-Leaf Let-
tuce with Maple-Wal-
nut Dressing, 351
Spinach Salad with Pears,
Walnuts and Warm
Mustard Vinaigrette,
334–35
Wheat berries
Chicken and Wheat Berry
Salad, 278–79
Sprouted Wheat-Berry
Bread, 400–401
Whipped cream, mock,
<u>315</u>
Whole-wheat flour
for baked goods, <u>304</u>
Whole-Grain Bagels,
117–19
Whole-Grain Cocoa Angel
Food Cake, 366–67
Whole-Grain Mandelbrot,
359–60
Whole-Wheat and Honey
Challah, 396–97
Whole-Wheat Cinnamon
Rolls, 414–16
Whole-Wheat French Bread,
399–400

Whole-wheat flour *(continued)*
  Whole-Wheat Monkey
      Bread, 395–96
  for yeast breads, 384, 385,
      391
Wild rice
  Minnesota Wild Rice Bread,
      406–7
  Roasted Chestnut and Wild
      Rice Soup, 292–93
Wonton wraps
  Wonton Chips,
      300–301

Y

Yams. *See also* Sweet potatoes
  Baked Yams with Nutmeg
      Cream, 318
  Mashed Potatoes with a
      Difference, 346

Old-Fashioned Chicken and
    Vegetable Stew,
    352–53
Yeast
  active dry, 385
  proofing, 386
Yeast breads. *See* Breads,
      yeast
Yogurt
  Cucumber and Yogurt
      Spread, 381–82

Z

Zucchini
  European Mixed Vegetable
      Salad, 347–48
  Vegetable Stuffed Bread,
      422–23
  Zucchini Spice Bread,
      361–62